C. Kordon   R.-C. Gaillard
Y. Christen (Eds.)

# Hormones and the Brain

With 53 Figures and 7 Tables

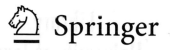 Springer

*Kordon, Claude,* Ph.D.
Institut Necker
156, Rue de Vaugirad
75015 Paris
France
e-mail: kordon@necker.fr

*Christen, Yves,* Ph.D.
Fondation IPSEN
Pour la Recherche Thérapeutique
24, rue Erlanger
75781 Paris Cedex 16
France
e-mail: yves.christen@ipsen.com

*Gaillard, Rolf-Christian,* M.D.
Dept. Medecine Interne
Div. Endocrinologie
Centre Hospitaier Universitaire Vadois
1011 Lausanne
Switzerland
e-mail: rolf.gaillard@chur.hospvd.ch

ISBN 3-540-21355-4   Springer-Verlag Berlin  Heidelberg  New York

Cataloging-in-Publication Data applied for Bibliographic information published by Die Deutsche Bibliothek
Die Deutsche Bibliothek lists this publication in the Deutsche Nationalbibliografie; detailed bibliographic data is available in the Internet at <http://dnb.ddb.de>.

Springer-Verlag is a part of Springer Science+Business Media

springeronline.com

© Springer-Verlag Berlin Heidelberg 2005
Printed in Germany

The use of general descriptive names, registered names, trademarks, etc. in this publications does not imply, even in the absence of a specific statement, that such names are exempt from the relevant protective laws and regulations and therefore free for general use.

Product liability: The publishers cannot guarantee the accuracy of any information about dosage and application contained in this book. In every individual case the user must check such information by consulting the relevant literature.

Production: PRO EDIT GmbH, 69126 Heidelberg, Germany
Cover design: design & production, 69121 Heidelberg, Germany
Typesetting: Satz & Druckservice, 69181 Leimen, Germany
Printed on acid-free paper         27/3150Re         5  4  3  2  1  0
SPIN: 10992654

# Contents

Activins and Inhibins:
Physiological Roles, Signaling Mechanisms and Regulation
*P.C. Gray, L.M. Bilezikjian, C.A. Harrison, E. Wiater, and W. Vale* . . . . . . . . . . .  1

Twins and the Fetal Origins Hypothesis: an Application to Growth Data
*D. Boomsma, G. Willemsen, E. de Geus, N. Kupper, D. Posthuma,*
*R. Ijzerman, B. Heijmans, E. Slagboom, L. Beem, and C. Dolan* . . . . . . . . . . . .  29

Towards Understanding the Neurobiology of Mammalian Puberty: Genetic,
Genomic and Proteomic Approaches
*S.R. Ojeda, A. Lomniczi, A. Mungenast, C. Mastronardi,*
*A.-S. Parent, C. Roth, V. Prevor, S. Heger, and H. Jung* . . . . . . . . . . . . . . . . . . . .  47

The Non-Genomic Action of Sex Steroids
*I. Joe, J.L. Kipp, and V.D. Ramirez* . . . . . . . . . . . . . . . . . . . . . . . . . . . . . . . . . . . . .  61

Mechanisms of Steroid Hormone Actions on Hypothalamic Nerve Cells:
Molecular and Biophysical Studies
Relevant for Hormone-Dependent Behaviors
*L.-M. Kow, N. Vasudevan, N. Devidze, A. Ragnauth, and D.W. Pfaff* . . . . . . . . .  73

Biological Effects and Markers of Exposure to Xenostroids
and Selective Estrogen Receptor Modulators (SERMs)
at the Hypothalamic-Pituitary Unit
*M. Tena-Sempere and E. Aguilar* . . . . . . . . . . . . . . . . . . . . . . . . . . . . . . . . . . . . .  79

Regulation of Neurosteroid Biosynthesis
by Neurotransmitters and Neuropeptides
*H. Vaudry, J.L. Do Rego, D. Beaujean-Burel, J. Leprince,*
*L. Galas, D. Larhammar, R. Fredriksson, V. Luu-The,*
*G. Pelletier, M.C. Tonon, and C. Delarue* . . . . . . . . . . . . . . . . . . . . . . . . . . . . . .  99

Progestins and Antiprogestins: Mechanisms of Action,
Neuroprotection and Myelination
*M. Schumacher, A. Ghoumari, R. Guennoun, F. Labombarda,*
*S.L. Gonzalez, M.C. Gonzalez Deniselle, C. Massaad, J. Grenier,*
*K.M. Rajkowski, F. Robert, EE. Baulieu, and A.F. De Nicola* . . . . . . . . . . . . . .  111

Rapid Effects of Estradiol on Motivated Behaviors
*J.B. Becker* ..................................................... 155

Behavioral Effects of Rapid Changes
in Aromatase Activity in the Central Nervous System
*J. Balthazart, M. Baillien, C.A. Cornil,*
*T.D. Charlier, H.C. Evrard, and G.F. Ball* .............................. 173

Modulatory of Endogenous Neuroprotection:
Estrogen, Corticotropin-Releasing Hormone and Endocannabinoids
*C. Behl* ......................................................... 201

Estrogens, Aging, and Neurodegenerative Diseases
*C.E. Finch, T. Morgan, and I. Rozovsky* ............................... 213

Hormones, Stress and Depression
*M.B. Müller and F. Holsboer* ......................................... 227

Subject Index ...................................................... 237

# Contributors

*Aguilar, Enrique*
Physiology Section, Department of Cell Biology, Physiology and Immunology,
Faculty of Medicine, University of Córdoba,
Avda. Menéndez Pidal s/n, 14004 Córdoba, Spain

*Baillien, Michelle*
Center for Cellular and Molecular Neurobiology,
Research Group in Behavioral Neuroendocrinology, University of Liège,
17 place Delcour , 4020 Liège, Belgium

*Ball, Gregory F.*
Department of Psychological and Brain Sciences, Johns Hopkins University,
Baltimore, MD 21218, USA

*Balthazart, Jacques*
Center for Cellular and Molecular Neurobiology, Research Group in Behavioral
Neuroendocrinology, University of Liège, 17 place Delcour , 4020 Liège, Belgium

*Baulieu, Etienne Emile*
INSERM U 488, 80 rue du Général Leclerc, 94276 Kremlin-Bicêtre, France

*Beaujean-Burel, Delphine*
European Institute for Peptide Research, Laboratory of Cellular and Molecular
Neuroendocrinology, INSERM U413, UA CNRS, University of Rouen,
76821 Mont-Saint Aignan, France

*Becker, Jill B.*
Psychology Department, Neuroscience Program and Reproductive Sciences
Program, 525 East University, Ann Arbor, MI 48109-1109, USA

*Beem, Leo*
Dept. of Biological Psychology, Vrije Universiteit, Van der Boechostraat 1,
1081 BT Amsterdam, The Netherlands

*Behl, Christian*
Institute for Physiological Chemistry and Pathobiochemistry,
Johannes Gutenberg University, Medical School, 55099 Mainz, Germany

*Bilezikjian, Louise M.*
Clayton Foundation Laboratories for Peptide Biology, The Salk Institute,
La Jolla, CA 92037, USA

*Boomsma, Dorret*
Dept. of Biological Psychology, Vrije Universiteit, Van der Boechorstraat 1,
1081 BT Amsterdam, The Netherlands

*Charlier, Thierry D.*
Center for Cellular and Molecular Neurobiology, Research Group in Behavioral
Neuroendocrinology, University of Liège, 17 place Delcour , 4020 Liège, Belgium

*Cornil, Charlotte A.*
Center for Cellular and Molecular Neurobiology, Research Group in Behavioral
Neuroendocrinology, University of Liège, 17 place Delcour , 4020 Liège, Belgium

*De Geus, Eco*
Dept. of Biological Psychology, Vrije Universiteit, Van der Boechorstraat 1,
1081 BT Amsterdam, The Netherlands

*Delarue, C*
European Institute for Peptide Research, Laboratory of Cellular and Molecular
Neuroendocrinology, INSERM U413, UA CNRS, University of Rouen,
76821 Mont-Saint-Aignan, France

*De Nicola, Alejandro F.*
Laboratory of Neuroendocrine Biochemistry,
Instituto de Biologia y Medicina Experimental,
University of Buenos Aires, Argentina

*Devidze, Nino*
Laboratory of Neurobiology and Behaviour, The Rockefeller University, Box 363,
1230 York Avenue, New York, NY 10021, USA

*Dolan, Conor*
Dept. of Psychology, Universiteit van Amsterdam, 1012 WX Amsterdam,
The Netherlands

*Do Rego, Jean-Luc*
European Institute for Peptide Research, Laboratory of Cellular and Molecular
Neuroendocrinology, INSERM U413, UA CNRS, University of Rouen,
76821 Mont-Saint-Aignan, France

*Evrard, Henry C.*
Center for Cellular and Molecular Neurobiology, Research Group in Behavioral
Neuroendocrinology, University of Liège, 17 place Delcour , 4020 Liège, Belgium

*Finch, Caleb E.*
Andrus Gerontology Center and Department of Biological Sciences,
University of Southern California, Los Angeles, CA 90089-0191, USA

*Fredriksson, Robert*
Department of Neuroscience, Unit of Pharmacology, Uppsala University,
75124 Uppsala, Sweden

*Galas, Ludovic*
European Institute for Peptide Research, Laboratory of Cellular and Molecular
Neuroendocrinology, INSERM U413, UA CNRS, University of Rouen,
76821 Mont-Saint-Aignan, France

*Ghoumari, Abdel*
INSERM U 488, 80 rue du Général Leclerc, 94276 Kremlin-Bicêtre, France

*Gonzalez, Susana L.*
Laboratory of Neuroendocrine Biochemistry,
Instituto de Biologia y Medicina Experimental,
University of Buenos Aires, Argentina

*Gonzalez Deniselle, Maria Claudia*
Laboratory of Neuroendocrine Biochemistry,
Instituto de Biologia y Medicina Experimental,
University of Buenos Aires, Argentina

*Gray, Peter C.*
Clayton Foundation Laboratories for Peptide Biology, The Salk Institute,
La Jolla, CA 92037, USA

*Grenier, J.*
INSERM U 488, 80 rue du Général Leclerc, 94276 Kremlin-Bicêtre, France

*Guennoun, Rachida*
INSERM U 488, 80 rue du Général Leclerc, 94276 Kremlin-Bicêtre, France

*Harrison, Craig A.*
Clayton Foundation Laboratories for Peptide Biology, The Salk Institute,
La Jolla, CA 92037, USA

*Heger, Sabine*
Department of Pediatrics, Division of Pediatric Endocronology,
University Children's Hospital, Schwanenweg 20, 24105 Kiel, Germany

*Heijmans, Bas*
Dept. of Molecular Epidemiology, Leiden University Medical Centre,
Leiden, The Netherlands

*Holsboer, Florian*
Max Planck Institute of Psychiatry, Kraepelinstr. 2-10, 80804 Munich, Germany

*Ijzerman, Richard*
Vrije Universiteit Medical Centre, Amsterdam, The Netherlands

*Joe, Ilkro*
Department of Molecular and Integrative Physiology,
University of Illinois at Urbana, IL 61801, USA

*Jung, Heike*
Lilly Deutschland GmbH, Niederlassung Bad Homburg, Saalburgstraße,
611350 Bad Homburg, Germany

*Kipp, Jingjing L.*
Department of Molecular and Integrative Physiology,
University of Illinois at Urbana, IL 61801, USA

*Kow, Lee-Ming*
Laboratory of Neurobiology and Behaviour, The Rockefeller University,
Box 363, 1230 York Avenue, New York, NY 10021, USA

*Kupper, Nina*
Dept. of Biological Psychology, Vrije Universiteit, Van der Boechorstraat 1,
1081 BT Amsterdam, The Netherlands

*Labombarda, Florencia*
Laboratory of Neuroendocrine Biochemistry,
Instituto de Biologia y Medicina Experimental,
University of Buenos Aires, Argentina

*Larhammar, Dan*
Department of Neuroscience, Unit of Pharmacology, Uppsala University,
75124 Uppsala, Sweden

*Leprince, Jerôme*
European Institute for Peptide Research, Laboratory of Cellular and Molecular Neuroendocrinology, INSERM U413, UA CNRS, University of Rouen, 76821 Mont-Saint-Aignan, France

*Lomniczi, Alejandro*
Division of Neuroscience, Oregon National Primate Research Center/Oregon Health and Science University, 505 N.W., 185th Avenue, Beaverton, Oregon 97006, USA

*Luu-The, Van*
Laboratory of Molecular Endocrinology and Oncology, Laval University Medical Center, Québec, Canada G1V 4G2

*Massaad, Charbel*
INSERM U 488, 80 rue du Général Leclerc, 94276 Kremlin-Bicêtre, France

*Mastronardi, Claudio*
Division of Neuroscience, Oregon National Primate Research Center/Oregon Health and Science University, 505 N.W., 185th Avenue, Beaverton, Oregon 97006, USA

*Morgan, Todd*
Andrus Gerontology Center and Department of Biological Sciences, University of Southern California, Los Angeles, CA 90089-0191, USA

*Müller, Marianne B.*
Max Planck Institute of Psychiatry, Kraepelinstr. 2-10, 80804 Munich, Germany

*Mungenast, Alison*
Division of Neuroscience, Oregon National Primate Research Center/Oregon Health and Science University, 505 N.W., 185th Avenue, Beaverton, Oregon 97006, USA

*Ojeda, Sergio R.*
Division of Neuroscience, Oregon National Primate Research Center/Oregon Health and Science University, 505 N.W., 185th Avenue, Beaverton, Oregon 97006, USA

*Parent, Anne-Simone*
Division of Neuroscience, Oregon National Primate Research Center/Oregon Health and Science University, 505 N.W., 185th Avenue, Beaverton, Oregon 97006, USA

*Pelletier, Georges*
Laboratory of Molecular Endocrinology and Oncology,
Laval University Medical Center, Québec, Canada G1V 4G2

*Pfaff, Donald W.*
Laboratory of Neurobiology and Behaviour, The Rockefeller University,
Box 363, 1230 York Avenue, New York, NY 10021, USA

*Posthuma, Danielle*
Dept. of Biological Psychology, Vrije Universiteit, Van der Boechorstraat 1,
1081 BT Amsterdam, The Netherlands

*Prevot, Vincent*
INSERM U422, Place de Verdun, 59045 Lille Cedex, France

*Ragnauth, Andre*
Laboratory of Neurobiology and Behaviour, The Rockefeller University,
Box 363, 1230 York Avenue, New York, NY 10021, USA

*Rajkowski, K.M.*
INSERM U 488, 80 rue du Général Leclerc, 94276 Kremlin-Bicêtre, France

*Ramirez, Victor D.*
Department of Molecular and Integrative Physiology,
University of Illinois at Urbana, IL 61801, USA

*Robert, Francoise*
INSERM U 488, 80 rue du Général Leclerc, 94276 Kremlin-Bicêtre, France

*Roth, Christian*
Division of Neuroscience, Oregon National Primate Research Center/Oregon
Health and Science University, 505 N.W., 185th Avenue, Beaverton,
Oregon 97006, USA

*Rozovsky, Irina*
Andrus Gerontology Center and Department of Biological Sciences,
University of Southern California, Los Angeles, CA 90089-0191, USA

*Schumacher, Michael*
INSERM U 488, 80 rue du Général Leclerc, 94276 Kremlin-Bicêtre, France

*Slagboom, Eline*
Dept. of Molecular Epidemiology, Leiden University Medical Centre,
Leiden, The Netherlands

*Tena-Sempere, Manuel*
Physiology Section, Department of Cell Biology, Physiology and Immunology,
Faculty of Medicine, University of Córdoba, Avda. Menéndez Pidal s/n,
14004 Córdoba, Spain

*Tonon, Marie-Christine*
European Institute for Peptide Research, Laboratory of Cellular and Molecular
Neuroendocrinology, INSERM U413, UA CNRS, University of Rouen,
76821 Mont-Saint-Aignan, France

*Vale, Wylie*
Clayton Foundation Laboratories for Peptide Biology, The Salk Institute,
La Jolla, CA 92037, USA

*Vasudevan, Nandini*
Penn State University, State College, PA, USA

*Vaudry, Hubert*
European Institute for Peptide Research, Laboratory of Cellular and Molecular
Neuroendocrinology, INSERM U413, UA CNRS, University of Rouen,
76821 Mont-Saint-Aignan, France

*Wiater, Ezra*
Clayton Foundation Laboratories for Peptide Biology, The Salk Institute,
La Jolla, CA 92037, USA

*Willemsen, Gonneke*
Dept. of Biological Psychology, Vrije Universiteit, Van der Boechorstraat 1,
1081 BT Amsterdam, The Netherlands

# Preface

*Claude Kordon, Rolf Gaillard, and Yves Christen*

## Pleiotypy and Ambiguity of Hormone Actions on the Brain

Increased awareness over recent years of the role of peripheral hormones in neuronal processes has led to define a 'humoral brain' concept. Most lipophilic and some hydrophilic hormones, although not directly involved in cell to cell communication within the brain (with the noticeable exception of neurosteroids, which are synthetized in brain cells themselves), can selectively cross the blood-brain barrier and affect a wide array of neurophysiological parameters, as early differenciation of brain connections, secretion of growth factors, or neurotransmitter activity.

Since the seventies, many efforts were made to map steroid hormone receptors in the brain, leading to important discoveries as the implication of estrogen and progesterone in reproductive functions and behaviour, or of adrenal steroids in memory and coping behaviour. Mapping studies uncovered however a few mismatches between the distribution of receptors and neuronal reponses to hormones. For instance, estradiol is known to affect dopamine neurotransmission in the nigro-striatal system, although the appropriate receptors have not been found there. In order to overcome this paradox, investigators were able to show that, in contrast to the traditional concept assigning a genomic site of action to steroid hormones, estradiol and progesterone are also able to act directly on neuronal membranes to induce instantaneous depolarization.

Many of these findings are reviewed in the present volume, based on presentations to the Conference *Hormones and the Brain* organized in December 8, 2003 by the IPSEN Foundation. Most contributors have made pioneer discoveries in the field. Given the complexity of the area, the meeting was restricted to brain actions of gonadal hormones – mostly estradiol, but also progesterone, testosterone and the non steroid hormones activin and inhibin. Neurosteroids, brain moieties related to gonadal steroids, were also addressed.

Pleiotypic actions of estradiol are summarized in figure 1. By its impact on discrete areas of the brain during embryogenesis or at early stages of post-natal development, the hormone can control the density of synaptic contacts (a process involved in the generation of sex dimorphism, among other effects), in communication between neurons and glial cells, and in formation of microtubules, an important step in neurogenesis.

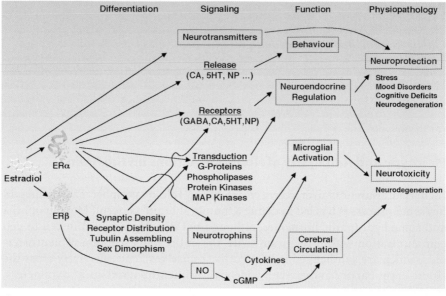

**Fig. 1.**

Another major effect of estrogens is to influence cell signaling. This involves multiple levels of action :

–  neurotransmitter release (which results from both genomic and membrane impacts of the hormone). A large number of neurotransmitters and neuropeptides are sensitive to estrogens, as dopamine, noradrenaline and serotonin, but also β-endorphin, corticotropin-releasing hormone, neuropeptide Y or somatostatin (Kordon et al. 1994).

–  regulation of expression of several classes of neurotransmitter and neuropeptide receptors. Interestingly, the hormone (but also inhibin) can operate molecular switches affecting the balance between receptor isotypes. For instance, an estradiol-induced shift in the balance between D1 and D2 dopamine receptors in the striatum can reverse the physiological response to dopamine, since both receptors act in opposite ways on cAMP accumulation (Maus et al. 1989). A similar situation has been observed in the case of several neuropeptide receptors, thus accounting for the discrepant responses of intact and ovariectomized animals to neuropeptide administration (Kordon et al. 1994).

–  transduction parameters, such as G proteins, phospholipases or various classes of protein kinases (for instance protein kinase C and MAP kinases) are also targets of estrogen effects. By modifying intracellular information processing, interference of estrogens with transduction adds one level of complexity to the central modulatory actions of hormones.

Functional implications of all above parameters are not only relevant for reproductive functions. They also concern behavioural effects of estrogens, accounting for the relative protection provided by estrogens against adverse effects of stress, mood disorders and cognitive deficits. As reviewed in this volume, gonadal hormones for instance control the mesolimbic dopaminergic tone underlying motivational processes, and thus parameters involved in addictive behaviour.

Finally, estrogens can influence the expression of neurotrophic factors and cytokines, or generation of free radicals as nitric oxyde in astrocytes or microglia, thereby affecting both neuroprotective and neurotoxic mechanisms. These actions account for effects of the hormone on the cerebral circulation and on microglial activation. This further illustrates the ambiguity of estrogen actions on the brain: depending upon the receptor isotype involved (ERα or ERβ), but also upon intensity and duration of exposure to the hormone, pleiotypic effects can result in either neuroprotective or neurotoxic processes, the latter favouring neurodegeneration. Recent epidemiological data from the NIH's Women's Health Initiative stressing increased risk of Alzheimer disease after long term estrogen medication are also consistent with this conclusion. In fact, the ambiguity of estrogen effects accounts for the wide discrepancies found in the literature with respect to the chronic therapeutic use of estradiol, and for the great difficulty in anticipating the ratio of actual benefits and adverse effects for the patients.

*Acknowledgment*
The editors want to thank J. Mervaillie for the organization of the meeting and M.-L. Gage and Elsa Guillermin for the editing of the book.

## References

Kordon C, Drouva SV, Martinez de la Escalera G, Weiner RI (1994) Role of classic and peptide neuromediators in the neuroendocrine regulation of luteinizing hormone and prolactin, in: Knobil E, Neill JD (eds) The Physiology of Reproduction (2nd edition). Raven Press, New York, pp. 1621–1661

Maus M, Bertrand P, Drouvas S, Rasolonjanahary R, Kordon C, Glowinski J, Premont J, Enjalbert A (1989) Differential modulation of D1 and D2 dopamine-sensitive adenylate cyclases by 17 beta-estradiol in cultured striatal neurons and anterior pituitary cells. J Neurochem 52: 410–418

# Activins and inhibins: Physiological roles, signaling mechanisms and regulation

*Peter C. Gray, Louise M. Bilezikjian, Craig A. Harrison, Ezra Wiater, and Wylie Vale[1]*

Activins and inhibins belong to the transforming growth factor β (TGF-β) superfamily, which also includes the TGF-β (Massague 1998), bone morphogenetic protein (BMP) (Wozney et al. 1988), growth and differentiation (GDF) and nodal-related families (Schier et al. 2000). In human there are now known to be 42 members of the TGF-β superfamily (reviewed in Shi et al. 2003). This review summarizes the physiological roles of activins and inhibins, focusing on activin actions in the central nervous system (CNS). In addition, we outline the molecular basis for activin signal transduction and regulation, emphasizing recent advances regarding the structural basis for ligand/receptor interactions and the roles of betaglycan and Cripto in attenuating activin signaling.

## Activins and inhibins

Inhibins are heterodimeric proteins composed of one α and one β subunit, linked by a disulfide bridge; activins are related dimers composed of two β subunits. Five β subunits have been reported (βA, βB, βC, βD, and βE), whereas only a single α subunit has been identified (Hotten et al. 1995; Mason et al. 1985; Oda et al. 1995). Thus, there is an extensive array of possible dimers; of these, βA-βA (activin-A), βA-βB (activin-AB), βB-βB (activin-B), α-βA (inhibin-A) and α-βB (inhibin-B) have been isolated as dimeric proteins and shown to be biologically active. The X-ray crystallographic analysis of TGF-β2 (Daopin et al. 1992; Schlunegger et al. 1992), BMP-7 (Griffith et al. 1996) and BMP-2 (Scheufler et al. 1999), along with the NMR structure of TGF-β1 (Archer et al. 1993), provide insights concerning the structure of members of the TGF-β superfamily, which belongs to the even larger Cystine Knot Superfamily (Vitt et al. 2001).

[1] Clayton Foundation Laboratories for Peptide Biology
The Salk Institute for Biological Studies, La Jolla, CA 92037

Kordon et al.
Hormones and the Brain
© Springer-Verlag Berlin Heidelberg 2005

## Physiological roles of activins and inhibins

Activins and inhibins were initially recognized for their important roles in the regulation of the anterior pituitary (reviewed in (Bilezikjian et al. 1992; De Kretser, et al. 1988; DeJong 1988; DePaolo et al.1991,; Mather et al. 1992; Vale et al. 1988)). Inhibins, which suppress the production of follicle stimulating hormone (FSH), were isolated in 1985 by several groups (Ling et al. 1985; Miyamoto et al. 1985; Rivier, et al. 1985; Robertson et al. 1985). The purification of activins was first reported a year later, based on their actions to stimulate FSH secretion from the anterior pituitary (Ling et al. 1986,; Vale et al. 1986).

Since their characterization, activins and inhibins have been demonstrated to exert a broad range of biological effects in various reproductive tissues. Mice null for activin/inhibin subunits and signaling components exhibit various reproductive anomalies (Matzuk et al. 1996). At the pituitary level in the rat, activin-B acts as a local autocrine factor to stimulate FSH production (Corrigan et al. 1991; Weiss et al. 1992) whereas gonadal inhibin reaches the pituitary through the circulation to suppress FSH production. Activins also suppress the secretion of growth hormone (GH), prolactin (PRL), and adrenocorticotropic hormone (ACTH) by the pituitary, but these actions are not blocked by inhibin (reviewed in (Bilezikjian et al. 1992). Locally produced activins and inhibins can modify hormone production in the gonads and placenta and can regulate ovarian and testicular gametogenesis (Hsueh et al. 1987; Mather et al. 1990; Shaha et al. 1989). Activins and inhibins have also been implicated in the progression to malignant prostate disease (Dowling et al. 2000) and endometriosis (Reis et al. 2001).

Activins and inhibins are pleiotropic hormones/growth factors with powerful actions on erythropoiesis (Broxmeyer et al. 1988; Eto et al. 1987; Hangoc et al. 1992; Lebrun et al. 1997; Yu et al. 1987), liver proliferation (Matzuk et al. 1994; Matzuk et al. 1992; Schwall et al. 1993b), immune function (Brosh et al. 1995), bone formation (Ogawa et al. 1992), skin morphogenesis and cutaneous wound repair (Beer et al. 2000), and angiogenesis (McCarthy et al. 1993). Activin has profound effects on early mesoderm development, axis formation, and cell fate determination (Asashima et al. 1990; Smith et al. 1990; Thomsen et al. 1990; van den Eijnden van Raaij et al.,1991), and activin receptors and endogenous activin-related ligands such as nodal are important determinants of vertebrate developmental steps, including mesoderm induction and establishment of left-right asymmetry (Levin et al. 1995; Ryan et al. 1998; Schier et al. 2000).

In comparison with inhibin-A and activin-A, little is known of the physiology of inhibin-B and activin-B. Mice with homozygous disruption of the *Inhba* locus (lacking activin-A and inhibin-A) demonstrate disruption of whisker, palate and tooth development, leading to neonatal lethality, whereas homozygous *Inhbb* (lacking activin-B and inhibin-B) null mice are viable, fertile and have eye defects (Chang et al. 2002). To better understand the functional relationship between activin-A and activin-B (63% amino acid identity between the two subunits), Brown et al. (2000) inserted the βB subunit gene into the *Inhba* locus. Activin-B protein was sufficient to rescue the craniofacial malformations and neonatal lethality of mice lacking activin-A. However, activin-B did not fully compensate for activin-A function, as illustrated by the novel phenotypes (somatic, testicular, genital and hair growth abnormalities) and decreased survival of the inhibin-B knock-in mice. These results suggest some functional differences between the activin-A and activin-B isoforms, which may extend to inhibin-A and inhibin-B. Although it has been shown that inhibin-A and -B associate with the same repertoire of binding proteins in TM4 Sertoli cells, there were differences in their potencies (Harrison et al. 2001). It is possible that such differences in the inhibin and activin isoforms extend to their physiological roles in the pituitary and gonads.

## Activin actions in the CNS

A role for activin signaling in the CNS has been indicated by studies demonstrating expression of activin/inhibin subunits (Meunier et al. 1988), activin receptors (Cameron et al. 1994; Funaba et al. 1997; Shoji et al. 1998) and regulatory proteins such as follistatin (Macconell et al. 1996) in multiple brain regions. Increased activin expression has also been observed during neocortical development (Andreasson et al. 1995). Although our understanding of activin functions in the CNS is still emerging, several roles of activin have been characterized, including its ability to regulate neuronal secretion, survival, growth and differentiation. In addition, there is recent evidence that activin plays a role in mediating immune functions in the CNS.

Several studies have provided evidence that activin regulates the function of hypothalamic neurons. Activin-containing cell bodies in the nucleus of the solitary tract (NTS) project to oxytocin-secreting neurons, and an increased oxytocin production was observed following intrahypothalamic injections of activin-A in vivo (Sawchenko et al. 1988). More recently, activin was shown to cause depolarization of supraoptic magnocellular neurosecretory cells, supporting a direct role for activin in control of neurohypophysial hormone release (Oliet et al. 1995). Activin increases corticotropin releasing factor (CRF) production following intrahypothalamic injections in vivo (Plotsky et al. 1991) and increases gonadotropin releasing factor (GnRH) production both in vitro (Calogero et al. 1998; Gonzalez-Manchon et al. 1991; MacConell et al. 1999) and in vivo (Lee et al. 1997). A role for activin in regulating GnRH levels in vivo is supported by the finding that activin betaA and follistatin immunostaining are closely associated with GnRH-positive neurons in the hypothalamus (MacConell, et al. 1998). Also, the activin type I receptor ALK4 is expressed in GnRH neurons and in hypothalamic areas of female rat (Prevot et al. 2000), and expression of hypothalamic activin type II receptors can be regulated by estradiol in vivo (Trudeau et al. 1996). Finally, there is evidence that activin acts in the hypothalamus to regulate appetite (Hawkins et al. 1995; Schwall et al. 1993a; Kubota et al. 2003).

Activin also regulates the growth, survival and differentiation of neurons. Early work showed that activin could promote the survival of embryonal carcinoma P19 cells, in addition to other neuronal cell lines (Schubert et al. 1990), while inhibiting proliferation of differentiated neuronal cells (Hashimoto et al. 1990). It was subsequently found that activin prevented neuronal differentiation of P19 cells (van den Eijnden-van Raaij et al. 1991). In a subsequent study, follistatin inhibited anchorage-independent growth of P19 cells in soft agar, whereas activin inhibited retinoic acid-stimulated P19 cell neural differentiation and proliferation (Hashimoto et al. 1992). Activin has also been shown to induce PC12 cell neuronal differentiation (Paralkar et al. 1992) and to promote astrocyte differentiation of CNS neural progenitors (Satoh et al. 2000). Activin stimulates somatostatin expression and differentiation of developing ciliary ganglion neurons (Coulombe, et al. 1993) and is produced by the targets of these neurons (Darland et al. 1995), suggesting that it may be a target cell differentiation signal. In addition, activin co-operates with FGF-2 to induce tyrosine hydroxylase expression in basal forebrain ventricular zone progenitor cells during embryogenesis, and activin treatment permitted neuronal survival and differentiation of these progenitor cells in vitro (Daadi et al. 1998). In summary, activin promotes neuronal survival and can act to promote or inhibit differentiation, depending on the cellular context.

An important advance has been the discovery of a neuroprotective role for activin in response to brain injury (reviewed in Alzheimer et al. 2002; Wankell et al. 2003). Brain lesions induced by kainate (Tretter et al. 1996), ischemia/hypoxia (Lai et al. 1996) or saline injection (Lai et al. 1997) result in a strong induction of activin βA subunit expression, suggesting a role for activin-A in response to brain injury. Induction of βA has also been observed in response to excitatory synaptic stimulation under conditions that generate long-term potentiation (LTP) (Andreasson et al. 1995; Inokuchi et al. 1996). These findings indicate that activin-A plays a role in response to excitotoxic neuronal damage or perhaps facilitates maintenance of LTP. Activin-A promotes survival of midbrain and hippocampal neurons in vitro (Iwahori et al. 1997; Krieglstein et al. 1995) and protects striatal and midbrain neurons against neurotoxic damage (Hughes et al. 1999; Krieglstein et al. 1995). In addition, activin-A reduces ischemic brain injury in neonatal rats (Wu et al. 1999). A role for activin in preventing neuronal cell death was expanded with the discovery that the neuroprotective effects of fibroblast growth factor (FGF) require induction of activin-A. It was found that activin-A was as effective as FGF-2 in preventing excitotoxic neuronal loss in the CA3 region of the hippocampus and that the activin inhibitor follistatin blocked the effects of FGF-2 while having no effects in the absence of FGF-2 treatment (Tretter et al. 2000). With regard to regulation of activin during the response to brain injury, follistatin-related gene (FLRG) is produced in astroglial cells in a TGF-β1-dependent manner and is induced following brain injury, providing a mechanism for TGF-β to regulate activin activity (Zhang et al. 2003). There is also evidence that bone morphogenetic proteins (BMPs) play a neuroprotective role. BMPRII and ALK2 mRNAs encoding BMP receptors are upregulated in dentate gyrus neurons following brain injury (Lewen et al. 1997). In addition, OP-1/BMP-7 (Lin, et al. 1999) and BMP-6 (Wang et al. 2001) have been shown to protect against neuronal death in models of ischemic injury.

The above findings indicate that members of the TGF-β superfamily, including activin-A and BMP-6 and BMP-7, may play complementary neuroprotective roles in response to brain injury and that their signaling pathways may provide useful therapeutic targets in treating human brain injuries such as stroke. The involvement of TGF-β family members has also been implicated in other CNS disorders. TGF-β isoforms and type II and type I TGF-β receptors were shown to be upregulated in macrophages, hypertrophic astrocytes and endothelial cells associated with multiple sclerosis lesions (De Groot et al. 1999) and in human glioma (Kjellman et al. 2000). Activin-A (Michel et al. 2003) and BMP-7 (Dattatreyamurty et al. 2001) are each present at high levels in cerebrospinal fluid (CSF), and it has been shown that bacterial infection of the CSF causes a 15-fold increase in activin-A levels within 24 hours, together with an increase in macrophages and microglia, indicating that activin participates in the CNS response to immune challenge and may mediate inflammatory processes in the brain (Michel et al. 2003).

## Activin signaling and the receptor serine kinase superfamily

The molecular basis of signal transduction by TGF-β superfamily members has been extensively characterized (reviewed in (Shi et al. 2003 and see Table 1). Like other TGF-β family members, activins exert their biological effects by interacting with two types of transmembrane receptors (type I and type II) with intrinsic serine/threonine kinase activities, called receptor serine kinases (RSKs; Shi et al. 2003). Following the characterization of the first vertebrate RSK by our group (Mathews et al. 1991), five type II receptors and seven type I receptors have now been identified in humans (Shi et al. 2003). Type I RSKs are referred to as ALK1 to 7, for Activin receptor-Like Kinases (Bassing et al. 1994; Ebner et al. 1993; ten Dijke et al. 1993, 1994a; Tsuchida et al. 1993, 1996). The receptor activation mechanism was first established for TGF-β, which was shown to bind its type II receptor (TβRII), leading to the recruitment, phosphorylation and activation of its type I receptor ALK5; (Wrana et al. 1992). A similar mechanism of ligand-mediated receptor assembly and type I receptor phosphorylation has been demonstrated for activin receptors, involving initial binding of activin to

ActRII or ActRIIB followed by recruitment, phosphorylation and activation of the type I receptor ALK4 (Attisano et al. 1996; Lebrun et al. 1997).

## Structural basis of ligand: receptor binding

The crystal structure of the ActRII extracellular domain (ECD) provided detailed information regarding sites predicted to be involved in receptor:ligand interactions (Greenwald et al. 1999), leading to our identification of a binding site on ActRII for activin-A and inhibin-A (Gray et al. 2000). With our collaborators, we have recently solved the crystal structure of the ActRII-ECD bound to BMP-7 and we showed that the amino acids on ActRII required for activin-A binding make up interfacial contacts between ActRII and BMP-7 and are required for BMP-7 binding (Greenwald et al. 2003). An allosteric conformational change was observed in BMP-7 in its predicted type I receptor binding site following binding to ActRII, which suggested a general model for cooperative type I/type II receptor assembly induced by BMPs (or activin) to form a hexameric complex containing the dimeric ligand, two type II receptors and two type I receptors (Greenwald et al. 2003). The structure of activin-A bound to the ActRIIB-ECD was also recently solved (Thompson et al. 2003) and was generally consistent with our previous findings regarding the activin-A binding site on ActRII (Gray et al. 2000). The structure of TGF-$\beta_3$ bound to the T$\beta$RII-ECD has also been solved (Hart, et al., 2002) and indicates, unexpectedly, that the TGF-$\beta$ binding interface with its type II receptor is very different from the corresponding interface of activin and BMP7 with ActRII (Greenwald et al. 2003). This finding suggests that, although activin and TGF-$\beta$ have a similar mechanism of receptor activation (Attisano et al. 1996; Lebrun et al. 1997; Wrana et al. 1992), they apparently have unrelated ligand-type II receptor interfaces (Greenwald et al. 2003). The crystal structure of BMP2 bound to the BMP type I receptor (ALK3-ECD) has also been solved (Kirsch et al. 2000). Using this structure as a guide, we recently identified an activin-A binding surface on the type I receptor ALK4-ECD that is overlapping but distinct from the corresponding binding site on ALK3 for BMP2 (Harrison et al. 2003). Regardless of the precise mechanism of receptor assembly by TGF-$\beta$ superfamily ligands, it has been generally established that, following receptor assembly, type II receptors phosphorylate type I receptors within a juxtamembrane cytoplasmic glycine- and serine-rich region called the GS domain, and this phosphorylation event activates the type I receptor kinase to initiate downstream signaling (Shi, et al., 2003).

**Table 1.** TGF-β superfamily signaling. The receptors, co-receptors and Smads involved in signaling by the indicated TGF ligands are shown.

| Ligand | Type II Receptor | Type I Receptor | Co-Receptor | Pathway Smad | Common Smad | Inhibitory Smad |
|---|---|---|---|---|---|---|
| Activin | ActRII<br>ActRIIB<br>ActRII | ALK4 (ACTRIB) | ? | Smad2<br><br>Smad3 | Smad4 | Smad7 |
| Inhibin | ActRIIB<br>BMPRII | ? | Betaglycan | ? | ? | ? |
| BMP-2<br>BMP-4<br>BMP-7<br>BMP-9 | ActRII<br>ActRIIB<br>BMPR II | ALK2 (ActRI)<br>ALK3 (BMPRIA)<br>ALK6 (BMPRIB) | ? | Smad1<br>Smad5<br>Smad8 | Smad4 | Smad6<br>Smad7 |
| TGF-β | TGF-βR II | ALK5 (TGF-βRI)<br>ALK1 (TSRI) | Betaglycan<br>Endoglin | Smad2<br>Smad3<br>Smad 1/5/8 | Smad4 | Smad7 |
| Nodal | ActRII<br>ActRIIB | ALK4<br>ALK7 | Cripto<br>(EGF-CFC) | Smad2<br><br>Smad3 | Smad4 | Smad7 |

## Smad Proteins

Based upon genetic studies in *Drosophila* and *Caenorhabditis elegans* (Savage et al. 1996; Sekelsky et al. 1995), a group of proteins now called Smads has been found to transduce RSK signals and mediate the regulation of target gene transcription by activin, TGF-β, and other superfamily members (Heldin et al. 1997; Massague 1998). The relationships of ligand/receptor/Smad are shown in Table 1. Structural and functional considerations allow their subdivision into three subfamilies: pathway-specific, common mediator, and inhibitory Smads. Activin signals are mediated by Smad2 and Smad3 through ALK4. Activation of a type I/ALK by its respective ligands and type II receptors triggers a transient association and phosphorylation of the pathway-specific Smads by the ALK at the last two serine residues in the C terminal SSXS motif (Heldin et al. 1997; Kretzschmar et al. 1997; Macias et al. 1996; Zhang et al. 1996). Activated pathway-specific Smads form hetero-oligomeric complexes with the common mediator Smad4, first discovered in humans as the pancreatic tumor suppressor gene, DPC4 (Hahn et al.,1996). This Smad complex translocates to the nucleus and activates transcription of target genes by either associating with DNA binding proteins or by binding DNA directly (Chen et al. 2002; Cordenonsi et al. 2003; Feng et al. 1998, 2002a,b; Janknecht, et al. 1998; Kang et al. 2003; Kim et al. 1997; Labbe et al. 1998; Song et al. 1998; Yingling et al. 1997; Zhang et al. 1998).

Two vertebrate inhibitory Smads have been identified, Smad6 and Smad7 (Imamura et al. 1997; Nakao et al.,1997), that lack the C-terminal SSXS motif found in the pathway specific Smads (Hayashi et al. 1997). Smad6 and Smad7 are inhibitors of Smad signaling and bind to ALKs to prevent phosphorylation and activation of the pathway-specific Smads by their respective type I receptor. In transfected cells, Smad7 inhibits transcriptional responses induced by either activin or TGF-β or by a constitutively active ALK4 (Bilezikjian et al. 2001; Chen et al. 1998; Lebrun et al. 1999; Nakao et al. 1997) and is induced by activin (Bilezikjian et al. 2001; Ishisaki et al. 1998). Thus, Smad7 may provide an intracellular feedback signal to restrain the effects of activin and TGF-β.

## Inhibin and its co-receptors

Inhibins are critical for the maintenance of normal function in many tissues, the best known being those of the reproductive axis. Inhibin opposes some but not all actions of activin. As testimony to the importance of inhibin as an antagonist of activin, mice deficient in the inhibin a subunit develop gonadal tumors and exhibit cachexia with severe weight loss and liver necrosis (Matzuk et al. 1992, 1994). Several models of inhibin antagonism of activin actions have been proposed. A proposed model of inhibin (αβ) action is that the β subunit binds to a type II activin receptor (ActRII or IIB) but, because the α subunit is unable to recruit a type I receptor, no signal is generated and access of activin to type II receptors is blocked (Xu et al., 1995). Inhibin has relatively low affinity for ActRII or ActRIIB in cells transfected with these type II receptors (Attisano et al. 1992; Mathews et al. 1991). Moreover, inhibin blocks activin effects with high potency in some systems but not others. Altogether, these observations suggest that alternative mechanisms may exist. Several groups, including us (Draper et al. 1998; Hertan et al. 1999; Lebrun et al. 1997), have reported evidence for the existence of an inhibin-binding protein (co-receptor). It has been proposed that such a co-receptor interacts with the α subunit of inhibin while the β subunit binds the type II receptor and stabilizes the type II activin receptor/inhibin complex and perhaps even generates a signal on its own.

## Betaglycan, an inhibin co-receptor

We recently identified betaglycan (BG; TGF-β type III receptor) as an inhibin-binding protein that facilitates the antagonism of activin signaling by inhibin-A

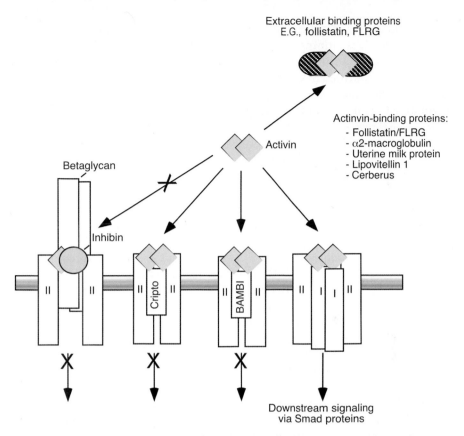

**Fig. 1.** Regulation of activin signaling. Several mechanisms by which activin signaling can be attenuated are illustrated (see text for details). These include blockade by activin-binding protein such as follistatin and interference with receptor assembly by inhibin/betaglycan, Cripto and BAMBI.

(Lewis et al. 2000). The proposed role of betaglycan is illustrated in Figure 1. Betaglycan is also known as the TGF-β type III receptor, and it binds TGF-β2 with higher affinity than TGF-β1 or TGF-β3. It has been proposed that betaglycan is an enhancer of TGF-β access to its own signaling type II receptor (Lopez-Casillas et al. 1993). Consistent with earlier work and the proposed mechanism of inhibin action described above, we have identified the presence of complexes comprising inhibin with endogenous betaglycan and ActRII. Lopez-Casillas and colleagues have confirmed our observation that betaglycan has high affinity for inhibin (Esparza-Lopez et al. 2001). Harrison et al. (2001) have purified several inhibin-binding cell surface proteins from mouse testicular cells and have reported that three of the proteins could be immunoprecipitated with antibodies to betaglycan. The additional bands do not react with antibodies to p120/InhBP, a protein identified by Woodruff and colleagues as a potential inhibin-binding protein. Woodruff and colleagues have reported that p120/InhBP, an ~120 kDa single membrane spanning protein that contains 12 immunoglobulin (Ig) domain repeats, is an inhibin-binding protein (Chong et al. 2000). Although this protein was purified based on its binding to inhibin-A (Chong et al. 2000), it was reported to enhance the biological response to inhibin-B but not inhibin-A (Bernard et al. 2001). By contrast, we observe that betaglycan markedly increases the functional response to both inhibin-A and inhibin-B.

Another proposed difference between the effects of the two putative inhibin receptors has been that p120/InhBP was reported to interact with ALK4 but not ActRII in a ligand-independent manner whereas betaglycan interacts with ActRII but does not recruit ALK4. Although the possibility that inhibin utilizes more than one mechanism to exert its antagonism is quite provocative and still warrants evaluation, further comparative re-examination of the function of betaglycan and p120/InhBP has led Woodruff and colleagues to conclude that betaglycan was more likely to fit the criteria of an inhibin receptor than InhBP/p120 (Bernard et al. 2001). This conclusion was further substantiated by their finding that InhBP/p120 did not bind inhibin A or B when expressed alone or in combination with activin receptors (Chapman et al. 2002). Finally, targeted disruption of the InhBP/p120 gene resulted in mice that appeared phenotypically normal with no apparent abnormalities in FSH regulation or reproductive function (Bernard et al. 2003). In summary, a growing body of evidence now indicates that InhBP/p120 protein is not involved in regulating inhibin function.

Betaglycan protein and mRNA are expressed in inhibin-responsive tissues with high expression levels in the rat hypothalamus, pituitary and gonads (MacConell et al. 2002). In the rat pituitary, betaglycan protein is expressed in the anterior and intermediate lobes and, importantly, we find that it co-localizes with LH in gonadotropes, consistent with a role for betaglycan in inhibin-mediated regulation of this cell type. Clearly, however, betaglycan is widely distributed and, in addition to its role as an inhibin co-receptor, plays important roles as a modulator of the action of TGF-β (Massague 1998).

## Inhibin blocks BMP signaling

Like other members of the TGF-β superfamily, BMPs signal through a complex of type II (ActRII, ActRIIB and BMPRII) and type I (ALK2, ALK3 and ALK6) RSKs (Table 1; Massague 1998). Unlike other TGF-β superfamily members, BMPs can initially bind to either the type I or type II receptor (ten Dijke et al. 1994b) and form an active signaling complex with both receptor components (Liu et al. 1995). The active BMP receptor complex leads to phosphorylation of Smad1, Smad5, and/or Smad8 and generates responses that are typically distinct from those initiated by activins and TGF-βs via Smad2 and Smad3 (Wrana et al. 2000). This pattern, however, is not universal and GDF-9 was reported to stimulate both inhibin-A and inhibin-B production in granulosa cells through Smad2 (Roh et al. 2003). In cells/tissues that respond to both types of ligands, the responses to activin/TGF-β are often distinct from, or even opposed by, BMPs such as reported for BMP-2 and BMP-7 (Heldin et al. 1997; Kimelman et al. 2000; Massague et al. 2000;Yamaguchi 1995).

Since BMPs signal via type II activin receptors, we hypothesized that inhibin might antagonize their signaling in a manner similar to its antagonism of activins. We have subsequently shown that inhibin does indeed block signaling by multiple BMPs in HepG2 cells and TM4 Sertoli cells and that the inhibin blockade is facilitated by betaglycan (Wiater et al. 2003). We further demonstrated that the ability of inhibin to block BMP effects on $C_2C_{12}$ cells is dependent on betaglycan expression (Wiater et al. 2003). The observation that inhibin in conjunction with betaglycan can block BMP signaling raises the possibility that inhibin, of either local or blood-borne origin might exert physiological actions that are much broader than previously appreciated.

## TGF-β superfamily members in the pituitary

As discussed above, members of the TGF-β family of growth and differentiation factors have been recently recognized as a class of important modulators of anterior pituitary function and organogenesis (Bilezikjian et al. 1992; Burns et al. 1993; Ericson et al. 1998; Mather et al. 1997; Treier et al. 1998; Vale et al. 1990; Woodruff 1998). Activins regulate the function of multiple pituitary cell types, including gonadotropes, somatotropes, corticotropes and lactotropes (Bilezikjian et al. 1990, 1991; Billestrup et al. 1990; Carroll et al. 1989). In contrast, the effects of TGF-β are limited to lactotropes (Abraham et al. 1998), whereas the effects of inhibin (Vale et al. 1990) and BMP-15 (Otsuka et al. 2002) appear to be gonadotrope specific. The central role of betaglycan in both the TGF-β and inhibin receptor complexes identifies this molecule as a key mediator of crosstalk between TGF-β superfamily members within the anterior pituitary. Indeed a recent report showed that TGF-β1 and TGF-β2 can modulate inhibin activity in LβT2 gonadotrope cells by decreasing the number of available betaglycan molecules essential for inhibin antagonism of activin activity (Ethier et al.2002). Thus, any examination of the role of betaglycan in inhibin's antagonism of activin must also address the potential disruption of TGF-β and BMP effects in the pituitary.

## Activin/TGF-β signaling pathway and cancer

Given their roles in regulating cell proliferation and differentiation, it is not surprising that disruptions or alterations in activin and TGF-β signaling have been observed in several types of human cancer (reviewed in Chen et al. 2002; Massague et al. 2000). Inactivating mutations in TβRII have been observed in colorectal and gastric carcinomas (Markowitz et al. 1995) and inactivation of ActRII was recently observed in gastrointestinal cancers (Hempen, et al., 2003). An inactivating mutation in TβRI (ALK5) occurs in one third of ovarian cancers observed (Wang et al., 2000) and ALK4 mutations have been described in pancreatic cancer, leading to the designation of ALK4 as a tumor suppressor gene (Su et al. 2001). The activin/TGF-β signaling pathway is also disrupted by mutations in Smad4 and Smad2. As mentioned above, Smad4 was originally identified as DPC4 (_deleted in pancreatic carcinoma locus 4_) and this gene is functionally absent in half of all pancreatic cancers (Hahn et al. 1996) and one third of colon carcinomas (Miyaki et al. 1999). Smad2 is also inactivated in a small proportion of colorectal cancers and lung cancers (Eppert et al. 1996, Uchida et al. 1996), whereas Smad3 levels were shown to be reduced in human gastric cancer tissues (Han et al. 2003) and Smad3[-/-] mice develop colorectal cancer (Zhu et al. 1998). In addition, it was recently shown that Smad7 but not Smad6, in conjunction with ras, caused malignant conversion in a mouse model for squamous cell carcinoma (Liu et al. 2003). Since Smad7 blocks Smad2/3 signaling but Smad6 does not, this result further indicates the importance of the Smad2/3 pathway in preventing tumorigenesis.

Interestingly, despite their antiproliferative effects, TGF-β and activin can also exacerbate the cancer phenotype under conditions in which cells have become refractory to Smad2/3-induced growth inhibition (Derynck et al. 2001; Wakefield et al. 2002). For example, increased production of TGF-β or activin by tumor cells that are no longer growth inhibited by Smad2/3 signals may lead to increased angiogenesis, decreased immune surveillance and/or an increase in the epithelial to mesenchymal transition (EMT) of tumor cells favoring tumor growth and spread (Derynck et al. 2001; Wakefield et al. 2002). There is evidence that the level of Smad2/3 signaling is an important determinant of whether there is an antiproliferative response or tumorigenic or prometastatic response (Nicolas et al. 2003; Tian et al. 2003). It is therefore important to further understand the molecular causes underlying reduced Smad2/3 signaling in tumor cells as well as the basis for the selective loss of the antiproliferative effects when Smad2/3 signaling is reduced (Derynck et al. 2001; Wakefield et al. 2002).

## Regulation of TGF-β ligand signaling by EGF-CFC proteins

Similar to activin, nodal (Schier 2003; Schier et al. 2000) and GDF-1/Vg1 (Cheng et al. 2003) have been shown to signal via the activin receptors ActRII/IIB and ALK4. Unlike activin, however, these TGF-β superfamily members require additional co-receptors from the *Epidermal Growth Factor-Cripto, FRL-1, Cryptic* (EGF-CFC) protein family to assemble type II and type I receptors and generate signals (Table 1) (Cheng, et al., 2003, Schier, 2003, Schier, A. F., et al., 2000). The EGF-CFC of extracellular signaling proteins includes human and mouse Cripto and Cryptic, Xenopus FRL-1 and zebrafish *one-eyed pinhead* (oep) (Saloman, et al., 2000, Schier, 2003, Shen, et al., 2000). EGF-CFC proteins act cell autonomously as GPI-anchored cell surface co-receptors but also have been shown to have activity when expressed as soluble proteins (Bianco, et al., 2002, Minchiotti, et al., 2001, Saloman, et al., 2000, Zhang, J., et al., 1998) or when released from the cell surface following enzymatic cleavage of their GPI anchor (Yan, et al., 2002). Genetic studies in zebrafish and mice have demonstrated that EGF-CFC proteins are essential for mesoderm and endoderm formation, cardiogenesis, and the establishment of left/right asymmetry during embryonic development (Schier, 2003, Schier, A. F., et al., 2000, Shen, et al., 2000). Targeted disruption of the Cripto gene in mice results in the absence of primitive streak formation and failure to form embryonic mesoderm (Ding, et al., 1998). This phenotype is very similar to that of mice lacking both ActRII and ActRIIB (Song, et al., 1999) or ALK4 (Gu, et al., 1998) or nodal (Conlon, et al., 1994, Zhou, et al., 1993), consistent with a nodal signaling pathway that requires activin receptors and Cripto (Schier, 2003, Schier, A. F., et al., 2000). Biochemical experiments have demonstrated that Cripto binds nodal via its EGF-like domain and ALK4 via its CFC domain (Yeo, et al., 2001) and Cripto mutants defective in nodal binding or ALK4 binding do not facilitate nodal signaling (Yan, et al., 2002, Yeo, et al., 2001). In summary, substantial evidence now indicates that nodal requires EGF-CFC proteins to assemble a functional receptor complex (Bianco, et al., 2002, Cheng, et al., 2003, Reissmann, et al., 2001, Yan, et al., 2002, Yeo, et al., 2001).

## Cripto is an oncogene and blocks activin signaling

Cripto is an oncogene and blocks activin signaling. Cripto was initially isolated as a putative oncogene from a human teratocarcinoma cell line (Ciccodicola, et al., 1989) and was subsequently shown to confer anchorage independent growth to NOG-8 mouse mammary epithelial cells (Ciardiello, et al., 1991). Cripto is expressed at high levels in multiple human tumors including those of breast, colon, stomach, pancreas, lung, ovary, endometrial, testis, bladder and prostate but it is absent or expressed at low levels in their normal counterparts (Salomon, et al., 2000). Cripto was recently identified as a primary target of Wnt/beta-catenin signals both in embryogenesis as well as in colon carcinoma cell lines and tissues (Morkel, et al., 2003) providing a basis for Cripto upregulation in tumors. It has been demonstrated that recombinant, soluble Cripto and a chemically synthesized 47 amino acid fragment spanning the EGF-like domain of Cripto (Lohmeyer, et al., 1997) can activate the mitogen activated protein kinase (MAPK) and phosphatidylinositol-3-kinase (PI3K) pathways (Saloman, et al., 2000). Cripto does not bind to ErbB family members, although [$^{125}$I]-Cripto specifically labeled mammary epithelial and breast cancer cell lines and formed crosslinked complexes with 60 kDa and 130 kDa membrane proteins (Bianco, et al., 1999). Although these putative Cripto receptor proteins have not been identified, the 60 kDa protein may have been ALK4 (Bianco, et al., 2002).

We and others have recently demonstrated that Cripto can antagonize activin signaling (see Figure 1; Adkins, et al. 2003; Gray et al. 2003), providing an additional mechanism by which Cripto may promote tumorigenesis (Shen 2003). We have shown that Cripto forms a complex with activin-A and type II activin receptors that is mutually exclusive with binding of activin-A to ALK4 (Gray et al. 2003). Our data indicated that the EGF-like domain of Cripto was required for activin-A binding to Cripto, whereas mutations in the CFC domain previously shown to block Cripto binding to ALK4 did not prevent activin-A binding to Cripto (Gray et al. 2003). We further showed that transfection of Cripto into HepG2 cells or 293T cells that otherwise do not express Cripto confers inhibition of activin-A signaling, and we have proposed a model in which Cripto blocks activin signaling by functionally excluding ALK4 from activin·ActRII/IIB complexes (Gray et al. 2003). In a related study, Adkins et al. (2003) reported direct binding of activin-B but not activin-A to Cripto using purified soluble proteins (i.e., soluble Cripto) in vitro (Adkins et al. 2003). They further demonstrated that a breast cancer cell line stably expressing Cripto was resistant to activin-B but not activin-A signaling relative to control cells (Adkins et al. 2003). Finally, they showed that a monoclonal antibody directed against the CFC domain of Cripto was able to block activin-B binding to Cripto in vitro, and this antibody also slowed Cripto-induced tumor growth in vivo (Adkins et al. 2003). Although mechanistic discrepancies remain to be resolved, these studies each support a novel role for Cripto in attenuating activin signaling.

## Follistatin and other activin modulators

Follistatins and follistatin-related proteins are important regulators of activin signaling (reviewed in Welt et al. 2002)) and were originally characterized as components of gonadal fluids with suppressive effects on pituitary FSH secretion (DePaolo et al.,1991; Michel et al. 1993; Phillips et al. 1998). As illustrated in Figure 1, follistatins are activin-binding proteins capable of inactivating and antagonizing all biological actions of activins (Bilezikjian et al. 1992; DePaolo et al. 1991; Michel et al. 1993; Phillips et al. 1998; Woodruff 1998). They are present in a wide range of tissues, often coinciding with the distribution of the inhibin β subunits, suggestive of their role as local buffers of activins (Michel et al. 1990; Shimasaki et al. 1989). Either null mutation (Matzuk et al. 1995) or over-expression (Guo et al. 1998) of the follistatin gene has provided clear evidence for the importance of follistatin in developmental processes, fertility and normal reproductive function.

Additional proteins are likely to play important roles in regulating activin's ability to bind its receptors and generate cellular responses (Fig. 1; Phillips 2000). Like follistatin, α2 macroglobulin is an extracellular activin-binding protein thought to play a dual role both in stabilizing activin in the circulation and targeting activin for degradation (Niemuller et al. 1995; Vaughan et al. 1992). Recently discovered activin-binding proteins with poorly characterized physiological roles in regulating activin signaling include Cerberus (Hsu et al. 1998), uterine milk protein (McFarlane et al. 1999) and lipovitellin 1 (Iemura et al.,1999). As discussed above, nodal is a TGF ligand that signals through an activin-like pathway via ActRII or ActRIIB and ALK4 but, unlike activin, nodal signaling is dependent on the presence of a member of the EGF-CFC family (Schier 2003; Schier 2000). Lefty/antivin proteins are TGF ligands that are nodal antagonists (Schier 2003; Schier 2000). Genetic evidence had indicated that Lefty/antivin proteins might act as competitive antagonists of nodal and activin signaling by binding directly to ActRII or IIB (Thisse et al. 1999). A recent study has shown, however, that Lefty antagonizes nodal but not activin by binding directly to EGF-CFC proteins (Cheng et al. 2004). At the level of the membrane, BAMBI (*B*MP and *a*ctivin *m*embrane-*b*ound *i*nhibitor) has been identified as a transmembrane pseudo type I receptor that lacks a kinase domain and, similar to what has been proposed for Cripto antagonism of activin (Adkins et al. 2003; Gray et al. 2003), forms inactive complexes with TGF-β family members to block their signaling (Fig. 1; Onichtchouk et al. 1999). BAMBI is co-expressed with BMP-4 during Xenopus embryogenesis and requires BMP signaling for its expression (Onichtchouk et al. 1999). The possible roles of BAMBI, Cripto and other related pseudo receptors in regulating activin signaling remain to be elucidated.

## Conclusions

In summary, TGF-β superfamily signaling and regulation are exquisitely complex. At each level, there is promiscuity, yet each ligand class relies on a unique combination of receptors/co-receptors and pathway-selective Smad proteins (see Table 1). For example, activins and BMPs share Type II activin receptors and signal via unique type I receptors and distinct Smads. On the other hand, activins and TGF-βs form complexes with distinct Type II and Type I receptors, yet phosphorylate the same Smads. Betaglycan apparently binds the inhibin α subunit, thereby preventing activin binding to Type II receptors that are instead bound to the β subunit of inhibin. Betaglycan binds TGF-βs and inhibins with opposing functional consequences, biasing the systems towards promoting TGF-β responses while inhibiting activin signaling. Cripto and other EGF-CFC family members add further to the intricacies of signaling regulation. These co-receptors are required for signaling by nodals but not activins and can instead antagonize activin signaling. Furthermore, EGF-CFC proteins are the target for Leftys, allowing selective blockade of nodals but not activins. In addition to cell surface events, numerous cytoplasmic and nuclear factors confer tissue-specific and context-dependent modulation of responses to these ligands (von Bubnoff et al. 2001). There are undoubtedly additional factors to be discovered that regulate components of the activin signaling pathway and determine sensitivity to activins and inhibins. Current evidence is most consistent with competitive antagonism at the level of cell surface receptors, although the possibility that inhibin generates independent intracellular signals cannot be ruled out.

Activin and other members of the TGF-β family play crucial developmental and functional roles in normal and diseased circumstances. Improved understanding of the molecules and mechanisms of signaling and counter-regulation will provide insight concerning reproductive physiology and pathophysiology. Furthermore, these studies will identify potential molecular targets for the development of therapeutic means for modulating fertility and managing medical disorders.

## References

Abraham EJ, Faught WJ, Frawley LS (1998) Transforming growth factor beta1 is a paracrine inhibitor of prolactin gene expression. Endocrinology 139:5174-5181

Adkins HB, Bianco C, Schiffer SG, Rayhorn P, Zafari M, Cheung AE, Orozco O, Olson D, De Luca A, Chen LL, Miatkowski K, Benjamin C, Normanno N, Williams KP, Jarpe M, LePage D, Salomon D, Sanicola M (2003) Antibody blockade of the Cripto CFC domain suppresses tumor cell growth in vivo. J Clin Invest 112:575-587

Alzheimer C, Werner S (2002) Fibroblast growth factors and neuroprotection. Adv Exp Med Biol 513:335-351

Andreasson K, Worley PF (1995) Induction of beta-A activin expression by synaptic activity and during neocortical development. Neurosci 69:781-796

Archer SJ, Bax A, Roberts AB, Sporn MB, Ogawa Y, Piez KA, Weatherbee JA, Tsang M, Lucas R, Zheng B-L, Wenker J, Torchia DA (1993) Transforming growth factor β1: secondary structure as determined by heteronuclear magnetic resonance spectroscopy. Biochem 32: 1164-1171

Asashima M, Nakano H, Shimada K, Kinoshita K, Ishii K, Shibai H, Ueno N (1990) Mesodermal induction in early amphibian embryos by activin A. Roux's Arch Dev Biol 198:330-335

Attisano L, Wrana JL, Cheifetz S, Massague J (1992) Novel activin receptors: distinct genes and alternative mRNA splicing generate a repertoire of serine/threonine kinase receptors. Cell 68:97-108

Attisano L, Wrana JL, Montalvo E, Massague J (1996) Activation of signalling by the activin receptor complex. Mol Cell Biol 16:1066-1073

Bassing CH, Yingling JM, Howe DJ, Wang T, He WW, Gustafson ML, Shah P, Donahoe PK, Wang X-F (1994) A transforming growth factor-β type I receptor that signals to activate gene expression. Science 263:87-89

Beer HD, Gassmann MG, Munz B, Steiling H, Engelhardt F, Bleuel K, Werner S (2000) Expression and function of keratinocyte growth factor and activin in skin morphogenesis and cutaneous wound repair. J Invest Dermatol Symp Proc 5:34-39.

Bernard DJ, Chapman SC, Woodruff TK (2001) Mechanisms of inhibin signal transduction. Recent Prog Horm Res 56:417-450.

Bernard DJ, Burns KH, Haupt B, Matzuk MM, Woodruff TK (2003) Normal reproductive function in InhBP/p120-deficient mice. Mol Cell Biol 23:4882-4891

Bianco C, Adkins HB, Wechselberger C, Seno M, Normanno N, De Luca A, Sun Y, Khan N, Kenney N, Ebert A, Williams KP, Sanicola M, Salomon DS (2002) Cripto-1 activates nodal- and ALK4-dependent and -independent signaling pathways in mammary epithelial Cells. Mol Cell Biol 22:2586-2597

Bianco C, Kannan S, De Santis M, Seno M, Tang CK, Martinez-Lacaci I, Kim N, Wallace-Jones B, Lippman ME, Ebert AD, Wechselberger C, Salomon DS (1999) Cripto-1 indirectly stimulates the tyrosine phosphorylation of erb B-4 through a novel receptor. J Biol Chem 274:8624-8629

Bianco C, Normanno N, De Luca A, Maiello MR, Wechselberger C, Sun Y, Khan N, Adkins H, Sanicola M, Vonderhaar B, Cohen B, Seno M, Salomon D (2002) Detection and localization of Cripto-1 binding in mouse mammary epithelial cells and in the mouse mammary gland using an immunoglobulin-cripto-1 fusion protein. J Cell Physiol 190:74-82

Bilezikjian LM, Corrigan AZ, Vale WW (1990) Activin-A modulates growth hormone secretion from cultures of rat anterior pituitary cells. Endocrinology 126:2369-2376

Bilezikjian LM, Blount AL, Campen CA, Gonzalez-Manchon C, Vale WW (1991) Activin-A inhibits proopiomelanocortin messenger RNA accumulation and adrenocorticotropin secretion of AtT20 cells. Mol Endocrinol 5:1389-1395

Bilezikjian LM, Vale WW (1992) Local extragonadal roles of activins. Trends Endocrinol Metab 3:218-223

Bilezikjian LM, Corrigan AZ, Blount AL, Chen Y, Vale WW (2001) Regulation and actions of smad7 in the modulation of activin, inhibin and TGFβ signaling in anterior pituitary cells. Endocrinology 142:1065-1072

Billestrup N, Gonzalez-Manchon C, Potter E, Vale WW (1990) Inhibition of somatotroph growth and GH biosynthesis by activin in vitro. Mol Endocrinol 4:356-362

Brosh N, Sternberg D, Honigwachs-Sha'anani J, Lee BC, Shav-Tal Y, Tzehoval E, Shulman LM, Toledo J, Hacham Y, Carmi P, Jiang W, Sasse J, Horn F, Burstein Y, Zipori D (1995) The plasmacytoma growth inhibitor restrictin-P is an antagonist of interleukin 6 and interleukin 11. J Biol Chem 270:29594-29600

Brown CW, Houston-Hawkins DE, Woodruff TK, Matzuk MM (2000) Insertion of Inhbb into the Inhba locus rescues the Inhba-null phenotype and reveals new activin functions. Nat Genet 25:453-457

Broxmeyer HE, Lu L, Cooper S, Schwall R, Mason AJ, Nikolics K (1988) Selective and indirect modulation of human multipotential and erythroid hematopoietc progenitor cell proliferation by recombinant human activin and inhibin. Proc Natl Acad Sci USA 85: 9052-9056

Burns G, Sarkar DK (1993) Transforming growth factor β1-like immunoreactivity in the pituitary gland of the rat: effect of estrogen. Endocrinology 133:1444-1449

Calogero AE, Burrello N, Ossino AM, Polosa P, D'Agata R (1998) Activin-A stimulates hypothalamic gonadotropin-releasing hormone release by the explanted male rat hypothalamus: interaction with inhibin and androgens. J Endocrinol 156:269-274

Cameron VA, Nishimura E, Mathews LS, Lewis KA, Sawchenko PE, Vale WW (1994) Hybridization histochemical localization of activin receptor subtypes in rat brain, pituitary, ovary and testis. Endocrinology 134:799-808

Carroll RS, Corrigan AZ, Gharib SD, Vale WW, Chin WW (1989) Inhibin, activin and follistatin: regulation of follicle-stimulating hormone messenger ribonucleic acid levels. Mol Endocrinol 3:1969-1976

Chang H, Brown CW, Matzuk MM (2002) Genetic analysis of the mammalian transforming growth factor-beta superfamily. Endocr Rev 23:787-823

Chapman SC, Bernard DJ, Jelen J, Woodruff TK (2002) Properties of inhibin binding to betaglycan, InhBP/p120 and the activin type II receptors. Mol Cell Endocrinol 196:79-93

Chen CR, Kang Y, Siegel PM, Massague J (2002) E2F4/5 and p107 as Smad cofactors linking the TGFbeta receptor to c-myc repression. Cell 110:19-32

Chen YG, Lui HM, Lin SL, Lee JM, Ying SY (2002) Regulation of cell proliferation, apoptosis, and carcinogenesis by activin. Exp Biol Med (Maywood) 227:75-87

Cheng SK, Olale F, Bennett JT, Brivanlou AH, Schier AF (2003) EGF-CFC proteins are essential coreceptors for the TGF-beta signals Vg1 and GDF1. Genes Dev 17:31-36

Cheng SK, Olale F, Brivanlou AH, Schier AF (2004) Lefty Blocks a Subset of TGFbeta Signals by Antagonizing EGF-CFC Coreceptors. PLoS Biol 2:E30

Chong H, Pangas SA, Bernard DJ, Wang E, Gitch J, Chen W, Draper LB, Cox ET, Woodruff TK (2000) Structure and expression of a membrane component of the inhibin receptor system [see comments]. Endocrinology 141:2600-2607

Ciardiello F, Dono R, Kim N, Persico MG, Salomon DS (1991) Expression of cripto, a novel gene of the epidermal growth factor gene family, leads to in vitro transformation of a normal mouse mammary epithelial cell line. Cancer Res 51:1051-1054

Ciccodicola A, Dono R, Obici S, Simeone A, Zollo M, Persico MG (1989) Molecular characterization of a gene of the 'EGF family' expressed in undifferentiated human NTERA2 teratocarcinoma cells. Embo J 8:1987-1991

Conlon FL, Lyons KM, Takaesu N, Barth KS, Kispert A, Herrmann B, Robertson EJ (1994) A primary requirement for nodal in the formation and maintenance of the primitive streak in the mouse. Development 120:1919-1928

Cordenonsi M, Dupont S, Maretto S, Insinga A, Imbriano C, Piccolo S (2003) Links between tumor suppressors. p53 is required for TGF-beta gene responses by cooperating with Smads. Cell 113:301-314

Corrigan AZ, Bilezikjian LM, Carroll RS, Bald LN, Schmelzer CH, Fendly BM, Mason AJ, Chin WW, Schwall RH, Vale WW (1991) Evidence for an autocrine role of activin B within rat anterior pituitary cultures. Endocrinology 128:1682-1684

Coulombe JN, Schwall R, Parent AS, Eckenstein FP, Nishi R (1993) Induction of somatostatin immunoreactivity in cultured ciliary ganglion neurons by activin in choroid cell-conditioned medium. Neuron 10:899-906

Daadi M, Arcellana-Panlilio MY, Weiss S (1998) Activin co-operates with fibroblast growth factor 2 to regulate tyrosine hydroxylase expression in the basal forebrain ventricular zone progenitors. Neuroscience 86:867-880

Daopin S, Piez KA, Ogawa Y, Davies DR (1992) Crystal structure of transforming growth factor-$\beta$2: an unusual fold for the superfamily. Science 257:369-373

Darland DC, Link BA, Nishi R (1995) Activin A and follistatin expression in developing targets of ciliary ganglion neurons suggests a role in regulating neurotransmitter phenotype. Neuron 15:857-866

Dattatreyamurty B, Roux E, Horbinski C, Kaplan PL, Robak LA, Beck HN, Lein P, Higgins D, Chandrasekaran V (2001) Cerebrospinal fluid contains biologically active bone morphogenetic protein-7. Exp Neurol 172:273-281.

De Groot CJ, Montagne L, Barten AD, Sminia P, Van Der Valk P (1999) Expression of transforming growth factor (TGF)-beta1, -beta2, and - beta3 isoforms and TGF-beta type I and type II receptors in multiple sclerosis lesions and human adult astrocyte cultures. J Neuropathol Exp Neurol 58:174-187

De Kretser DM, Robertson DM, Risbridger GP, Hedger MP, McLachlan RI, Burger HG, Findlay JK (1988) Inhibin and related peptides. Prog Endocrinol 13-23

DeJong FH (1988) Inhibin. Physiol Rev 68:555-607

DePaolo LV, Bicsak TA, Erickson GF, Shimasaki S, Ling N (1991) Follistatin and activin: a potential intrinsic regulatory system within diverse tissues. Proc Soc Exp Biol Med 198: 500-512

Derynck R, Akhurst RJ, Balmain A (2001) TGF-beta signaling in tumor suppression and cancer progression. Nat Genet 29:117-129

Ding J, Yang L, Yan YT, Chen A, Desai N, Wynshaw-Boris A, Shen MM (1998) Cripto is required for correct orientation of the anterior-posterior axis in the mouse embryo. Nature 395:702-707

Dowling CR, Risbridger GP (2000) The role of inhibins and activins in prostate cancer pathogenesis. Endocr Relat Cancer 7:243-256.

Draper LB, Matzuk MM, Roberts V, Cox E, Weiss J, Mather JP, Woodruff TK (1998) Identification of an inhibin receptor in gonadal tumors from inhibin alpha-subunit knockout mice. J Biol Chem 273:398-403

Ebner R, Chen R-H, Shum L, Lawler S, Zioncheck TF, Lee A, Lopez AR, Derynck R (1993) Cloning of type I TGF-β receptor and its effect on TGF-β binding to the type II receptor. Science 260:1344-1348

Eppert K, Scherer SW, Ozcelik H, Pirone R, Hoodless P, Kim H, Tsui LC, Bapat B, Gallinger S, Andrulis IL, Thomsen GH, Wrana JL, Attisano L (1996) MADR2 maps to 18q21 and encodes a TGFbeta-regulated MAD-related protein that is functionally mutated in colorectal carcinoma. Cell 86:543-552

Ericson J, Norlin S, Jessell TM, Edlund T (1998) Integrated FGF and BMP signaling controls the progression of progenitor cell differentiation and the emergence of pattern in the embryonic anterior pituitary. Development 125:1005-1015

Esparza-Lopez J, Montiel JL, Vilchis-Landeros M, Okadome T, Miyazono K, Lopez-Casillas F (2001) Ligand binding and functional properties of betaglycan, a co-receptor of the transforming growth factor-{beta} superfamily. Specialized binding sites for transforming growth factor-beta and inhibin A. J Biol Chem 18:14588-14596

Ethier JF, Farnworth PG, Findlay JK, Ooi GT (2002) Transforming growth factor-beta modulates Inhibin A bioactivity in the LbetaT2 gonadotrope cell line by competing for binding to betaglycan. Mol Endocrinol 16:2754-2763

Eto Y, Tsuji T, Takezawa M, Takano S, Yokogawa Y, Shibai H (1987) Purification and characterization of erythroid differentiation factor (EDF) isolated from human leukemia cell line THP-1. Biochem Biophys Res Commun 142:1095-1103
Mol Cell 9:133-143.

Feng XH, Zhang Y, Wu RY, Derynck R (1998) The tumor suppressor Smad4/DPC4 and transcriptional adaptor CBP/p300 are coactivators for smad3 in TGF-beta-induced transcriptional activation. Genes Dev 12:2153-2163

Feng XH, Lin X, Derynck R (2000) Smad2, Smad3 and Smad4 cooperate with Sp1 to induce p15(Ink4B) transcription in response to TGF-beta. Embo J 19:5178-5193.

Feng XH, Liang YY, Liang M, Zhai W, Lin X (2002) Direct interaction of c-Myc with Smad2 and Smad3 to inhibit TGF-beta-mediated induction of the CDK inhibitor p15(Ink4B) Mol Cell 9:133-143

Funaba M, Murata T, Fujimura H, Murata E, Abe M, Torii K (1997) Immunolocalization of type I or type II activin receptors in the rat brain. J Neuroendocrinol 9:105-111

Gonzalez-Manchon C, Bilezikjian LM, Corrigan AZ, Mellon PL, Vale WW (1991) Activin-A modulates gonadotropin-releasing hormone secretion from a gonadotropin-releasing hormone-secreting neuronal cell line. Neuroendocrinology 54:373-377

Gray PC, Greenwald J, Blount AL, Kunitake KS, Donaldson CJ, Choe S, Vale W (2000) Identification of a Binding Site on the Type II Activin Receptor for Activin and Inhibin. J Biol Chem 275:3206-3212

Gray PC, Harrison CA, Vale W (2003) Cripto forms a complex with activin and type II activin receptors and can block activin signaling. Proc Natl Acad Sci USA 100:5193-5198

Greenwald J, Fischer WH, Vale WW, Choe S (1999) Three-finger toxin fold for the extracellular ligand-binding domain of the type II activin receptor serine kinase. Nat Struct Biol 6:18-22

Greenwald J, Groppe J, Gray P, Wiater E, Kwiatkowski W, Vale W, Choe S (2003) The BMP7/ActRII extracellular domain complex provides new insights into the cooperative nature of receptor assembly. Mol Cell 11:605-617

Griffith DL, Keck PC, Sampath TK, Rueger DC, Carlson WD (1996) Three-dimensional structure of recombinant human osteogenic protein 1: structural paradigm for the transforming growth factor beta superfamily. Proc Natl Acad Sci U S A 93:878-883

Gu Z, Nomura M, Simpson BB, Lei H, Feijen A, van den Eijnden-van Raaij J, Donahoe PK, Li E (1998) The type I activin receptor ActRIB is required for egg cylinder organization and gastrulation in the mouse. Genes Dev 12:844-857

Guo Q, Kumar TR, Woodruff T, Hadsell LA, DeMayo FJ, Matzuk MM (1998) Overexpression of mouse follistatin causes reproductive defects in transgenic mice. Mol Endocrinol 12: 96-106

Hahn SA, Schutte M, Hoque AT, Moskaluk CA, da Costa LT, Rozenblum E, Weinstein CL, Fischer A, Yeo CJ, Hruban RH, Kern SE (1996) DPC4, a candidate tumor suppressor gene at human chromosome 18q21.1. Science 271:350-353

Han SU, Kim HT, Seong DH, Kim YS, Park YS, Bang YJ, Yang HK, Kim SJ (2003) Loss of the Smad3 expression increases susceptibility to tumorigenicity in human gastric cancer. Oncogene 23(7): 1333-1341

Hangoc G, Carow CE, Schwall R, Mason AJ, Broxmeyer HE (1992) Effects invivo of recombinant human inhibin on myelopoiesis in mice. Exp Hematol 20:1243-1246

Harrison CA, Farnworth PG, Chan KL, Stanton PG, Ooi GT, Findlay JK, Robertson DM (2001) Identification of specific inhibin a-binding proteins on mouse leydig (tm3) and sertoli (tm4) cell lines. Endocrinology 142:1393-1402.

Harrison CA, Gray PC, Koerber SC, Fischer W, Vale W (2003) Identification of a functional binding site for activin on the type I receptor ALK4. J Biol Chem 278: 21129-21135

Hart PJ, Deep S, Taylor AB, Shu Z, Hinck CS, Hinck AP (2002) Crystal structure of the human TbetaR2 ectodomain–TGF-beta3 complex. Nat Struct Biol 9:203-208

Hashimoto M, Kondo S, Sakurai T, Etoh Y, Shibai H, Muramatsu M (1990) Activin/EDF as an inhibitor of neural differentiation. Biochem Biophys Res Commun 173:193-200

Hashimoto M, Nakamura T, Inoue S, Kondo T, Yamada R, Eto Y, Sugino H, Muramatsu M (1992) Follistatin is a developmentally regulated cytokine in neural differentiation. J Biol Chem 267:7203-7206

Hawkins RL, Inoue M, Mori M, Torii K (1995) Effect of inhibin, follistatin, or activin infusion into the lateral hypothalamus on operant behavior of rats fed lysine deficient diet. Brain Res 704:1-9

Hayashi H, Abdollah S, Qiu Y, Cai J, Xu YY, Grinnell BW, Richardson MA, Topper JN, Gimbrone J, M.A., Wrana JL, Falb D (1997) The MAD-related protein Smad7 associates with the TGFbeta receptor and functions as an antagonist of TGFb signaling. Cell 89: 1165-1173

Heldin CH, Miyazono K, ten Dijke P (1997) TGF-beta signalling from cell membrane to nucleus through SMAD proteins. Nature 390:465-471

Hempen PM, Zhang L, Bansal RK, Iacobuzio-Donahue CA, Murphy KM, Maitra A, Vogelstein B, Whitehead RH, Markowitz SD, Willson JK, Yeo CJ, Hruban RH, Kern SE (2003) Evidence of selection for clones having genetic inactivation of the activin A type II receptor (ACVR2) gene in gastrointestinal cancers. Cancer Res 63:994-999

Hertan R, Farnworth PG, Fitzsimmons KL, Robertson DM (1999) Identification of high affinity binding sites for inhibin on ovine pituitary cells in culture. Endocrinology 140: 6-12

Hotten G, Neidhart H, Schneider C, Pohl J (1995) Cloning of a new member of the TGF-beta family: putative new activin beta-C chain. Biochem Biophys Res Commun 206:608-613

Hsu DR, Economides AN, Wang X, Eimon PM, Harland RM (1998) The Xenopus dorsalizing factor Gremlin identifies a novel family of secreted proteins that antagonize BMP activities. Mol Cell 1:673-683

Hsueh AJW, Bicsak TA, Vaughan J, Tucker E, Rivier J, Vale WW (1987) Heterodimers and homodimers of inhibin subunits have different paracrine action in the modulation of luteinizing hormone-stimulated androgen biosynthesis. Proc Natl Acad Sci USA 84: 5082-5086

Hughes PE, Alexi T, Williams CE, Clark RG, Gluckman PD (1999) Administration of recombinant human Activin-A has powerful neurotrophic effects on select striatal phenotypes in the quinolinic acid lesion model of Huntington's disease. Neuroscience 92:197-209

Iemura S, Yamamoto TS, Takagi C, Kobayashi H, Ueno N (1999) Isolation and characterization of bone morphogenetic protein-binding proteins from the early Xenopus embryo. J Biol Chem 274:26843-26849

Imamura T, Takase M, Nishihara A, Oeda E, Hanai J, Kawabata M, Miyazono K (1997) Smad6 inhibits signalling by the TGF-beta superfamily. Nature 389:622-626

Inokuchi K, Kato A, Hiraia K, Hishinuma F, Inoue M, Ozawa F (1996) Increase in activin beta A mRNA in rat hippocampus during long-term potentiation. FEBS Lett 382:48-52

Ishisaki A, Yamato K, Nakao A, Nonaka K, Ohguchi M, tenDijke P, Nishihara T (1998) Smad7 is an activin-inducible inhibitor of activin-induced growth arrest and apoptosis in mouse B cells. J Biol Chem 273:24293-24296

Iwahori Y, Saito H, Torii K, Nishiyama N (1997) Activin exerts a neurotrophic effect on cultured hippocampal neurons. Brain Res 760:52-58

Janknecht R, Wells NJ, Hunter T (1998) TGF-beta-stimulated cooperation of Smad proteins with the coactivators CBP/p300. Genes Dev 12:2114-2119

Kang Y, Chen CR, Massague J (2003) A self-enabling TGFbeta response coupled to stress signaling: Smad engages stress response factor ATF3 for Id1 repression in epithelial cells. Mol Cell 11:915-926

Kim J, Johnson K, Chen HJ, Carroll S, Laughon A (1997) Drosophila Mad binds to DNA and directly mediates activation of vestigial by Decapentaplegic. Nature 388:304-308

Kimelman D, Griffin KJ (2000) Vertebrate mesendoderm induction and patterning. Curr Opin Genet Dev 10:350-356

Kirsch T, Sebald W, Dreyer MK (2000) Crystal structure of the BMP-2-BRIA ectodomain complex. Nat Struct Biol 7:492-496

Kjellman C, Olofsson SP, Hansson O, Von Schantz T, Lindvall M, Nilsson I, Salford LG, Sjogren HO, Widegren B (2000) Expression of TGF-beta isoforms, TGF-beta receptors, and SMAD molecules at different stages of human glioma. Int J Cancer 89:251-258

Kretzschmar M, Liu F, Hata A, Doody J, Massague J (1997) The TGF-beta family mediator Smad1 is phosphorylated directly and activated functionally by the BMP receptor kinase. Genes Dev 11:984-995

Krieglstein K, Suter-Crazzolara C, Fischer WH, Unsicker K (1995) TGF-beta superfamily members promote survival of midbrain dopaminergic neurons and protect them against MPP+ toxicity. Embo J 14:736-742

Kubota K, Suzuki M, Yamanouchi K, Takahashi M, Nishihara M (2003) Involvement of activin and inhibin in the regulation of food and water intake in the rat. J Vet Med Sci 65:237-242

Labbe E, Silvestri C, Hoodless PA, Wrana JL, Attisano L (1998) Smad2 and Smad3 positively and negatively regulate TGF beta-dependent transcription through the forkhead DNA-binding protein FAST2. Mol Cell 2:109-120

Lai M, Sirimanne E, Williams CE, Gluckman PD (1996) Sequential patterns of inhibin subunit gene expression following hypoxic-ischemic injury in the rat brain. Neuroscience 70: 1013-1024

Lai M, Gluckman P, Dragunow M, Hughes PE (1997) Focal brain injury increases activin betaA mRNA expression in hippocampal neurons. Neuroreport 8:2691-2694

Lebrun J-J, Vale WW (1997) Activin and inhibin have antagonistic effects on ligand-dependent heterodimerization of the type I and type II activin receptors and human erythroid differentiation. Mol Cell Biol 17:1682-1691

Lebrun J-J, Takabe K, Chen Y, Vale WW (1999) Roles of pathway-specific and inhibitory Smads in activin receptor signaling. Mol Endocrinol 13:15-23

Lee S, Rivier CL (1997) Effect of repeated activin-A treatment on the activity of the hypothalamic-pituitary-gonadal axis of the adult male rat. Biol Reprod 56:969-975

Levin M, Johnson RL, Stern CD, Kuehn M, Tabin C (1995) A molecular pathway determining left-right asymmetry in chick embryogenesis. Cell 82:803-814

Lewen A, Soderstrom S, Hillered L, Ebendal T (1997) Expression of serine/threonine kinase receptors in traumatic brain injury. Neuroreport 8:475-479

Lewis KA, Gray PC, Blount AL, MacConell LA, Wiater E, Bilezikjian LM, Vale W (2000) Betaglycan binds inhibin and can mediate functional antagonism of activin signaling. Nature 404:411-414

Lin SZ, Hoffer BJ, Kaplan P, Wang Y (1999) Osteogenic protein-1 protects against cerebral infarction induced by MCA ligation in adult rats. Stroke 30:126-133

Ling N, Ying SY, Ueno N, Esch F, Denoroy L, Guillemin R (1985) Isolation and partial characterization of a Mr 32,000 protein with inhibin activity from porcine follicular fluid. Proc Natl Acad Sci USA 82:7217-7221

Ling N, Ying SA, Ueno N, Shimasaki S, Esch F, Hotta M, Guillemin R (1986) Pituitary FSH is released by a heterodimer of the b-subunits from the two forms of inhibin. Nature 321: 779-782

Liu F, Ventura F, Doody J, Massague J (1995) Human type II receptor for bone morphogenic proteins (BMPs): extension of the two-kinase receptor model to the BMPs. Mol Cell Biol 15:3479-3486

Liu X, Lee J, Cooley M, Bhogte E, Hartley S, Glick A (2003) Smad7 but not Smad6 cooperates with oncogenic ras to cause malignant conversion in a mouse model for squamous cell carcinoma. Cancer Res 63:7760-7768

Lohmeyer M, Harrison PM, Kannan S, DeSantis M, O'Reilly NJ, Sternberg MJ, Salomon DS, Gullick WJ (1997) Chemical synthesis, structural modeling, and biological activity of the epidermal growth factor-like domain of human cripto. Biochemistry 36:3837-3845

Lopez-Casillas F, Wrana JL, Massague J (1993) Betaglycan presents ligand to the TGF beta signaling receptor. Cell 73:1435-1444.

MacConell LA, Barth S, Roberts VJ (1996) Distribution of follistatin messenger ribonucleic acid in the rat brain: implications for a role in the regulation of central reproductive functions. Endocrinology 137:2150-2158

MacConell LA, Widger AE, Barth-Hall S, Roberts VJ (1998) Expression of activin and follistatin in the rat hypothalamus: anatomical association with gonadotropin-releasing hormone neurons and possible role of central activin in the regulation of luteinizing hormone release. Endocrine 9:233-241

MacConell LA, Lawson MA, Mellon PL, Roberts VJ (1999) Activin A regulation of gonadotropin-releasing hormone synthesis and release in vitro. Neuroendocrinology 70: 246-254

MacConell LA, Leal A, Vale W (2002) The distribution of betaglycan protein and mRNA in rat brain, pituitary and gonads: Implications for a role in inhibin-mediated reproductive functions. Endocrinology 143:1066-1075

Macias SM, Abdollah S, Hoodless PA, Pirone R, Attisano L, Wrana JL (1996) MADR2 is a substrate of the TGFbeta receptor and its phosphorylation is required for nuclear accumulation and signaling. Cell 87:1215-1224

Markowitz S, Wang J, Myeroff L, Parsons R, Sun L, Lutterbaugh J, Fan RS, Zborowska E, Kinzler KW, Vogelstein B (1995) Inactivation of the type II TGF-beta receptor in colon cancer cells with microsatellite instability. Science 268:1336-1338

Mason AJ, Hayflick JS, Ling N, Esch F, Ueno N, Ying SY, Guillemen R, Niall H, Seeburg PH (1985) Complementary DNA sequences of ovarian follicular fluid inhibin show precursor structure and homology with transforming growth factor-beta. Nature 318:659-663

Massague J (1998) TGF-$\beta$ signal transduction. Annu Rev Biochem 67:753-791

Massague J, Chen Y-C (2000) Controlling TGF-$\beta$ signaling. Genes Dev 14:627-644

Massague J, Wotton D (2000) Transcriptional control by the TGF-beta/Smad signaling system. Embo J 19:1745-1754

Massague J, Blain SW, Lo RS (2000) TGFbeta signaling in growth control, cancer, and heritable disorders. Cell 103:295-309

Mather JP, Attie KM, Woodruff TK, Rice GC, Phillips DM (1990) Activin stimulates spermatogonial proliferation in germ-sertoli cell cocultures from immature rat testis. Endocrinology 127:3206-3214

Mather JP, Moore A, Li RH (1997) Activins, inhibins, and follistatins: further thoughts on a growing family of regulators. Proc Soc Exp Biol Med 215:209-222

Mather JP, Woodruff TK, Krummen LA (1992) Paracrine regulation of reproductive function by inhibin and activin. Proc Soc Exp Biol Med 201:1-15

Mathews LS, Vale WW (1991) Expression cloning of an activin receptor, a predicted transmembrane serine kinase. Cell 65:973-982

Matzuk MM, Finegold MJ, Su JGJ, Hsueh AJW, Bradley A (1992) Alpha-inhibin is a tumor-suppressor gene with gonadal specificity in mice. Nature 366:313-319

Matzuk MM, Finegold MJ, Mather JP, Krummen L, Lu H, Bradley A (1994) Development of cancer cachexia-like syndrome and adrenal tumors in inhibin-deficient mice. Proc Natl Acad Sci USA 91:8817-8821

Matzuk MM, Lu N, Vogel H, Sellheyer K, Roop DR, Bradley A (1995) Multiple defects and perinatal death in mice deficient in follistatin. Nature 374:360-363

Matzuk MM, Kumar TR, Shou W, Coerver KA, Lau AL, Behringer RR, Finegold MJ (1996) Transgenic models to study the roles of inhibins and activins in reproduction, oncogenesis, and development. Recent Prog Horm Res 51:123-54; discussion 155-157

McCarthy SA, Bicknell R (1993) Inhibition of vascular endothelial cell growth by Activin-A. J Biol Chem 268:23066-23071

McFarlane JR, Foulds LM, O'Connor AE, Phillips DJ, Jenkin G, Hearn MT, de Kretser DM (1999) Uterine milk protein, a novel activin-binding protein, is present in ovine allantoic fluid. Endocrinology 140:4745-4752

Meunier H, Rivier C, Evans RM, Vale WW (1988) Gonadal and extra gonadal expression of inhibin $\alpha$, $\beta_A$ and $\beta_B$ subunits in various tissues predicts diverse functions. Proc Natl Acad Sci USA 85:247-251

Michel U, Albiston A, Findlay JK (1990) Rat follistatin: gonadal and extragonadal expression and evidence for alternative splicing. Biochem Biophys Res Commun 173:401-407

Michel U, Farnworth P, Findlay JK (1993) Follistatins: more than follicle-stimulating hormone suppressing proteins. Mol Cellul Endocrinol 91:1-11

Michel U, Gerber J, A EOC, Bunkowski S, Bruck W, Nau R, Phillips DJ (2003) Increased activin levels in cerebrospinal fluid of rabbits with bacterial meningitis are associated with activation of microglia. J Neurochem 86:238-245

Minchiotti G, Manco G, Parisi S, Lago CT, Rosa F, Persico MG (2001) Structure-function analysis of the EGF-CFC family member Cripto identifies residues essential for nodal signalling. Development 128:4501-4510

Miyaki M, Iijima T, Konishi M, Sakai K, Ishii A, Yasuno M, Hishima T, Koike M, Shitara N, Iwama T, Utsunomiya J, Kuroki T, Mori T (1999) Higher frequency of Smad4 gene mutation in human colorectal cancer with distant metastasis. Oncogene 18:3098-3103

Miyamoto K, Hasegawa Y, Fukuda M, Nomura M, Igarashi M, Kangawa K, Matsuo H (1985) Isolation of porcine follicular fluid inhibin of 32K daltons. Biochem Biophys Res Commun 129:396-403

Morkel M, Huelsken J, Wakamiya M, Ding J, van de Wetering M, Clevers H, Taketo MM, Behringer RR, Shen MM, Birchmeier W (2003) Beta-catenin regulates Cripto- and Wnt3-dependent gene expression programs in mouse axis and mesoderm formation. Development 130:6283-6294

Nakao A, Afrakhte M, Moren A, Nakayama T, Christian JL, Heuchel R, Itoh S, Kawabata M, Heldin NE, Heldin CH, ten Dijke P (1997) Identification of Smad7, a TGFbeta-inducible antagonist of TGF-beta signalling. Nature 389:631-635

Nicolas FJ, Hill CS (2003) Attenuation of the TGF-beta-Smad signaling pathway in pancreatic tumor cells confers resistance to TGF-beta-induced growth arrest. Oncogene 22:3698-3711

Niemuller CA, Randall KJ, Webb DJ, Gonias SL, LaMarre J (1995) Alpha 2-macroglobulin conformation determines binding affinity for activin A and plasma clearance of activin A/alpha 2-macroglobulin complex. Endocrinology 136:5343-5349

Oda S, Nishimatsu S, Murakami K, Ueno N (1995) Molecular cloning and functional analysis of a new activin beta subunit: a dorsal mesoderm-inducing activity in Xenopus. Biochem Biophys Res Commun 210:581-588

Ogawa Y, Schmidt DK, Nathan RM, Armstrong RM, Miller KL, Sawamura SJ, Ziman JM, Erickson KL, Deleon ER, Rosen DM, al e (1992) Bovine bone activin enhances bone morphogenetic protein-induced ectopic bone formation. J Biol Chem 267:14233-14237

Oliet SH, Plotsky PM, Bourque CW (1995) Effects of activin-A on neurons acutely isolated from the rat supraoptic nucleus. J Neuroendocrinol 7:661-663

Onichtchouk D, Chen YG, Dosch R, Gawantka V, Delius H, Massague J, Niehrs C (1999) Silencing of TGF-beta signalling by the pseudoreceptor BAMBI. Nature 401:480-485

Otsuka F, Shimasaki S (2002) A novel function of bone morphogenetic protein-15 in the pituitary: selective synthesis and secretion of FSH by gonadotropes. Endocrinology 143:4938-4941

Paralkar VM, Weeks BS, Yu YM, Kleinman HK, Reddi AH (1992) Recombinant human bone morphogenetic protein 2B stimulates PC12 cell differentiation: potentiation and binding to type IV collagen. J Cell Biol 119:1721-1728

Phillips DJ (2000) Regulation of activin's access to the cell: why is mother nature such a control freak? Bioessays 22:689-696.

Phillips DJ, deKretser DM (1998) Follistatin: A multifunctional regulatory protein. Front Neuroendocrinol 19:287-322

Plotsky PM, Kjaer A, Sutton SW, Sawchenko PE, Vale WW (1991) Central activin administration modulates corticotropin-releasing hormone and adrenocorticotropin secretion. Endocrinology 128:2520-2525

Prevot V, Bouret S, Croix D, Takumi T, Jennes L, Mitchell V, Beauvillain JC (2000) Evidence that members of the TGFbeta superfamily play a role in regulation of the GnRH neuroendocrine axis: expression of a type I serine-threonine kinase receptor for TGRbeta and activin in GnRH neurones and hypothalamic areas of the female rat. J Neuroendocrinol 12:665-670

Reis FM, Di Blasio AM, Florio P, Ambrosini G, Di Loreto C, Petraglia F (2001) Evidence for local production of inhibin A and activin A in patients with ovarian endometriosis. Fertil Steril 75:367-373.

Reissmann E, Jornvall H, Blokzijl A, Andersson O, Chang C, Minchiotti G, Persico MG, Ibanez CF, Brivanlou AH (2001) The orphan receptor ALK7 and the Activin receptor ALK4 mediate signaling by Nodal proteins during vertebrate development. Genes Dev 15:2010-2022

Rivier J, Spiess J, McClintock R, Vaughan J, Vale W (1985) Purification and partial characterization of inhibin from porcine follicular fluid. Biochem Biophys Res Commun 133:120-127

Robertson DM, Foulds LM, Leversha L, Morgan FJ, Hearn MT, Burger HG, Wettenhall RE, de Kretser DM (1985) Isolation of inhibin from bovine follicular fluid. Biochem Biophys Res Commun 126:220-226

Roh JS, Bondestam J, Mazerbourg S, Kaivo-Oja N, Groome N, Ritvos O, Hsueh AJ (2003) Growth differentiation factor-9 stimulates inhibin production and activates Smad2 in cultured rat granulosa cells. Endocrinology 144:172-178

Ryan AK, Blumberg B, Rodriguez-Esteban C, Yonei-Tamura S, Tamura K, Tsukui T, de la Pe—a J, Sabbagh W, Greenwald J, Choe S, Norris DP, Robertson EJ, Evans RM, Rosenfeld MG, Izpis'a Belmonte JC (1998) Pitx2 determines left-right asymmetry of internal organs in vertebrates. Nature 394:545-551

Salomon DS, Bianco C, Ebert AD, Khan NI, De Santis M, Normanno N, Wechselberger C, Seno M, Williams K, Sanicola M, Foley S, Gullick WJ, Persico G (2000) The EGF-CFC family: novel epidermal growth factor-related proteins in development and cancer. Endocr Relat Cancer 7:199-226.

Satoh M, Sugino H, Yoshida T (2000) Activin promotes astrocytic differentiation of a multipotent neural stem cell line and an astrocyte progenitor cell line from murine central nervous system. Neurosci Lett 284:143-146

Savage C, Das P, Finelli AL, Townsend SR, Sun CY, Baird SE, Padgett RW (1996) Caenorhabditis elegans genes sma-2, sma-3, and sma-4 define a conserved family of transforming growth factor beta pathway components. Proc Natl Acad Sci USA 93:790-794

Sawchenko PE, Plotsky PM, Pfeiffer W, Cunningham ET, Jr., Vaughan J, Rivier J, Vale WW (1988) Inhibin β in central neural pathways involved in the control of oxytocin secretion. Nature 334:615-617

Scheufler C, Sebald W, Hulsmeyer M (1999) Crystal structure of human bone morphogenetic protein-2 at 2.7 A resolution. J Mol Biol 287:103-115

Schier AF (2003) Nodal signaling in vertebrate development. Annu Rev Cell Dev Biol 19:589-621

Schier AF, Shen MM (2000) Nodal signalling in vertebrate development. Nature 403:385-389

Schlunegger MP, Gr,tter MG (1992) An unusual feature revealed by the crystal structure at 2.2 ≈ resolution of human transforming growth factor-β2. Nature 358:430-434

Schubert D, Kimura H, LaCorbiere M, Vaughan J, Karr D, Fischer WH (1990) Activin is a nerve cell survival molecule. Nature 344:868-870

Schwall RH, Jakeman LB, Altar CA (1993a) Hypothalamic infusion of activin A increases water consumption and urine volume in the rat. Neuroendocrinology 57:510-516

Schwall RH, Robbins K, Jardieu P, Chang L, Lai C, Terrell TG (1993b) Activin induces cell death in hepatocytes in vivo and in vitro. Hepatology 18:347-356

Sekelsky JJ, Newfeld SJ, Raftery LA, Chartoff EH, Gelbart WM (1995) Genetic characterization and cloning of mothers against dpp, a gene required for decapentaplegic function in Drosophila melanogaster. Genetics 139:1347-1358

Shaha C, Morris PL, Chen CLC, Vale W, Bardin CW (1989) Immunostainable inhibin subunits are in multiple types of testicular cells. Endocrinology 125:1941-1950

Shen MM, Schier AF (2000) The EGF-CFC gene family in vertebrate development. Trends Genet 16:303-309

Shen MM (2003) Decrypting the role of Cripto in tumorigenesis. J Clin Invest 112:500-502

Shi Y, Massague J (2003) Mechanisms of TGF-beta signaling from cell membrane to the nucleus. Cell 113:685-700

Shimasaki S, Koga M, Buscaglia ML, Simons DM, Bicsak TA, Ling N (1989) Follistatin gene expression in the ovary and extragonadal tissues. Mol Endocrinol 3:651-659

Shoji H, Nakamura T, van den Eijnden-van Raaij AJ, Sugino H (1998) Identification of a novel type II activin receptor, type IIA-N, induced during the neural differentiation of murine P19 embryonal carcinoma cells. Biochem Biophys Res Commun 246:320-324

Smith JC, Price BMJ, Van Nimmen K, Huylebroeck D (1990) Identification of a potent Xenopus mesoderm-inducing factor as a homologue of activin A. Nature 345:729-731

Song CZ, Siok TE, Gelehrter TD (1998) Smad4/DPC4 and Smad3 mediate transforming growth factor-beta (TGF-beta) signaling through direct binding to a novel TGF-beta-responsive element in the human plasminogen activator inhibitor-1 promoter. J Biol Chem 273:29287-29290

Song J, Oh SP, Schrewe H, Nomura M, Lei H, Okano M, Gridley T, Li E (1999) The type II activin receptors are essential for egg cylinder growth, gastrulation, and rostral head development in mice. Dev Biol 213:157-169

Su GH, Bansal R, Murphy KM, Montgomery E, Yeo CJ, Hruban RH, Kern SE (2001) ACVR1B (ALK4, activin receptor type 1B) gene mutations in pancreatic carcinoma. Proc Natl Acad Sci U S A 98:3254-3257.

ten Dijke P, Ichijo H, Franzen P, Schulz P, Saras J, Toyoshima H, Heldin CH, Miyazono K (1993) Activin receptor-like kinases: a novel subclass of cell-surface receptors with predicted serine/threonine kinase activity. Oncogene 8:2879-2887

ten Dijke P, Yamashita H, Ichijo H, Franzen P, Laiho M, Miyazono K, Heldin CH (1994a) Characterization of type I receptors for transforming growth factor- beta and activin. Science 264:101-104

ten Dijke P, Yamashita H, Sampath TK, Reddi AH, Estevez M, Riddle DL, Ichijo H, Heldin CH, Miyazono K (1994b) Identification of type I receptors for osteogenic protein-1 and bone morphogenetic protein-4. J Biol Chem 269:16985-16988

Thisse C, Thisse B (1999) Antivin, a novel and divergent member of the TGFbeta superfamily, negatively regulates mesoderm induction. Development 126:229-240

Thompson TB, Woodruff TK, Jardetzky TS (2003) Structures of an ActRIIB:activin A complex reveal a novel binding mode for TGF-beta ligand:receptor interactions. Embo J 22:1555-1566

Thomsen G, Woolf T, Whitman M, Sokol S, Vaughan J, Vale W, Melton D (1990) Activins are expressed early in Xenopus embryogenesis and can induce axial mesoderm and anterior structures. Cell 63:485-493

Tian F, DaCosta Byfield S, Parks WT, Yoo S, Felici A, Tang B, Piek E, Wakefield LM, Roberts AB (2003) Reduction in Smad2/3 signaling enhances tumorigenesis but suppresses metastasis of breast cancer cell lines. Cancer Res 63:8284-8292

Treier M, Gleiberman AS, O'Connell SM, Szeto DP, McMahon JA, McMahon AP, Rosenfeld MG (1998) Multistep signaling requirements for pituitary organogenesis in vivo. Genes Dev 12:1691-1704

Tretter YP, Munz B, Hubner G, ten Bruggencate G, Werner S, Alzheimer C (1996) Strong induction of activin expression after hippocampal lesion. Neuroreport 7:1819-1823

Tretter YP, Hertel M, Munz B, ten Bruggencate G, Werner S, Alzheimer C (2000) Induction of activin A is essential for the neuroprotective action of basic fibroblast growth factor in vivo. Nat Med 6:812-815

Trudeau VL, Pope L, de Winter JP, Hache RJ, Renaud LP (1996) Regulation of activin type-II receptor mRNA levels in rat hypothalamus by estradiol in vivo. J Neuroendocrinol 8: 395-401

Tsuchida K, Mathews LS, Vale WW (1993) Cloning and characterization of a transmembrane serine kinase that acts as an activin type I receptor. Proc Natl Acad Sci USA 90:11242-11246

Tsuchida K, Sawchenko PE, Nishikawa SI, Vale WW (1996) Molecular cloning of a novel type I receptor serine/threonine kinase for the TGFβ superfamily from rat brain. Mol Cell Neurosci 7:467-478

Uchida K, Nagatake M, Osada H, Yatabe Y, Kondo M, Mitsudomi T, Masuda A, Takahashi T (1996) Somatic in vivo alterations of the JV18-1 gene at 18q21 in human lung cancers. Cancer Res 56:5583-5585

Vale W, Rivier J, Vaughan J, McClintock R, Corrigan A, Woo W, Karr D, Spiess J (1986) Purification and characterization of an FSH releasing protein from porcine ovarian follicular fluid. Nature 321:776-779

Vale W, Hsueh A, Rivier C, Yu J (1990) The inhibin/activin family of growth factors. In: Roberts AB (eds) Peptide growth factors and their receptors, Handbook of experimental pharmacology. Springer-Verlag, Heidelberg, pp 211-248

van den Eijnden van Raaij AJ, van Achterberg TA, van der Kruijssen CM, Piersma AH, Huylebroeck D, de Laat SW, Mummery CL (1991) Differentiation of aggregated murine P19 embryonal carcinoma cells is induced by a novel visceral endoderm-specific FGF-like factor and inhibited by activin A. Mech Dev 33:157-165

Vaughan JM, Vale W (1992) a2-macroglobulin is a binding protein of inhibin and activin. Endocrinology 132:2038-2050

Vitt UA, Hsu SY, Hsueh AJ (2001) Evolution and classification of cystine knot-containing hormones and related extracellular signaling molecules. Mol Endocrinol 15:681-694.

von Bubnoff A, Cho KW (2001) Intracellular BMP signaling regulation in vertebrates: pathway or network? Dev Biol 239:1-14.

Wakefield LM, Roberts AB (2002) TGF-beta signaling: positive and negative effects on tumorigenesis. Curr Opin Genet Dev 12:22-29

Wang D, Kanuma T, Mizunuma H, Takama F, Ibuki Y, Wake N, Mogi A, Shitara Y, Takenoshita S (2000) Analysis of specific gene mutations in the transforming growth factor-beta signal transduction pathway in human ovarian cancer. Cancer Res 60:4507-4512

Wang Y, Chang CF, Morales M, Chou J, Chen HL, Chiang YH, Lin SZ, Cadet JL, Deng X, Wang JY, Chen SY, Kaplan PL, Hoffer BJ (2001) Bone morphogenetic protein-6 reduces ischemia-induced brain damage in rats. Stroke 32:2170-2178.

Wankell M, Werner S, Alzheimer C (2003) The roles of activin in cytoprotection and tissue repair. Ann NY Acad Sci 995:48-58

Weiss J, Harris PE, Halvorson LM, Crowley J, W.F., Jameson JL (1992) Dynamic regulation of follicle-stimulating hormone-beta messenger ribonucleic acid levels by activin and Gonadotropin-Releasing hormone in perifused rat pituitary cells. Endocrinology 131:1403-1408

Welt C, Sidis Y, Keutmann H, Schneyer A (2002) Activins, inhibins, and follistatins: from endocrinology to signaling. A paradigm for the new millennium. Exp Biol Med (Maywood) 227:724-752

Wiater E, Vale W (2003) Inhibin is an antagonist of bone morphogenetic protein signaling. J Biol Chem 278:7934-7941

Woodruff TK (1998) Regulation of cellular and system function by activin. Biochem Pharmacol 55:953-963

Wozney JM, Rosen V, Celeste AJ, Mitsock LM, Whitters MJ, Kriz RW, Hewick RM, Wang EA (1988) Novel regulators of bone formation: molecular clones and activities. Science 242:1528-1534

Wrana JL, Attisano L (2000) The Smad pathway. Cytokine Growth Factor Rev 11:5-13

Wrana J, Attisano L, Carcamo J, Zentella A, Doody J, Laiho M, Wang X-F, Massague J (1992) Mechanism of activation of the TGF-b receptor. Nature 370:341-347

Wu DD, Lai M, Hughes PE, Sirimanne E, Gluckman PD, Williams CE (1999) Expression of the activin axis and neuronal rescue effects of recombinant activin A following hypoxic-ischemic brain injury in the infant rat. Brain Res 835:369-378

Xu JM, McKeehan K, Matsuzaki K, McKeehan WL (1995) Inhibin antagonizes inhibition of liver cell growth by activin by a dominant-negative mechanism. J Biol Chem 270:6308-6313

Yamaguchi A (1995) Regulation of differentiation pathway of skeletal mesenchymal cells in cell lines by transforming growth factor-beta superfamily. Semin Cell Biol 6:165-173

Yan YT, Liu JJ, Luo Y, E C, Haltiwanger RS, Abate-Shen C, Shen MM (2002) Dual roles of Cripto as a ligand and coreceptor in the nodal signaling pathway. Mol Cell Biol 22:4439-4449

Yeo C, Whitman M (2001) Nodal signals to Smads through Cripto-dependent and Cripto-independent mechanisms. Mol Cell 7:949-957

Yingling JM, Datto MB, Wong C, Frederick JP, Liberati NT, Wang XF (1997) Tumor suppressor Smad4 is a transforming growth factor beta-inducible DNA binding protein. Mol Cell Biol 17:7019-7028

Yu J, Shao L, Lemas V, Yu AL, Vaughan J, Rivier J, Vale W (1987) The role of FSH releasing protein and inhibin in erythrodifferentiation. Nature 330:765-767

Zhang G, Ohsawa Y, Kametaka S, Shibata M, Waguri S, Uchiyama Y (2003) Regulation of FLRG expression in rat primary astroglial cells and injured brain tissue by transforming growth factor-beta 1 (TGF-beta 1). J Neurosci Res 72:33-45

Zhang J, Talbot WS, Schier AF (1998) Positional cloning identifies zebrafish one-eyed pinhead as a permissive EGF-related ligand required during gastrulation. Cell 92:241-251

Zhang Y, Feng X, We R, Derynck R (1996) Receptor-associated Mad homologues synergize as effectors of the TGF-beta response. Nature 383:168-172

Zhang Y, Feng XH, Derynck R (1998) Smad3 and Smad4 cooperate with c-Jun/c-Fos to mediate TGF-beta-induced transcription. Nature 394:909-913

Zhou X, Sasaki H, Lowe L, Hogan BL, Kuehn MR (1993) Nodal is a novel TGF-beta-like gene expressed in the mouse node during gastrulation. Nature 361:543-547

Zhu Y, Richardson JA, Parada LF, Graff JM (1998) Smad3 mutant mice develop metastatic colorectal cancer. Cell 94:703-714

# Twins and the fetal origins hypothesis: An application to growth data

*Dorret Boomsma[1], Gonneke Willemsen[1], Eco de Geus[1], Nina Kupper[1], Danielle Posthuma[1], Richard IJzerman[2], Bas Heijmans[3], Eline Slagboom[3], Leo Beem[1], and Conor Dolan[4]*

## Summary

The Barker hypothesis states that size at birth is negatively associated with disease risk later in life. Numerous studies have tested and confirmed this hypothesis in singletons. Using twin (or sibling) data, several extensions of the Barker hypothesis may be considered:

1. Within pairs, is the smallest twin also the one with the highest disease risk later in life? Since twins (or siblings) come from the same family, this test controls for any shared family effects, such as maternal nutrition, parental education or socio-economic status.
2. A second extension compares associations of differences in size at birth with differences in disease risk in monozygotic (MZ) and dizygotic (DZ) twin pairs. If associations of difference scores are larger in DZ than in MZ twin pairs, this is taken as evidence that the association is mediated by genetic factors.
3. These two methods can be considered as alternative approaches to the full bivariate analysis of MZ and DZ twin data. Using a bivariate structural equation model, the correlation between two traits can be decomposed into genetic and environmental correlations.

We address some statistical questions regarding the relation of difference scores (within MZ and DZ pairs) and genetic and environmental correlations. We show that the comparison of associations between MZ and DZ difference scores does not necessarily provide clear-cut answers to the question of how the relation of size at birth and later outcome is mediated.

We present an empirical application to data on stature, birth weight and height assessed in a large sample of Dutch adult MZ and DZ twin pairs. There is a significant association between size at birth (both weight and length) and

---

[1] Dept of Biological Psychology, Vrije Universiteit, Van der Boechorststraat 1, 1081 BT Amsterdam, The Netherlands
[2] Vrije Universiteit Medical Centre, Amsterdam, The Netherlands
[3] Dept of Molecular Epidemiology, Leiden University Medical Centre, Leiden, The Netherlands
[4] Dept of Psychology, Universiteit van Amsterdam, The Netherlands

Kordon et al.
Hormones and the Brain
© Springer-Verlag Berlin Heidelberg 2005

later stature. Within MZ and DZ twin pairs, the largest/heaviest twin at birth is the one who is tallest later in life. Using a bivariate structural equation model, we show that the association of birth length/weight and adult stature is explained by shared genes as well as by correlated common family and unique environmental influences.

## Introduction

The "fetal origins" or "Barker" hypothesis states that body size at birth is negatively associated with cardiovascular disease risk later in life. Numerous studies have tested the Barker hypothesis in singletons, and evidence has accumulated that low birth weight is indeed associated with an increased risk of cardiovascular disease and that this association may be mediated by the association of low birth weight with blood pressure, insulin resistance, diabetes, plasma lipids, fibrinogen or hypothalamic-pituitary-adrenal axis activity (see, e.g., Phillips 2002 and the accompanying papers in the November issue of Trends in Endocrinology and Metabolism 2002).

One of the explanations for these associations, the "programming" hypothesis, states that poor intrauterine growth leads to metabolic changes that have adverse effects on cardiovascular risk and cardiovascular risk factors in later life. In testing this hypothesis, birth weight and /or height are often used as surrogate measures of fetal nutrition (Barker 1995, 1998; Barker et al. 1989; but see also Paneth and Susser 1995; Huxley et al. 2002).

If the Barker hypothesis is tested in genetically related subjects instead of unrelated cases (small size at birth) and controls, it becomes possible to conduct several explicit tests that might explain the association between size at birth and later outcome variables. The fetal origins hypothesis explains the association solely in terms of a causal mechanism, with poor prenatal growth leading to later adverse effects, although it is recognized that the strength of the association can be modified by genotype (Barker 2002, 2003) or later childhood growth (e.g., Eriksson et al. 2003).

Several alternative explanations of the Barker hypothesis may be considered if data from at least two offspring from the same family are available. The offspring can consist of siblings or twin pairs. In this paper we focus on the analysis of data from monozygotic (MZ) and dizygotic (DZ) twins, but the principles apply to sibling data as well. In a simple and straightforward analysis, one can test if the twin or sibling with the smallest size at birth is also the sibling with the highest disease risk later in life. Since twins and siblings come from the same family, this test controls for any shared family effects such as parental education, diet and socio-economic status (SES) and may control for lifestyle factors like nutrition and smoking during a twin pregnancy.

A second test, usually employed for twin data, is to look at the association of differences in size at birth within pairs with later differences in, for example, blood pressure, cholesterol levels, stature or BMI. This test is carried out separately for MZ and DZ twins. If the association of difference scores is larger in DZ twins than in MZ twins, this is taken as evidence that the relation of size at birth and later outcome is mediated by genetic factors. Differences between trait values of MZ twins can only be influenced by environmental factors that are unique to individuals. Differences between trait values of DZ twins are influenced both by environmental factors and by non-shared genetic factors. The association of difference scores for two traits such as size at birth and blood pressure is therefore expected to be larger in DZ twins if the part of the association is mediated by genetic factors.

The analyses of difference scores within pairs can be considered an alternative approach to a full bivariate analysis of MZ and DZ twin data, in which the complete distribution of scores for size at birth and for later outcome is modeled using covariance analysis or structural equation modeling. In this last approach the covariance, or correlation, between size at birth and later outcome is decomposed into genetic and environmental correlations, which may be tested for significance. An association of birth weight with, for example, adult stature can arise because environmental factors that influence birth weight also are of importance for stature later in life, or because genes that influence birth weight also influence measures later in life. Such effects are referred to as pleiotropic genetic effects.

In this chapter we focus on data obtained in MZ and DZ twins and address the question of what the relationship is between size at birth and stature later in life. Adult stature is reliably obtained by self-report, is determined mostly by genetic factors, and is associated with disease risk (McCarron et al. 2002; Silvertoinen et al. 2003). We examine the association within MZ and DZ pairs and determine the genetic and environmental correlations between size at birth and stature through genetic covariance analysis. We look at the usefulness of analyzing difference scores and present an algebraic derivation for their expectations.

## Methods

### Participants

The Netherlands Twin Register (NTR) has collected longitudinal data by mailed survey every two to three years in adolescent and adult twins and their family members. The twin families were recruited through city councils in 1990/1991. In 1990 all city councils in The Netherlands were asked for the names and addresses of twins aged between 13 and 20 years. Of the 720 city councils that were approached, 252 gave a positive response and supplied 4,036 addresses of twin families. Between 1991 and 1993, additional addresses were obtained for 1,987 twin families. These included addresses from several of the larger cities. In the past 10 years, we have also recruited adult twins through city councils and have asked adult twins to register with the NTR in our yearly newsletter (Boomsma et al. 2002a).

Survey studies of health, lifestyle, personality and psychopathology have taken place in 1991, 1993, 1995, 1997 and 2000. A sixth survey is ongoing. A total of 8,219 twins participated in the first five surveys (3,226 twins participated once; 1,717 twice, 1,490 three times, 1,212 four times and 574 twins participated five times). Socioeconomic status (SES) for twins and siblings who are over 25 years (and most of whom have finished their education) is low in 22.1%, middle in 43.8% and high in 34.1% of the sample. Smoking behavior of twins and religious background of the participating families is comparable to that in the Dutch population (Boomsma et al. 1994, 1999).

For same-sex twin pairs, zygosity was determined from questions about physical similarity and confusion of the twins by family members, friends and strangers. For 804 same-sex twin pairs, information on zygosity based on DNA polymorphisms was also available. Agreement between zygosity diagnoses from survey and DNA data was 98%.

## Measures

In all surveys, participants were asked about their current height and weight. The 1991 and 1993 surveys asked the mothers of twins, and in 1993 also the fathers, about the children's birth weight and height and gestational age. In 1993, 1995 and 2000, participants were asked about their own birth weight and height (but not gestational age). Extreme birth weights were checked by sending a response card to the participants and/or by phoning them. These participants were asked again for their birth weight and also were asked to indicate the source of the information, e.g., parents or hospital records.

For the definition of birth weight (BW), the following algorithm was used: if BW for twins was consistent across longitudinal surveys and consistent with parental report, this value was taken. If BW was not consistent over time, we took the values from the response cards when individuals indicated they checked BW with official records or with parents. Finally, if twins and parents gave different answers, but answers were consistent over time, we took BW as reported by the parents when within normal range (800-4500 grams); if not, we used the twin data. Similarly, for birth length the consistency across time and across parents and twins was checked. When twin data did not agree with the report of the parents, we used parental reports.

In this paper, we look at stature after age 20 years as the outcome variable in later life. Body height was obtained from all surveys between 1991 and 2000.

**Table 1.** Descriptive statistics for gestational age, year of birth, birth weight, birth length, and height for mono- and dizygotic twins (separately for males and females).

|      |      | GA | BYR | BW1 | BW2 | BL1 | BL2 | Height1 | Height2 |
|------|------|------|------|------|------|------|------|------|------|
| MZM | Mean | 36.1 | 1974.2 | 2555.8 | 2509.2 | 47.8 | 47.2 | 182.9 | 182.5 |
|      | SD | 3.15 | 3.10 | 543.73 | 547.94 | 3.00 | 2.99 | 7.77 | 7.24 |
|      | N | 252 | 252 | 230 | 230 | 157 | 154 | 237 | 235 |
| DZM | Mean | 36.7 | 1973.9 | 2681.9 | 2626.4 | 47.9 | 48.2 | 183.2 | 183.2 |
|      | SD | 2.92 | 2.93 | 529.31 | 564.65 | 2.81 | 3.03 | 6.70 | 6.67 |
|      | N | 213 | 213 | 196 | 187 | 131 | 126 | 200 | 191 |
| MZF | Mean | 36.5 | 1974.4 | 2454.8 | 2425.1 | 46.8 | 46.9 | 169.5 | 169.4 |
|      | SD | 2.99 | 2.92 | 524.44 | 502.23 | 2.93 | 2.93 | 6.00 | 6.09 |
|      | N | 384 | 384 | 351 | 355 | 261 | 257 | 358 | 363 |
| DZF | Mean | 36.6 | 1973.8 | 2599.1 | 2464.3 | 47.4 | 47.2 | 170.7 | 170.0 |
|      | SD | 3.19 | 3.09 | 521.38 | 542.16 | 2.78 | 3.13 | 6.29 | 6.76 |
|      | N | 278 | 278 | 252 | 253 | 164 | 173 | 256 | 258 |
| DZMF | Mean | 36.7 | 1974.3 | 2699.4 | 2555.4 | 48.4 | 47.6 | 184.4 | 171.0 |
|      | SD | 3.03 | 3.19 | 554.87 | 556.68 | 2.68 | 3.03 | 7.05 | 6.62 |
|      | N | 235 | 235 | 190 | 216 | 129 | 148 | 193 | 224 |
| DZFM | Mean | 36.8 | 1973.9 | 2586.6 | 2665.4 | 47.5 | 48.2 | 171.3 | 183.4 |
|      | SD | 3.17 | 2.90 | 511.12 | 560.54 | 2.88 | 2.78 | 6.23 | 7.32 |
|      | N | 219 | 219 | 203 | 173 | 124 | 107 | 206 | 177 |

GA, gestational age; BYR, year of birth of twins; BW1 and BW 2, birth weight for oldest (firstborn) and youngest twin; BL1 and BL2, birth lengths; Height1 and Height 2, body height between ages 20 and 40 years; MZ, monozygotic: DZ, dizygotic; F, females; M, males; N, number of pairs for GA and BYR and number of individuals for the other traits.

Height data were only included when height was obtained at 20 years or older. Most individuals completed more than one survey. Differences in height across the questionnaires were checked and height data were discarded when there was no consistency across surveys and when differences were larger than 5 cm (for 44 of 5,994 twins). For a number of participants, height was also measured during experimental protocols. When measured height was available for age 20 years or older, this value was used in the analyses instead of self-reported height (793 of 5,994 twins). The correlation between self-reported and measured height was 0.93 (Silventoinen et al. 2003). Height data after age 20 years were available for 5,950 twins (3,406 pairs; 2,544 complete and 862 incomplete pairs).

There were 4,451 twins for whom gestational age was reported by the mother in 1991 and 1993 (2,215 complete and 21 incomplete pairs). The twins were born between 1966 and 1980, so that for, a large number of these twins, stature after age 20 years had to come from surveys carried out after 1993. For these twins, height after age 20 years was available for 2,904 twins (from 1,320 complete and 264 incomplete pairs). For the analyses of birth length (reported by mother) and adult stature, there were 1,932 twins (from 836 complete and 260 incomplete pairs) and for the analysis of birth weight and stature, there were 2,862 twins (from 1,280 complete and 282 incomplete pairs) with data on these phenotypes. Table 1 gives the number of observations for each phenotype per sex by zygosity group.

## Statistical analyses

As a first approach, we compared the stature of the twins with the lowest birth weight or length within each pair with the stature of their co-twins (who had the highest birth weight or length).

Paired $t$- tests were used to test if these differences in later stature were significant (Spss 11). For these analyses, twin pairs had to be excluded when the birth weight or length of the twins within a pair was the same. Also, because of the known sex differences in both birth size and adult stature, data from opposite sex twin pairs (who are always dizygotic) were discarded.

We derived the expectations for the variances and covariances of the differences in birth size and stature within MZ and DZ twins in terms of genetic and environmental variances for these traits and obtained the expectation for the association of the traits in terms of genetic and environmental correlations between them.

Bivariate modeling of the covariance between size at birth and adult stature was carried out with a standard software package for covariance structure analysis (Mx; Neale et al. 2003).

The data from MZ and DZ twins were used to decompose the variance in birth size and stature into a contribution of the additive effects of many genes, common environmental influences that are shared by twins (such as effects of household, socioeconomic level, or diet) and unique environmental influences that are not shared by twins (such as illness, but also measurement errors). Genetic influences are correlated 1 in MZ and 0.5 in DZ twins. Common environmental effects are perfectly correlated in both MZ and DZ pairs. Unique environmental influences are uncorrelated in both types of twins. For a summary of the twin method, the various assumptions, and the plausibility of these assumptions see, for example, Kendler and Eaves (1986), Neale and Cardon (1992), Martin et al. (1997), Plomin et al. (2001), and Boomsma et al. (2002b).

Twin correlations for the different sex by zygosity groups (e.g., MZ female, DZ opposite sex pairs) give a first impression of the genetic and environmental influences on size at birth and stature. If the traits are influenced by genetic variation, we expect the correlations between members of MZ pairs to be larger than the correlations between members of DZ pairs. If the DZ correlation is larger than half the MZ correlation, this is evidence that shared environment contributes to twin resemblance, in addition to shared genes.

The analysis is based on the general model: $P = G + C + E$; where P stands for the observed phenotype and G, C and E for the latent (unobserved) genetic, common and unique environmental influences, respectively. Common environment refers to those environmental influences that are shared by members from the same household and that make them resemble each other. Unique environment refers to all non-genetic factors (including measurement error) that are unique to an individual and cause differences between family members. We assume there is no interaction or correlation between genotype and environment.

The variance (V) of a univariate phenotype can be decomposed as: $V(P) = V(G) + V(C) + V(E)$, assuming that genotype and environment are uncorrelated. The proportions of genetic and environmental variance in the phenotype (i.e., V(G), V(C) and V(E) divided by V(P)) are often referred to as $h^2$ (heritability), $c^2$ and $e^2$.

In case of a bivariate phenotype, the correlation between traits, e.g., X and Y, can be decomposed as: $r(x,y) = h_x h_y \, r(g) + c_x c_y \, r(c) + e_x e_y \, r(e)$ , where r(g), r(c) and r(e) represent the genetic and the two environmental correlations between X and Y. These correlations are weighted by the square roots of the heritabilities of X and Y and by the square roots of $c^2$ and $e^2$ to obtain the phenotypic correlation between X and Y.

To obtain estimates of genetic, common environmental, and unique environmental variances and correlations, the 4x4 variance-covariance matrix of birth size and stature for twin 1 and twin 2 was analyzed. A saturated bivariate model also known as a triangular decomposition (Neale and Cardon 1992) was fitted to the data. First, we fitted a model with additive genetic, common environmental and unique environmental influences (ACE model), including sex differences in these parameter estimates. Next, we tested if the genetic and environmental correlations between birth size and stature could be constrained to be equal for males and females. Finally, we tested whether these correlations were significantly different from zero. Likelihood-ratio tests were used to test the fit of a more constrained versus a less constrained model, with the degrees of freedom (df) for the test equal to the number of (linearly independent) equalities or the number of parameters constrained to be zero. To make optimal use of all available data, the analyses were performed on raw data using the maximum likelihood estimation procedure for raw data analysis in Mx. The individual values for birth weight, length and stature were corrected for the possible effects of sex, birth year and gestational age.

## Results

There was an association between stature and birth weight for males (N = 1208) and females (N = 1634). In males, the correlation was 0.22 and the regression coefficient (cm per kg) was 2.8. In females, the correlation was 0.24 and the regression coefficient also was 2.8. There was an association between stature and birth length in both males (N = 804) and females (N = 1128). The correlation in males was 0.30 and the regression coefficient (per cm) was 0.74. In females, the correlation was 0.27 and the regression coefficient was 0.56. All these associations were statistically significant.

Correlations of gestational age and birth weight were 0.50 (N=1208) and 0.54 (N=1634) in males and females. Correlations of gestational age and birth length were 0.43 (N= 804) and 0.43 (N=1128) in males and females.

Table 1 gives descriptive statistics for gestational age (GA), birth year, birth length and weight and adult stature for MZ and DZ twins, separately for males and females. There were no differences in gestational age or year of birth between the six groups (p > .10). For the other variables, a 2-way ANOVA with sex and zygosity was carried out (separately for first- and second-born twins). There were significant differences between MZ and DZ twins for birth weight (p > .000, both in first- and second-born twins), for birth length (p = .012/.000 in first- and second-born twins) and stature (p=.022/.085), with DZ twins being taller and heavier. The differences between the sexes for all three traits were also significant, but there were no interactions between sex and zygosity.

Table 2 summarizes the differences within MZ and DZ same-sex twin pairs for birth length and weight and stature. For birth weight, a difference of around 300 grams in MZ pairs is associated with a 0.9 cm (males) and 0.8 cm (females) difference in adult stature. In the DZ pairs, there is a somewhat larger difference in birth weight within pairs, but only in DZ females is this associated with a larger difference in stature (1.7 cm) than was observed in the MZ pairs. For birth length, a difference of around 1.75 cm in MZ twins is associated with a difference in adult stature of around 0.8 cm. In DZ twins, the differences between pairs in birth length and adult stature are even larger: a nearly 2 cm difference in birth length is associated with a 1.8 (males) and 3.2 cm (females) difference in adult stature.

These simple t-tests for paired observations are straightforward and informative. They confirm that, within families, differences between twins in size at birth are associated with later differences in adult stature. This finding implies that the association between size at birth and adult stature cannot entirely be explained by differences in parental social economic status that influence both size at birth and adult height.

There are some disadvantages to this approach: data from opposite sex pairs are discarded and data from twin pairs in which both members have the same

**Table 2A.** Average values for birth weight (BW) and for height after age 20 in same-sex twins with the highest and smallest birth weight within a pair (pairs in which twins had equal birth weights were excluded).

|  | MZM | DZM | MZF | DZF |
|---|---|---|---|---|
| N (pairs) | 197 | 166 | 309 | 215 |
| BW max | 2670 | 2833 | 2586 | 2727 |
| BW min | 2368 | 2466 | 2296 | 2350 |
| Difference in BW | 303 | 366 | 290 | 377 |
| t (p) | 16.11 (.00) | 14.15 (.00) | 18.62 (.00) | 17.30 (.00) |
| | | | | |
| Height for BW max | 182.8 | 183.6 | 169.7 | 171.2 |
| Height for BW min | 181.9 | 182.9 | 168.9 | 169.5 |
| Difference in height | 0.9 | 0.7 | 0.8 | 1.7 |
| t (p) | 4.67 (.00) | 1.29 (.2) | 6.26 (.00) | 3.81 (.00) |

**Table 2B.** Average values for birth length (BL) and for height after age 20 in same-sex twins with the highest and smallest birth length within a pair (pairs in which twins had equal birth lengths were excluded).

|  | MZM | DZM | MZF | DZF |
|---|---|---|---|---|
| N (pairs) | 99 | 87 | 158 | 108 |
| BL max | 48.0 | 49.1 | 47.6 | 48.2 |
| BL min | 46.2 | 47.0 | 45.9 | 46.3 |
| Difference in BL | 1.8 | 2.1 | 1.7 | 1.9 |
| t (p) | 13.64 (.00) | 16.34 (.00) | 17.26 (.00) | 15.45 (.00) |
| | | | | |
| Height for BL max | 183.2 | 183.9 | 170.1 | 171.6 |
| Height for BL min | 182.5 | 182.1 | 169.2 | 168.4 |
| Difference in height | 0.7 | 1.8 | 0.9 | 3.2 |
| t (p) | 2.66 (.00) | 2.45 (.02) | 5.09 (.00) | 5.71 (.00) |

birth weight (or length) cannot be used (there were 70 pairs with the same birth weight and 226 with equal birth length).

The second, widely used approach to analyzing within-family effects uses regression analysis to analyze the relationship of differences within pairs in size at birth with differences in adult stature. We did not employ this approach for

**Table 3.** Expectations for variances difference scores within monozygotic (MZ) and dizygotic (DZ) twin pairs for traits Y and X, and for the covariance and regression of the difference scores. Expectations are expressed as functions of the environmental variances Var(E) and the genetic variances Var(G) of the two traits and the environmental and genetic covariances between them.

| Statistic | MZ expectation | DZ expectation |
|---|---|---|
| Variance D(Y) | 2Var(Ey) | Var(Gy) + 2Var(Ey) |
| Variance D(X) | 2Var(Ex) | Var(Gx) + 2Var(Ex) |
| Covariance [D(Y),D(X)] | 2Cov(Ex,Ey) = 2r(e)[SD(Ex)*SD(Ey)] | 2Cov(Ex,Ey) + Cov(Gx,Gy) = 2r(e)[SD(Ex)*SD(Ey)] + r(g) [SD(Gx)*SD(Gy)] |
| Regression [D(Y),D(X)] | Cov(Ex,Ey) /Var (Ey) | 2Cov(Ex,Ey) + Cov(Gx,Gy) / 2Var(Ey) + Var(Gy) |

the analysis of the empirical data because it cannot provide clear-cut answers to the question of how the association between birth size and stature is mediated.

Table 3 provides a summary of the expectations in MZ and DZ twins (or siblings) of the variances of difference scores, their co-variances and regressions. These expectations are given in terms of the variance of the genetic and environmental factors that influence two phenotypes labeled X and Y and the genetic and environmental correlations between these two phenotypes. As can be seen, in MZ twin pairs, the variances and covariances of difference scores are a function of the unique environmental variances and the environmental correlation between the two traits X and Y. In DZ twins, the variances and covariances of difference scores are a function of both the genetic and the unique environmental variances and of the genetic and the environmental correlations between X and Y. These expectations make clear that the common practice of estimating and comparing the regressions of difference scores in MZ and DZ twin pairs is only of limited value if one wants to draw conclusions about the etiology of the association between X and Y.

For example, assume that the genetic and unique environmental variances for trait Y are both unity (Var (Gy) = Var (Ey) 1, i.e., a heritability of 50% for trait Y). Then, the regression of difference scores in MZ pairs equals cov (Ex,Ey), whereas in DZ pairs this regression equals  2/3 cov (Ex,Ey) + 1/3 cov (Gx, Gy). If the covariance of Ex and Ey is equal to the covariance of Gx and Gy, then the regression coefficients of MZ and DZ are the same, but there is still genetic mediation of the association between X and Y. To put this a bit more generally (regardless of the heritability of Y, as long as it is not zero): there always is a combination of values for the covariance of Ex and Ey and the covariance of Gx and Gy that leads to the same regression coefficients in MZ and DZ twins, whereas there still is genetic mediation of the association between X and Y. If Y is a heritable trait, but the covariance of Gx and Gy is zero, then the regression in DZ is even smaller than in MZ twins. It seems safe to state, however, that if the regression in DZ twins is larger than that in MZ twins, this implies that pleiotropic genes mediate at least part of the association between X and Y.

The only approach that makes optimal use of all data and that leads to an unambiguous conclusion about the etiology of the association of two traits is a full genetic analysis of the bivariate distribution of X and Y (i.e., size at birth and stature). We used this approach to model the birth weight and stature and the birth length and stature data collected in Dutch MZ and DZ twin pairs. All data, including those from "incomplete pairs" (for whom, e.g., stature was available in one twin but not in the co-twin) were analyzed, using the raw data likelihood estimator in Mx, which handles data from studies in which part of the sample has missing data. The bivariate analysis supplies estimates of the heritabilities of birth weight, height and stature and of the correlations between genetic (G), common environmental (C) and unique environmental (E) factors that influence these traits.

Table 4 summarizes the correlations between twins for birth weight and length and adult height. For height, both in males and in females, the twin correlations are substantially higher in MZ pairs than in DZ twin pairs, indicating that most of the variance in height in the Dutch population is due to genetic factors. For birth weight and length, the twin correlations show another pattern: both MZ and DZ correlations are high, although the MZ correlations are still somewhat larger than the correlations in the DZ groups. This pattern indicates that common environmental factors will explain a large proportion of the variance in birth weight and length. As we have seen, gestational age is highly correlated with both variables, and because it is (nearly) always the same in twins from the same pair, this is one of the common environmental influences shared by twins.

Two series of bivariate genetic analyses were carried out: for birth weight and adult stature (Table 5A) and for birth length and stature (Table 5B). We began with fitting a full model with sex differences in all parameter estimates, i.e., in genetic and environmental variances and correlations. Next, we tested if the genetic and environmental correlations could be constrained to be equal for males and females. The non-significant decrease in likelihood in Tables 5A and 5B (twice the difference in likelihoods is distributed as $\chi^2$) indicates that this constraint is allowed. Estimates for genetic, common environmental, and unique environmental correlations between birth weight and adult stature were 0.19, 1.00 and 0.36, respectively. The tests of constraining one, or all, of these correlations at zero are given in Table 5A and show that they are all significant. The proportions of variance in birth weight (corrected for gestational age and birth year) explained by genes, common environment and unique environment were 0.23/0.25, 0.38/0.41 and 0.39/0.34 (in males/females, respectively). For adult stature, these proportions were 0.90/0.90, 0.03/0.01 and 0.07/0.08. Applying the

**Table 4.** Twin correlations for stature in all participants aged 20-40 years and in a subsample with data on gestational age, and twin correlations for birth weight and height.

|      | Height | N   | Height* | N   | BW   | N   | BL   | N   |
| ---- | ------ | --- | ------- | --- | ---- | --- | ---- | --- |
| MZM  | 0.89   | 330 | 0.93    | 220 | 0.75 | 212 | 0.82 | 135 |
| DZM  | 0.47   | 233 | 0.50    | 178 | 0.60 | 172 | 0.73 | 108 |
| MZF  | 0.90   | 647 | 0.93    | 337 | 0.71 | 327 | 0.83 | 233 |
| DZF  | 0.49   | 386 | 0.47    | 236 | 0.61 | 232 | 0.77 | 149 |
| DZMF | 0.47   | 270 | 0.49    | 182 | 0.68 | 176 | 0.76 | 118 |
| DZFM | 0.40   | 252 | 0.45    | 164 | 0.70 | 158 | 0.74 | 93  |

* Height in subsample with data on gestational age; BW/BL, birth weight/length;
  N, number of pairs; MZ, monozygotic; DZ, dizygotic; M, male; F; female

**Table 5A.** Bivariate analysis of birth weight and stature: log-likelihoods (LL) for the full and reduced models; tests of constraining genetic, common environmental and unique environmental correlations at zero.

|                                               | -2LL     | # parameters | $\Delta\chi^2$ | p    |
| --------------------------------------------- | -------- | ------------ | ------ | ---- |
| Full ACE model                                | 33905.04 | 26           | -      |      |
| Full model, no sex differences in correlations | 33906.96 | 23           | 1.92   | 0.58 |
| No r(c)                                        | 33912.74 | 22           | 7.70   | 0.00 |
| No r(g)                                        | 33911.83 | 22           | 6.79   | 0.00 |
| No r(e)                                        | 33982.21 | 22           | 77.17  | 0.00 |
| No correlation                                | 34109.26 | 20           | 204.22 | 0.00 |

**Table 5B.** Bivariate analysis of birth length and stature: log-likelihoods (LL) for the full and reduced models; tests of constraining genetic, common environmental and unique environmental correlations at zero.

|                                               | -2LL     | # parameters | $\Delta\chi^2$ | p    |
| --------------------------------------------- | -------- | ------------ | ------ | ---- |
| Full ACE model                                | 26292.72 | 26           | -      |      |
| Full model, no sex differences in correlations | 26294.21 | 23           | 1.49   | 0.68 |
| No r(c)                                        | 26299.31 | 22           | 6.59   | 0.01 |
| No r(g)                                        | 26317.50 | 22           | 24.78  | 0.00 |
| No r(e)                                        | 26356.79 | 22           | 64.07  | 0.00 |
| No correlation                                | 26517.17 | 20           | 224.45 | 0.00 |

**Table 6.** Decomposition of the correlations between birth weight (BW) and adult stature and between birth length (BL) and adult stature for males and females.

|  | Phenotypic correlation | Proportion explained by G | Proportion explained by C | Proportion explained by E |
|---|---|---|---|---|
| BW, males | 0.22 | 0.34 | 0.43 | 0.23 |
| BW, females | 0.24 | 0.40 | 0.32 | 0.28 |
| BL, males | 0.30 | 0.68 | 0.16 | 0.16 |
| BL, females | 0.27 | 0.42 | 0.38 | 0.20 |

G, genetic influences; C, common environmental influences; E, unique environmental influences.

formula [$r(g) \, h_x h_y + r(c) \, c_x c_y + r(e) \, e_x e_y = r(x,y)$] for the decomposition of the phenotypic correlation between birth weight and stature in males, we get: $0.19\sqrt{0.23}\sqrt{0.90} + 1.0\sqrt{0.38}\sqrt{0.03} + 0.39\sqrt{0.39}\sqrt{0.07} = 0.25$. Thus, in males, about 34% (i.e., $19\sqrt{0.23}\sqrt{0.90}/0.25$) of the observed correlation can be ascribed to genetic pleiotropy. About 43% of the correlation comes from correlated common environmental factors and 23% from correlated unique environmental factors. Table 6 gives a complete summary of the proportions of the correlation between birth weight and stature that are explained by correlated genetic and environmental influences.

The analyses for birth length and adult stature also showed the estimates for genetic, common, and unique environmental correlations to be significant (Table 5B). These correlations were estimated at 0.59, 0.40 and 0.41, respectively. The lower part of Table 6 summarizes the proportions of the observed correlations that are explained by these correlations.

## Discussion

We saw correlations of 0.22-0.24 between birth weight and adult stature. Allison et al. (1995) observed a similar correlation of 0.24 for birth weight with adult height in a Minnesota twin sample aged 28 to 52 years. Allison et al. (1995) analyzed the intra-pair differences in MZ twins and found these differences to be associated with differences in adult height. They concluded that intrauterine environmental influences on birth weight have an enduring impact on adult height and that the intrauterine period is a critical period for the development of height. They did not model the birth weight–stature data in the DZ twin pairs from their sample. We also found differences in birth weight within MZ pairs to be associated with later differences in height and observed these differences in DZ twins as well. Bivariate analyses of the birth weight-stature relationship showed that 30 to 40% of the association was explained by correlated genetic influences. Another 30 to 40% of the association was explained by correlated common environmental influences, and the remainder of the association was due to correlated unique environmental factors.

The correlation between birth length and adult stature was 0.30 in Dutch adult males and 0.27 in females. This relationship was mediated by pleiotropic genetic effects, as well as by correlated common and unique environmental influences.

It is important to note that both types of environmental factors could be interpreted as evidence for the fetal origins hypothesis, which explains the association in terms of a causal mechanism with poor prenatal growth leading to later adverse effects. Unique environmental factors could be related to intrauterine differences experienced by the heavy and light twin, respectively, of twin pairs who are discordant for birth weight. These factors would reflect the variance in intrauterine conditions within the same mother across fetuses. Common environmental influences could be related to intrauterine differences experienced by both twins from a pair. These factors would reflect the variance in intrauterine conditions across different mothers. The evidence from the bivariate analyses for the presence of pleiotropic genetic effects indicates that there are genetic polymorphisms that influence variation in size at birth and have an influence on later variation in stature. Polymorphisms in, for example, the genes for insulin-like growth factor-I (Vaessen et al. 2002), or the insulin-like growth factor-I receptor (Abuzzahab et al. 2003) that are associated with low birth weight might be examples of such pleiotropic genetic effects. Interestingly, the polymorphism in the gene for insulin-like growth factor-I has also been shown to influence susceptibility to diabetes and cardiovascular disease in later life.

Several large-scale epidemiological studies (e.g., Rich-Edwards et al. 1995; Yarnell et al. 1992; McCarron et al. 2002) have reported an inverse association between adult height and (cardiovascular) mortality in males and females from Europe and the United States. Similar associations were found in young-adult Japanese (Miura et al. 2001) and in a large sample of middle-aged South Korean male civil servants (Song et al. 2003). Miura et al. observed an inverse relation of birth weight and height with blood pressure and serum cholesterol levels. Song et al. observed an inverse association between height and all-cause mortality. There was little evidence, however, of associations with coronary heart disease. The strongest inverse associations were with death from stroke, respiratory disease, and external causes. These findings suggest that factors operating in early life, which influence fetal growth and height, also influence future cardiovascular health. The lack of an association between height and coronary heart disease in the Song et al. study suggests that additional factors may be required for short stature to translate into increased coronary heart disease risk.

In an earlier study of adolescent Dutch twins (Ijzerman et al. 2001a), we found that the association between size at birth and stature is also significant during puberty. Most of the association in this earlier study was due to genetic factors influencing both size at birth and stature during puberty. The correlation between common environmental factors was not significant, which might be due to the fact that this adolescent sample was small (160 pairs).

Pictilainen et al. (2001, 2002) examined tracking of birth length and weight in a large sample of Finnish twin adolescents and when they were aged 16 and 18 years. Height in adolescence was predicted by both length and weight at birth. Bivariate analyses showed that the association (r = 0.39 in boys and 0.36 in girls) of birth length and stature at age 16 years was explained by genetic and environmental correlations. The estimates in males and females were, respectively, 0.36/0.32 for the genetic correlations, 0.74/0.75 for common environmental correlations and 0.25/0.40 for unique environmental correlations. In our data from Dutch adult twins, the genetic correlation of birth length and height was somewhat higher (0.59) and the correlations of common environmental factors somewhat lower (0.40) than in the Finnish adolescent sample. The estimate for the correlation between unique environmental factors was roughly the same (0.41). This finding may indicate that the etiology of the association shifts during puberty and young adulthood towards a larger genetic component. In fact, this is also the conclusion that is suggested by Pietilainen et al. (2002).

It has been questioned whether differences in birth size in twins are a suitable model for differences in birth weight in general, because intrauterine growth in twins is different from that in singletons (Doyle et al. 1999). However, associations of birth weight with, e.g., blood pressure (Ijzerman et al. 2000) or serum lipids (Ijzerman et al. 2001b) in twins are similar to those in singletons. Although intrauterine growth in twins may be different from that in singletons, the associations between birth weight and these traits in twins suggest that differences in birth weight in twins can be used as a model for differences in birth weight in singletons.

Using stature as an example, we have demonstrated how the predictions of the fetal origins hypothesis, i.e., that size at birth is negatively associated with disease risk later in life, can be tested in twins. Moreover, using a twin design offers the clear-cut advantage over the singleton case-control approach of yielding an answer to the question of which factors mediate the association of size at birth and later outcome variables. Analyzing the bivariate distribution of size at birth and later outcome variables gives estimates of the genetic pleiotropic, common and unique environmental contributions to the observed association. We have shown that the comparison of outcome variables within pairs discordant for size at birth gives an indication of whether common environmental effects are of importance. If the smallest twin at birth is also the one with the highest disease risk later in life, this suggests that household effects, or effects of socio-economic class cannot explain the entire association. This approach does not make full use of all data. Data from opposite-sex twins or siblings are usually discarded as are data from pairs with the same birth weight or height.

Expectations for difference scores within MZ and DZ twin pairs (please note that the expectations for siblings are the same as those for DZ twin pairs) and for the regression of difference scores on each other indicate that this commonly used approach is of limited value. It cannot provide an unequivocal solution to the problem of how the association of birth size with later outcome variables is mediated. Only when the regression coefficients of differences in birth size on differences in later variables are larger in DZ than in MZ twin pairs is it safe to conclude that the association is mediated (in part) by genetic factors.

Estimates of the relative size of these genetic pleiotropic influences, and of the contribution of correlated common and unique environmental factors, may be obtained from the full bivariate analysis of the covariance structure in twin pairs.

## Acknowledgments

Most of the data collection was funded by the Netherlands Organization for Scientific Research (NWO 575-25-006, 904-61-090, 904-61-193, 985-10-002). We also acknowledge the GenomEUtwin project supported by the European Union (Contract No. QLG2-CT-2002-01254).

## References

Abuzzahab MJ, Schneider A, Goddard A, Grigorescu F, Lautier C, Keller E, Kiess W, Klammt J, Kratzsch J, Osgood D, Pfaffle R, Raile K, Seidel B, Smith RJ, Chernausek SD; Intrauterine Growth Retardation (IUGR) Study Group (2003) IGF-I receptor mutations resulting in intrauterine and postnatal growth retardation. N Engl J Med 349:2211-2222

Allison DB, Paultre F, Heymsfield SB, Pi-Sunyer FX (1995) Is the intra-uterine period really a critical period for the development of adiposity? Int J Obes Relat Metab Disord 19:397-402

Barker DJP (1995) Fetal origins of coronary heart disease. BMJ 311:171-174

Barker DJ (ed) (1998) Mothers, babies and health in later life. Sidcup. Kent: Churchill Livingstone

Barker DJ (2002) Fetal programming of coronary heart disease. Trends Endocrinol Metab 13: 364-368

Barker DJ (2003) The developmental origins of adult disease. Eur J Epidemiol 18:733-736

Barker DJ, Osmond C, Golding J, Kuh D, Wadsworth ME (1989). Growth in utero, blood pressure in childhood and adult life, and mortality from cardiovascular disease. BMJ 298:564-567

Boomsma DI, Koopmans JR, Doornen LJP van, Orlebeke JF (1994) Genetic and social influences on starting to smoke: a study of Dutch adolescent twins and their parents, Addiction 89:219-226

Boomsma DI, Geus EJC de, Baal GCM van, Koopmans JR (1999) Religious upbringing reduces the influence of genetic factors on disinhibition: Evidence for interaction between genotype and environment, Twin Res 2:115-125

Boomsma DI, Vink JM, van Beijsterveldt TC, de Geus EJ, Beem AL, Mulder EJ, Derks EM, Riese H, Willemsen GA, Bartels M, van den Berg M, Kupper NH, Polderman TJ, Posthuma D, Rietveld MJ, Stubbe JH, Knol LI, Stroet T, van Baal GC (2002a) Netherlands Twin Register: a focus on longitudinal research. Twin Res 5: 401-406

Boomsma DI, Busjahn A, Peltonen L (2002b) The classical twin study and beyond. Nat Genet Rev 3: 872-882

Doyle D, Leon D, Morton S, de Stavola B (1999) Twins and the fetal origins hypothesis. Patterns of growth retardation differ in twins and singletons. BMJ 319:517-518

Eriksson JG, Forsen TJ, Osmond C, Barker DJ (2003) Pathways of infant and childhood growth that lead to type 2 diabetes. Diab Care 26:3006-3010

Huxley R, Neil A, Collins R (2002) Unravelling the fetal origins hypothesis: is there really an inverse association between birthweight and subsequent blood pressure? Lancet 360: 659-665

Ijzerman RG, Stehouwer CD, Boomsma DI (2000) Evidence for genetic factors explaining the birth weight-blood pressure relation: analysis in twins. Hypertension 36:1008-1012

Ijzerman RG, Stehouwer CDA, Weissenbruch MM van, Geus EJC de, Boomsma DI (2001a) Intra-uterine and genetic influences on the relationship between size at birth and height in later life: analysis in twins. Twin Res 4:337-343

Ijzerman RG, Stehouwer CD, van Weissenbruch MM, de Geus EJ, Boomsma DI (2001b) Evidence for genetic factors explaining the association between birth weight and LDL cholesterol, and possible intrauterine factors influencing the association between birth weight and HDL cholesterol: analysis in twins. J Clin Endocrinol Metab 86:5479-5484

Kendler KS, Eaves LJ (1986) Models for the joint effect of genotype and environment on liability to psychiatric illness. Am J Psychiat 143:279-289

Martin N, Boomsma D, Machin G. (1997) A twin-pronged attack on complex traits. Nature Genet 17:387-392

McCarron P, Okasha M, McEwen J, Smith GD (2002) Height in young adulthood and risk of death from cardiorespiratory disease: a prospective study of male former students of Glasgow University, Scotland. Am J Epidemiol 155:683-687

Miura K, Nakagawa H, Tabata M, Morikawa Y, Nishijo M, Kagamimori S (2001) Birth weight, childhood growth, and cardiovascular disease risk factors in Japanese aged 20 years. Am J Epidemiol 153:783-789

Neale M, Cardon L (1992) Methodology for genetic studies of twins and families. Dordrecht: Kluwer Academic Publishers

Neale MC, Boker SM, Xie G, Maes, HH (2003) Mx: Statistical modeling. 6th Edition. Richmond, VA, Department of Psychiatry

Paneth N, Susser M (1995) Early origins of coronary heart disease (the "Barker hypothesis"). BMJ 310:411-412

Phillips D (2002) Endocrine programming and fetal origins of adult disease. Trends Endocrinol Metab 13:363

Pietilainen KH, Kaprio J, Rasanen M, Winter T, Rissanen A, Rose RJ (2001) Tracking of body size from birth to late adolescence: contributions of birth length, birth weight, duration of gestation, parents' body size, and twinship. Am J Epidemiol 154:21-29

Pietilainen KH, Kaprio J, Rasanen M, Rissanen A, Rose RJ (2002) Genetic and environmental influences on the tracking of body size from birth to early adulthood. Obes Res 10:875-884

Plomin, R, DeFries JC, McClearn GE, McGuffin P (2001) Behavioral genetics. 4th Edition. New York: Worth Publishers

Rich-Edwards JW, Manson JE, Stampfer MJ, Colditz GA, Willett WC, Rosner B, Speizer FE, Hennekens CH (1995)  Height and the risk of cardiovascular disease in women. Am J Epidemiol 142:909-917

Silventoinen K, Sammalisto S, Perola M, Boomsma DI, Cornes BK, Davis C, Dunkel L, De Lange M, Harris JR, Hjelmborg JV, Luciano M, Martin NG, Mortensen J, Nistico L, Pedersen NL, Skytthe A, Spector TD, Stazi MA, Willemsen G, Kaprio J (2003) Heritability of adult body height: a comparative study of twin cohorts in eight countries. Twin Res 6: 399-408

Song YM, Smith GD, Sung J (2003) Adult height and cause-specific mortality: a large prospective study of South Korean men. Am J Epidemiol 158:479-485

Vaessen N, Janssen JA, Heutink P, Hofman A, Lamberts SW, Oostra BA, Pols HA, van Duijn CM (2002) Association between genetic variation in the gene for insulin-like growth factor-I and low birthweight. Lancet 359:1036-1037

Yarnell JW, Limb ES, Layzell JM, Baker IA (1992) Height: a risk marker for ischaemic heart disease: prospective results from the Caerphilly and Speedwell Heart Disease Studies. Eur Heart J 13:1602-1605

# Towards Understanding the Neurobiology of Mammalian Puberty: Genetic, Genomic and Proteomic Approaches

*Sergio R. Ojeda, Alejandro Lomniczi, Alison Mungenast, Claudio Mastronardi, Anne-Simone Parent, Christian Roth, Vincent Prevot[1], Sabine Heger[2], and Heike Jung[3]*

## Summary

The pubertal activation of gonadotropin hormone-releasing hormone (GnRH) release in rodents and primates is brought about by coordinated changes in excitatory and inhibitory inputs to GnRH neurons. These inputs include both transsynaptic and glia-to-neuron communication pathways. Using cellular and molecular approaches in combination with transgenic animal models and high throughput procedures for gene discovery, we are beginning to gain insights into the basic mechanisms underlying this dual transsynaptic/glial control of GnRH secretion, and hence, the initiation of mammalian puberty. The results thus far obtained suggest that the initiation of puberty requires reciprocal neuron-glia communication involving excitatory amino acids and growth factors, changes in synaptic make-up and glia-neuron adhesiveness, and the transcriptional regulation of genes required for the normal function of both neurons and glial cells involved in the control of GnRH secretion.

## Introduction

Puberty is initiated by central events that are set in motion independently of gonadal influences (Ojeda and Urbanski, 1994; Plant, 1994; Terasawa and Fernandez, 2001). The net outcome of these events is a synchronized increase in pulsatile gonadotropin hormone-releasing hormone (GnRH) release into the portal vasculature that links the hypothalamus to the pituitary gland. Upon delivery to the pituitary gland, GnRH stimulates the secretion and synthesis of

Division of Neuroscience, Oregon National Primate Research Center/Oregon Health & Science University, 505 N.W. 185th Avenue, Beaverton, Oregon

[1] Present address: INSERM U422, Place de Verdum, 59045 Lille cedex, France
[2] Present address: Department of Pediatrics, Division of Pediatric Endocrinology, University Children's Hospital, Schwanenweg 20, 24105 Kiel, Germany
[3] Present address: Lilly Deutschland GmvbH, Niederlassung Bad Homburg, Saalburgstrabe, 611350 Bad Homburg, Germany

Kordon et al.
Hormones and the Brain
© Springer-Verlag Berlin Heidelberg 2005

luteinizing hormone (LH) and follicle stimulating hormone (FSH), which in turn act on the gonads to promote their development and stimulate the secretion of sex steroids and peptidergic hormones.

It is now clear that the pubertal activation of pulsatile GnRH secretion is brought about by functional changes that occur in neuronal and astroglial networks connected to GnRH neurons. These changes include a coordinated decrease in gamma-amino butyric acid GABAergic inhibition, an increase in glutamatergic stimulation, and the activation of reciprocal glial-neuronal communication mechanisms (reviewed in Ojeda and Terasawa, 2002). In this article we discuss some new findings pertaining to each component of this tripartite control mechanism. For a more detailed discussion of the subject, the reader is referred to previous review articles (Ojeda and Terasawa, 2002; Plant, 2002; Terasawa and Fernandez, 2001).

## The transsynaptic control of GnRH neurons

It is well established that GABAergic neurons provide a tonic inhibitory input to GnRH neurons and that this inhibition is lifted at the time of puberty (see, for instance, Mitsushima et al., 1994; Mitsushima et al., 1996). GABA mainly uses $GABA_A$ receptors to reduce GnRH secretion (Mitsushima et al., 1994), as puberty is strikingly advanced in female monkeys when these receptors are blocked (Keen et al., 1999). For many years, it has been assumed that the inhibitory effect of GABA on GnRH secretion is directly exerted on GnRH neurons. However, the recent use of transgenic mice expressing green fluorescent protein specifically in GnRH neurons, in combination with electrophysiological and molecular approaches, led to the conclusion that this inhibitory GABAergic tone is not exerted directly on GnRH neurons, because they respond to $GABA_A$ receptor stimulation with excitation throughout postnatal development (DeFazio et al., 2002). These experiments showed that GABA excites GnRH neurons due to the presence of high intracellular chloride concentrations and that these high chloride levels result from a combination of two factors: the presence of the neuron-specific potassium-chloride cotransporter NKCC1, which transports chloride into the cell, and the absence of two chloride transporters that cause chloride extrusion – the voltage-gated chloride channel, CLC-2, and the chloride-extruding potassium/chloride cotransporter, KCC-2 (DeFazio et al., 2002). Because GnRH neurons also express $GABA_B$ receptors, which mediate a direct GABAergic inhibitory signal of GnRH neuronal activity (Lagrange et al., 1995), the conclusion was reached that the direct, GABA receptor-dependent regulation of GnRH secretion is provided by a balance between an excitatory input mediated by $GABA_A$ receptors and an inhibitory tone mediated by $GABA_B$ receptors. These findings also made it obvious that the inhibitory $GABA_A$

receptor-mediated effects on GnRH secretion are exerted on neuronal systems other than the GnRH neuronal network itself.

Glutamatergic neurotransmission is the predominant mode of transsynaptic excitation used by hypothalamic neurons (van den Pol and Trombley, 1993). Activation of glutamate receptors of the N-methy –D-aspartate (NMDA) class accelerates the initiation of puberty in both rats and monkeys (Plant et al., 1989; Urbanski and Ojeda, 1987). Because GnRH neurons contain NMDA receptors (Gore, 2001; Ottem et al., 2002) it would appear that at least part of the stimulatory effect of glutamate on GnRH release is exerted directly on GnRH neurons. Many of these neurons also contain kainate glutamate receptors (Eyigor and Jennes, 1997). Activation of kainate receptors increases GnRH and LH release (Donoso et al., 1990; Price et al., 1978); therefore, it can be concluded that glutamatergic neurons utilize both NMDA and kainate receptors to facilitate GnRH secretion. The widespread expression of both NMDA and kainate receptors throughout the hypothalamus suggests that glutamate stimulates GnRH secretion via activation of these two classes of receptors expressed on both GnRH neurons and neurons associated with the GnRH neuronal network.

Important for the understanding of this excitatory input is the identification of upstream components involved in the control of glutamate release. In recent experiments (Lee BJ, Lomniczi A, and Ojeda SR, unpublished), we observed that Nell-2, a neuron-specific gene containing EGF-like repeats and a thrombospodin-like motif (Matsuhashi et al., 1995; Watanabe et al., 1996), is selectively expressed in glutamatergic neurons throughout the brain. Nell-2 is present in the synaptosomal fraction of brain neurons; when expressed in neuronal cells, it facilitates glutamate release, indicating that it functions as a positive regulator of glutamatergic transmission. Because blockade of Nell-2 synthesis using antisense oligonucleotides resulted in delayed puberty, it would appear that Nell-2 is a required component of the glutamate-dependent activational process leading to the initiation of puberty.

## The glial control of GnRH neurons

Glial cells regulate GnRH secretion via plastic rearrangements and direct cell-cell communication. Growth factors contributing to these processes include the transforming growth factor beta 1 and 2 (TGFβs), insulin-like growth factor I (IGF-I), basic fibroblast growth factor (bFGF), and the family of epidermal growth factor (EGF)-related polypeptides (for a recent review, see Ojeda et al., 2003). Herein we will discuss only our work with the latter family of growth factors.

It is now well established that the EGF relatives, transforming growth factor alpha (TGFα) and neuregulins (NRGs), are produced in hypothalamic astrocytes and stimulate GnRH release via a cell-cell signaling mechanism that requires astrocyte-astrocyte communication (reviewed in Ojeda et al., 2000). TGFα and NRGs bind to erythroblastosis B (erbB) receptors (erbB-1 and erbB-4, respectively) located on the cell membrane of astroglial cells and elicit the release of chemical messengers that act directly on GnRH neurons to stimulate GnRH secretion. Prostaglandin $E_2$ ($PGE_2$) is one of these messengers (Ma et al., 1997; Ma et al., 1999).

The importance of astrocytic erbB-1 receptors in the control of female sexual development has been demonstrated using various approaches. Thus, either the pharmacological blockade of erbB-1 receptors in the median eminence (Ma et al., 1992), or a point mutation of the erbB-1 gene (Apostolakis et al., 2000) results in delayed puberty. Conversely, transgenic mice expressing the human TGFα gene under the control of an inducible promoter (Ma et al., 1994) and rats carrying intrahypothalamic grafts of cells genetically engineered to secrete TGFα (Rage et al., 1997) show an acceleration of the pubertal process. This latter finding and the demonstration of a rich network of astroglial cells containing TGFα and its erbB-1 receptor in two human hypothalamic hamartomas associated with sexual precocity (Jung et al., 1999) suggest that a focal increase in TGFα production near GnRH neurons may suffice to hasten the advent of puberty.

Relevant to this concept is the recent demonstration (Prevot et al., 2002) of an involvement of the glial erbB-1 signaling system in the regulation of tanycyte plasticity. Tanycytes, an ependymoglial cell type of the median eminence (Kozlowski and Coates, 1985), are thought to regulate GnRH release during the estrous cycle by undergoing plastic changes that alternatively allow or prevent direct access of the GnRH nerve terminals to the portal vasculature (reviewed in Prevot, 2003). In the study by Prevot et al. (2003), tanycytes were found to express erbB1 and erbB2, two of the four members of the erbB receptor family, and respond to TGFα with receptor phosphorylation, release of $PGE_2$, and a $PGE_2$-dependent increase in the release of $TGF\beta_1$, a growth factor previously implicated in the glial control of GnRH secretion (Melcangi et al., 1995). Blockade of either erbB1 receptor signal transduction or prostaglandin synthesis prevented the stimulatory effect of TGFα on both PGE2 and $TGF\beta_1$ release. Time-lapse studies revealed that, while TGFα promotes tanycytic outgrowth, $TGF\beta_1$ elicits retraction of tanycytic processes. However, both systems are functionally related, because prolonged exposure of tanycytes to TGFα resulted in focal tanycytic retraction and this effect was abolished by immunoneutralization of $TGF\beta_1$ action, indicating that the retraction was due to TGFα-induced $TGF\beta_1$ formation. These results demonstrated that erbB1-mediated signaling in tanycytes results in plastic changes that, involving $PGE_2$ and $TGF\beta_1$ as downstream effectors, mimic the morphological plasticity displayed by tanycytes during the hours encompassing the preovulatory surge of GnRH.

In addition to TGFα, hypothalamic astrocytes produce NRGs, which act via activation of erbB-3 and erbB-4 receptors. As in the case of erbB-1, ligand binding results in the recruitment of the co-receptor erbB-2 (for a review, see Hackel et al., 1999). Hypothalamic astrocytes express the erbB-2 and erbB-4 genes but do not contain erbB-3 (Ma et al., 1999), indicating that NRG signaling in these cells is exclusively mediated by erbB-4/erbB-2 complexes. During female sexual development, the hypothalamic content of erbB-2 and erbB-4 mRNA increases both at the end of juvenile development, when circulating sex steroid levels are still low, and then further during the hours preceding the first preovulatory surge of gonadotropins (Ma et al., 1999). This latter increase can be reproduced by treating immature rats with a combination of estradiol and progesterone; thus sit can be attributed to the peripubertal increase in circulating steroid levels (Ma et al., 1999).

As in the case of erbB-1, the importance of erbB-2 and erbB-4 receptors in the control of female puberty has been defined by using molecular and genetic approaches. For instance, *in vivo* disruption of hypothalamic erbB-2 receptor synthesis via intraventricular infusion of an antisense oligodeoxynucleotide directed against erbB-2 mRNA resulted in a striking delay of female puberty (Ma et al., 1999). Because these experiments did not define if the delay was caused by disruption of erbB-1/erbB-2 or erbB-4/erbB-2 signaling, experiments using transgenic mice were carried out to functionally dissect both systems apart and define the physiological importance of the NRG-dependent signaling system in the initiation of puberty. The animals used overexpress, in an astrocyte-specific fashion, a truncated erbB-4 protein that, lacking the intracellular domain, acts as a dominant negative receptor to block the signaling capability of the intact receptor (Prevot et al., 2003). The mutant animals exhibited a reduction in plasma gonadotropin levels and delayed puberty, deficiencies that were attributed to a disrupted ability of hypothalamic astrocytes to respond to NRGs with the production of substances able to stimulate GnRH release. Because astrocytic erbB-4/erbB-2 signaling was disrupted in the face of an apparently normal erbB-1 function, these findings established the importance of an intact astrocytic erbB-4 signaling system for the normal initiation of pubertal process. Mutant mice suffering from a combined deficiency of erbB-1 and erbB-4 receptors showed a further delay in the onset of puberty and a dramatic reduction in fertility (Prevot V, Lomniczi A, Ojeda SR, unpublished data), indicating that both the astrocytic erbB-1 and erbB-4 signaling systems are required to facilitate GnRH release during sexual development; thus, both are important for the timely initiation of female puberty.

What are the cellular proteins affected by the disruption of erbB4 signaling in the developing hypothalamus? Although cDNA array-based studies in our laboratory are aimed at identifying those genes affected by the loss of erbB4 function, it is also important to study the actions of the relevant genes at the protein level. Differences in mRNA levels may not necessarily reflect differential protein expression (Ideker et al., 2001) and give little indication of how protein activity may be modulated by post-translation modifications such as phosphorylation or proteolytic cleavage. Recently, the field of comparative proteomics has undergone technological advances that allow relatively simple, high-throughput approaches to examining differences in protein expression and regulation in tissues (Tao and Aebersold, 2003). To identify proteins that might be affected by the disruption of astrocytic erbB-4 signaling, we compared protein expression profiles in the hypothalamus of wild-type mice and mutant DN-erbB4 animals, using the newly developed method (Gygi et al., 1999) of isotope-coded affinity tag (ICAT) microcapillary liquid chromatography tandem mass-spectrometry (µLC-MS/MS). The results of this study revealed that protein levels of SynCAM, an immunoglobulin-like adhesion molecule recently described to play a critical role in homophilic adhesion and synapse formation and function (Biederer et al., 2002), were strikingly decreased in the hypothalamus of DN-erbB4 mice (Mungenast et al., 2003). SynCAM has been previously described as "tumor-suppressor in lung cancer-1" (TSLC1; Kuramochi et al., 2001) and "immunoglobulin superfamily4" (IGSF-4; Gomyo et al., 1999). SynCAM protein expression in the rat brain increases over the first three postnatal weeks (Biederer et al., 2002), the major period of synaptogenesis. The decrease in SynCAM expression that occurs following the loss of astrocytic erbB4 receptor function is exciting because it raises the intriguing possibility that a single astrocytic signaling system involved in glia-to-neuron communication may play a fundamental role in controlling synaptic assembly and synaptic communication in the neuroendocrine brain. If a functional erbB4 receptor is necessary for the expression and/or function of SynCAM, this could provide a link between erbB4 signaling and neuronal excitability during the onset of puberty.

This possibility notwithstanding, additional studies revealed that SynCAM is present not only in GnRH neurons (GT1-7 cell line) but also in hypothalamic astrocytes (Mungenast et al., 2003). SynCAM mRNA expression was reduced in the DN-erbB4 mouse astrocytes compared to wild-type controls. Sequencing of SynCAM-containing PCR products revealed that of the six possible alternate splice forms of the SynCAM mRNA, the same isoforms are present in both GT1-7 cells and hypothalamic astrocytes. Because SynCAM is a homophilic adhesion molecule (Biederer et al., 2002), the occurrence of the same isoforms in these two cells types suggests that SynCAM-mediated adhesion is an intrinsic component of GnRH neuron-astrocyte communication.

## The coordination of neuronal and glial facilitatory inputs to GnRH neurons

Recent studies have shown that neuronal systems using excitatory amino acids for neurotransmission activate the astrocytic erbB signaling system (Dziedzic et al., 2003). We showed that hypothalamic astrocytes express metabotropic receptors (mGluRs) of the mGluR5 subtype and ionotropic alpha-amino-3-hydroxy-5-methyl-4-isoxazolepropionic acid (AMPA) receptors containing the subunits GluR2 and 3. These receptors are physically associated not only with their respective clustering/interacting proteins, Homer and PICK-1, but also with erbB-1 and erbB-4 receptors. Combined metabotropic/AMPA receptor activation resulted in mobilization of erbB receptors to the cell surface and association of TGFα and NRGs with their respective receptors on the cell membrane. Phosphorylation of erbB receptors occurred, indicating that glutamate stimulation of astrocytes facilitates the interaction of erbB receptors with their TGFα/NRG ligands. This ligand-dependent activation requires a metalloproteinase activity that promotes the cleavage of both TGFα and NRGs mature forms from their respective precursors, making them available for interaction with their receptors (Dziedzic et al., 2003). In the case of TGFα, the enzyme involved is a metalloproteinase termed TACE (tumor necrosis factor alpha converting enzyme) or ADAM-17 (a disintegrin and metalloproteinase-17; Peschon et al., 1998). Concomitant activation of AMPA and metabotropic receptors enhances TACE activity in hypothalamic astrocytes, and TACE activity increases in the median eminence at the time of the first preovulatory surge of gonadotropins (Lomniczi and Ojeda, 2003), suggesting that an enhanced TGFα ectodomain shedding from cells near GnRH nerve terminals is a required component of the neuron-glia signaling process controlling GnRH release. Consistent with this view, blockade of TACE activity targeted to the median eminence resulted in a striking delay of puberty in female rats (Lomniczi and Ojeda, 2003).

## A global view of the hypothalamic changes in gene expression that occur during female puberty

Although a number of genes have been implicated in the central process that controls sexual development in higher primates (for review, see Ojeda and Terasawa, 2002; Plant, 2002), progress towards identifying the gene networks that, operating within the hypothalamus, are ultimately responsible for setting in motion the pubertal process has been hampered by the lack of global, high-throughput approaches. We have begun to use cDNA arrays not only to identify some of these gene networks but also to define the existence of region-specific changes in gene expression that occur in the hypothalamus at critical windows of primate sexual development. Puberty in primates is accompanied by profound changes in cortical synaptic connectivity and neuronal morphology (e.g., the adolescent "pruning" of cortical neurons; Huttenlocher, 1984). Similar plastic changes also occur in the hypothalamus (Perera and Plant, 1997). By comparing gene expression profiles between these two brain regions, we are identifying those changes that are specific to the neuroendocrine brain, those that are common to the hypothalamus and cerebral cortex, and those that are specific to the cerebral cortex and that consequently may be related to the establishment of adult cognitive functions, and not to the neuroendocrine control of reproductive development.

Using these two brain regions, we have interrogated 8,500 genes by comparing the gene expression profiles of juvenile female monkeys to those of animals initiating puberty and to monkeys more advanced in the process, but still far from the first ovulation. Strict criteria were applied to identify genes exhibiting increased or decreased expression at puberty. First, each comparison was done using duplicate arrays. Because each array contained duplicate spots per probe, each gene target was investigated four times. Since we compared a total of eight peripubertal animals with control juvenile animals, each gene was investigated a total of 32 times across pubertal development. Only those changes detected in five of the eight comparisons were accepted for further analysis. The data were analyzed using Omniviz software for merging and the J-Express analysis package for K-means clustering.

According to these criteria, we found that, among the 8,500 genes interrogated, the expression of only 68 genes increased in the hypothalamus at the time of puberty. Even fewer (18 genes) showed a decreased expression in peripubertal monkeys as compared with the juvenile group. Overall, a substantial portion of the genes with increased expression at puberty encoded proteins involved in signaling, transcriptional regulation, and cell-cell communication. Importantly, the increased pubertal expression of most of these genes was selective to the hypothalamus, as no significant changes were detected in the cerebral cortex.

These results provide support for the concept that the onset of puberty requires not only concerted changes in gene transcription and intracellular signaling cascades but also the activation of cell-cell communication pathways that may be critical for both neuron-to-neuron and glial-neuronal information transfer. Two genes showing a consistent increase in expression throughout the pubertal process deserve special mention, because they illustrate the concept that changes in transcriptional regulation might represent a key upstream component of the cascade of events that controls the pubertal process. One of them is a gene provisionally termed chromosome 14 open reading frame 4 (C14ORF4; Rampazzo et al., 2000). The peripubertal changes in C14ORF4 mRNA levels detected by the arrays (Betz et al., 1996) were validated by RealTime PCR experiments, which in addition showed the occurrence of similar changes during puberty in the female rat (Heger S, Mastronardi C, Ojeda, SR, unpublished). Because of this finding, C14ORF4 was initially termed IAP-1 (increasing at puberty), but we now propose to name it EAP-1 (enhanced at puberty-1) to avoid confusion with the family of inhibitors of apoptosis. EAP-1 is an intronless gene encoding a 796-amino acid proline-rich protein endowed with polyglutamine and polyalanine tracks in addition to a RING finger motif at the C-terminus (Rampazzo et al., 2000). Because the EAP-1 gene sequence also includes a nuclear localization sequence,

EAP-1 might participate in transcriptional regulation (Rampazzo et al., 2000). As the acronym "RING" (a Really Interesting New Gene) indicates, proteins endowed with a RING finger domain seem to have a diversity of fascinating functions, most of which are just beginning to be elucidated. The picture now emerging depicts RING finger proteins as crucial components of a variety of cellular processes such as ubiquitination, regulation of gene transcription, signal transduction and DNA repair (for a review, see Freemont, 2000). EAP-1 is different from many other members of the family in at least two regards: 1) its RING finger domain is located near the carboxy terminus instead of the amino terminus, and 2) it contains a nuclear localization signal suggestive of a role in the regulation of gene expression. Within the hypothalamus, EAP-1 mRNA levels are most abundant in neurons of the arcuate and ventromedial nuclei, a region of the primate hypothalamus that not only contains GnRH neurons but also houses some of the most prominent neuronal systems involved in the dual excitatory/inhibitory transsynaptic control of GnRH secretion – including those that always excite (glutamatergic), either excite or inhibit (GABAergic, NPY), or always inhibit (proenkephalin) the GnRH neuronal network (Weiner et al., 1988). The presence of EAP-1 within this functional network raises the exciting possibility that one of the functions of EAP-1 in the control of reproductive function is to coordinate the activity of genes that, operating within both excitatory and inhibitory neuronal subsets, are required for the normal activity of each individual subset.

The other gene found to be expressed at higher levels in the hypothalamus during primate puberty is a gene known as thyroid transcription factor-1 (TTF-1), T/ebp or Nkx-2.1. TTF-1 is a homeodomain gene of the Nkx family of homeodomain genes (Harvey, 1996). During embryonic development, TTF-1 is selectively expressed in the diencephalon (Lazzaro et al., 1991). After birth, its expression becomes restricted to select neuronal and glial subsets of the hypothalamus, such as proenkephalinergic neurons of the lateral ventromedial nucleus, GnRH neurons themselves, and cells of the median eminence. In this region, TTF-1 mRNA colocalizes with erbB-2 mRNA in tanycytes and tanycytic astrocytes (Lee et al., 2001). Lesions of the anterior hypothalamus that induce sexual precocity in rodents result in increased TTF-1 mRNA levels in neurons surrounding the lesion site (Lee et al., 2001). That this increase may be relevant to the advent of puberty is suggested by the observation that the hypothalamic content of TTF-1 mRNA increases transiently before the initiation of normal puberty, preceding the pubertal increase in gonadal steroid secretion. This assumption is supported by the results of recent studies showing a delay in puberty and disruption of reproductive function in mice in which expression of the TTF-1 gene was conditionally deleted from neurons using Cre-loxP technology (Mastronardi C, Smiley, G, Kusakabe T, Kawagushi A, Ojeda SR and Kimura S, unpublished results). TTF-1 may serve as an upstream coordinator of gene activity within the hypothalamus during neuroendocrine development, because it increases the transcriptional activity of both erbB-2 and GnRH, two genes required for the initiation of puberty, while decreasing transcription of the proenkephalin gene (Lee et al., 2001), which, as indicated earlier, works in concert with the GABAergic system to restrain the pubertal process. Thus TTF-1 appears to epitomize a group of controlling genes that, arranged in a hierarchical network and operating within diverse neuronal and glial subsets of the hypothalamus, coordinate the cell-cell communication events that lead to the initiation of puberty.

## Conclusions

The aforementioned observations suggest that activation of GnRH secretion at puberty requires the coordinated activation of transsynaptic and astroglial regulatory systems. Two key neuronal systems of this process are those that utilize glutamate and GABA as neurotransmitters. Astroglial cells facilitate GnRH secretion via pathways initiated by growth factors that act directly and indirectly on GnRH neurons to stimulate neurosecretion. The EGF family of growth factors and their erbB receptors are crucial components of the glia-to-neuron communication pathway used by hypothalamic glial cells to facilitate GnRH release. The integrity of this signaling system is not only important for the normalcy of glia-neuronal communication but it also appears to be required for maintaining adequate levels of expression of at least one protein (SynCAM) involved in synaptic organization. A pathway involved in coordinating the facilitatory transsynaptic and astroglial inputs to GnRH neurons has been identified and shown to be initiated by neurons that, using glutamate for neurotransmission, activate erbB signaling in glial cells. Finally, two genes (EAP-1 and TTF-1) have been implicated as components of the upstream regulatory hierarchy controlling those cellular events required for the synchronized changes in neuronal/glial transcriptional activity underlying the initiation of puberty.

## Acknowledgments

This research was supported by NIH grants HD-25123, NICHD/NIH through cooperative U54 HD18185-16 as part of the Specialized Cooperative Centers Program in Reproduction Research, and RR00163 for the operation of the Oregon Regional Primate Center. V.P. was in part supported by a grant from the Institut National de la Sante et de la Recherche Medicale (Paris, France); S.H, C.R and H.J were in part supported by fellowships provided by the European Society for Pediatric Endocrinology (ESPE). We also thank our collaborators Suzanne Moenter (University of Virginia, Charlottesville), Gabriel Corfas (Harvard

Medical School, Boston), Shioko Kimura (National Cancer Institute, NIH, Bethesda), Rudy Aebersold and S.S Chen (Institute for Systems Biology, Seattle), and Byung Ju Lee (University of Ulsan, South Korea).

# References

Apostolakis EM, Garai J, Lohmann JE, Clark JH, O'Malley BW (2000) Epidermal growth factor activates reproductive behavior independent of ovarian steroids in female rodents. Mol Endocrinol 14: 1086-1098

Betz WJ, Mao F, Smith CB (1996) Imaging exocytosis and endocytosis. Curr Opin Neurobiol 6: 365-371

Biederer T, Sara Y, Mozhayeva M, Atasoy D, Liu X, Kavalali ET, Südhof TC (2002) SynCAM, a synaptic adhesion molecule that drives synapse assembly. Science 297: 1525-1531

DeFazio RA, Heger S, Ojeda SR, Moenter SM (2002) Activation of A-type g-aminobutyric acid receptors excites gonadotropin-releasing hormone neurons. Mol Endocrinol 16: 2872-2891

Donoso AO, López FJ, Negro-Vilar A (1990) Glutamate receptors of the non-N-methyl-D-aspartic acid type mediate the increase in luteinizing hormone releasing hormone release by excitatory amino acid *in vitro*. Endocrinology 126: 414-420

Dziedzic B, Prevot V, Lomniczi A, Jung H, Cornea A, Ojeda SR (2003) Neuron-to-glia signaling mediated by excitatory amino acid receptors regulates erbB receptor function in astroglial cells of the neuroendocrine brain. J Neurosci 23: 915-926

Eyigor O, Jennes L (1997) Expression of glutamate receptor subunit mRNAs in gonadotropin-releasing hormone neurons during the sexual maturation of the female rat. Neuroendocrinology 66: 122-129

Freemont PS (2000) Ubiquitination: RING for destruction? Curr Biol 10: R84-R87

Gomyo H, Arai Y, Tanigami A, Murakami Y, Hattori M, Hosoda F, Arai K, Aikawa Y, Tsuda H, Hirohashi S, Asakawa S, Shimizu N, Soeda E, Sakaki Y, Ohki M (1999) A 2-Mb sequence-ready contig map and a novel immunoglobulin superfamily gene IGSF4 in the LOH region of chromosome 11q23.2. Genomics 62: 139-146

Gore AC (2001) Gonadotropin-releasing hormone neurons. NMDA receptors, and their regulation by steroid hormones across the reproductive life cycle. Brain Res Rev 37: 235-248

Gygi SP, Rist B, Gerber SA, Turecek F, Gelb MH, Aebersold R (1999) Quantitative analysis of complex protein mixtures using isotope-coded affinity tags. Nature Biotechnol 17: 994-999

Hackel PO, Zwick E, Prenzel N, Ullrich A (1999) Epidermal growth factor receptors: critical mediators of multiple receptor pathways. Curr Opin Cell Biol 11: 184-189

Harvey RP (1996) *NK-2* homeobox genes and heart development. Dev Biol 178: 203-216

Huttenlocher PR (1984) Synapse elimination and plasticity in developing human cerebral cortex. Am J Ment Defic 88: 488-496

Ideker T, Thorsson V, Ranish JA, Christmas R, Buhler J, Eng JK, Bumgarner R, Goodlett DR, Aebersold R, Hood L (2001) Integrated genomic and proteomic analyses of a systematically perturbed metabolic network. Science 292: 929-934

Jung H, Carmel P, Schwartz MS, Witkin JW, Bentele KHP, Westphal M, Piatt JH, Costa ME, Cornea A, Ma YJ, Ojeda SR (1999) Some hypothalamic hamartomas contain transforming growth factor alpha, a puberty-inducing growth factor, but not luteinizing hormone-releasing hormone neurons. J Clin Endocrinol Metab 84: 4695-4701

Keen KL, Burich AJ, Mitsushima D, Kasuya E, Terasawa E (1999) Effects of pulsatile infusion of the GABAA receptor blocker bicuculline on the onset of puberty in female rhesus monkeys. Endocrinology 140: 5257-5266

Kozlowski GP, Coates PW (1985) Ependymoneuronal specializations between LHRH fibers and cells of the cerebroventricular system. Cell Tissue Res 242: 301-311

Kuramochi M, Fukuhara H, Nobukuni T, Kanbe T, Maruyama T, Ghosh HP, Pletcher M, Isomura M, Onizuka M, Kitamura T, Sekiya T, Reeves RH, Murakami Y (2001) *TSLC1* is a tumor-suppressor gene in human non-small-cell lung cancer. Nature Genet 27: 427-430

Lagrange AH, Ronnekleiv OK, Kelly MJ (1995) Estradiol-17b and m-opioid peptides rapidly hyperpolarize GnRH neurons: A cellular mechanism of negative feedback? Endocrinology 136: 2341-2344

Lazzaro D, Price M, De Felice M, Di Lauro R (1991) The transcription factor TTF-1 is expressed at the onset of thyroid and lung morphogenesis and in restricted regions of the foetal brain. Development 113: 1093-1104

Lee BJ, Cho GJ, Norgren R, Junier M-P, Hill DF, Tapia V, Costa ME, Ojeda SR (2001) TTF-1, a homeodomain gene required for diencephalic morphogenesis, is postnatally expressed in the neuroendocrine brain in a developmentally regulated and cell-specific fashion. Mol Cell Neurosci 17: 107-126

Lomniczi A, Ojeda SR (2003) Hypothalamic tumor necrosis factor-a converting enzyme (TACE) activity is involved in the control of female sexual development. Program No 709 7, 2003 Abstract Viewer Washington, DC: Society for Neuroscience, 2003 Online

Ma YJ, Junier M-P, Costa ME, Ojeda SR (1992) Transforming growth factor alpha (TGFα) gene expression in the hypothalamus is developmentally regulated and linked to sexual maturation. Neuron 9: 657-670

Ma YJ, Dissen GA, Merlino G, Coquelin A, Ojeda SR (1994) Overexpression of a human transforming growth factor alpha (TGFα) transgene reveals a dual antagonistic role of TGFα in female sexual development. Endocrinology 135: 1392-1400

Ma YJ, Berg-von der Emde K, Rage F, Wetsel WC, Ojeda SR (1997) Hypothalamic astrocytes respond to transforming growth factor alpha with secretion of neuroactive substances that stimulate the release of luteinizing hormone-releasing hormone. Endocrinology 138: 19-25

Ma YJ, Hill DF, Creswick KE, Costa ME, Ojeda SR (1999) Neuregulins signaling via a glial erbB2/erbB4 receptor complex contribute to the neuroendocrine control of mammalian sexual development. J Neurosci 19: 9913-9927

Matsuhashi S, Noji S, Koyama E, Myokai F, Ohuchi H, Taniguchi S, Hori K (1995) New gene, nel, encoding a $M_r$ 93 K protein with EGF-like repeats is strongly expressed in neural tissues of early stage chick embryos. Dev Dyn 203: 212-222

Melcangi RC, Galbiati M, Messi E, Piva F, Martini L, Motta M (1995) Type 1 astrocytes influence luteinizing hormone-releasing hormone release from the hypothalamic cell line GT1-1: Is transforming growth factor-b the principle involved? Endocrinology 136: 679-686

Mitsushima D, Hei DL, Terasawa E (1994) Gamma-aminobutyric acid is an inhibitory neurotransmitter restricting the release of luteinizing hormone-releasing hormone before the onset of puberty. Proc Natl Acad Sci USA 91: 395-399

Mitsushima D, Marzban F, Luchansky LL, Bruich AJ, Keen KL, Durning M, Golos TG, Terasawa E (1996) Role of glutamic acid decarboxylase in the prepubertal inhibition of the luteinizing hormone releasing hormone release in female rhesus monkeys. J Neurosci 16: 2563-2573

Mungenast AE, Parent A, Chen SS, Goodlett D, Aebersold R, Corfas G, Ojeda SR (2003) The synaptic adhesion molecule SynCAM is associated with ERBB4 dysregulation in the hypothalamus of mice with a delayed onset of puberty. Program No 281 20, 2003 Abstract Viewer Washington, DC: Society for Neuroscience, 2003 Online

Ojeda SR, Terasawa E (2002) Neuroendocrine regulation of puberty. In: Pfaff D, Arnold A, Etgen A, Fahrbach, S, Moss R, Rubin R (eds) Hormones, brain and behavior. Vol. 4. Elsevier, New York, pp 589-659

Ojeda SR, Urbanski HF (1994) Puberty in the rat. In: Knobil E, Neill JD (eds) The physiology of reproduction. 2nd Edition, Vol. 2. Raven Press, New York, pp 363-409

Ojeda SR, Ma YJ, Lee BJ, Prevot V (2000) Glia-to-neuron signaling and the neuroendocrine control of female puberty. Rec Prog Horm Res 55: 197-224

Ojeda SR, Prevot V, Heger S, Lomniczi A, Dziedzic B, Mungenast A (2003) Glia-to neuron signaling and the neuroendocrine control of female puberty. Ann Med 35: 244-255

Ottem EN, Godwin JG, Petersen SL (2002) Glutamatergic signaling through the N-methyl-D-aspartate receptor directly activates medial subpopulations of luteinizing hormone-releasing hormone (LHRH) neurons, but does not appear to mediate the effects of estradiol on LHRH gene expression. Endocrinology 143: 4837-4845

Perera AD, Plant TM (1997) Ultrastructural studies of neuronal correlates of the pubertal reaugmentation of hypothalamic gonadotropin-releasing hormone (GnRh) release in the rhesus monkey (*Macaca mulatta*). J Comp Neurol 385: 71-82

Peschon JJ, Slack JL, Reddy P, Stocking KL, Sunnarborg SW, Lee DC, russell WE, Castner BJ, Johnson RS, Fitzner JN, Boyce RW, Nelson N, Koslosky CJ, Wolfson MF, Rauch CT, Cerretti DP, Paxton RJ, March CJ, Black RA (1998) An essential role for ectodomain shedding in mammalian development. Science 282: 1281-1284

Plant TM (1994) Puberty in primates. In: Knobil E, Neill J (eds) The physiology of reproduction. 2nd Edition, Vol. 2. Raven Press, New York, pp 453-485

Plant TM (2002) Neurophysiology of puberty. J Adolesc Health 31: 185-191

Plant TM, Gay VL, Marshall GR, Arslan M (1989) Puberty in monkeys is triggered by chemical stimulation of the hypothalamus. Proc Natl Acad Sci USA 86: 2506-2510

Prevot V (2002) Glial-neuronal-endothelial interactions are involved in the control of GnRH secretion. J Neuroendocrinol 14: 247-255

Prevot V, Cornea A, Mungenast A, Smiley G, Ojeda SR (2003) Activation of erbB-1 signaling in tanycytes of the median eminence stimulates transforming growth factor $\beta_1$ release via prostaglandin $E_2$ production and includes cell plasticity. J Neurosci 23:10622-10632

Prevot V, Rio C, Cho GJ, Lomniczi A, Heger S, Neville CM, Rosenthal NA, Ojeda SR, Corfas G (2003) Normal female sexual development requires neuregulin-erbB receptor signaling in hypothalamic astrocytes. J Neurosci 23: 230-239

Price MT, Olney JW, Cicero TJ (1978) Acute elevations of serum luteinizing hormone induced by kainic acid, N-methyl aspartic acid or homocystic acid. Neuroendocrinology 26: 352-358

Rage F, Hill DF, Sena-Esteves M, Breakefield XO, Coffey RJ, Costa ME, McCann SM, Ojeda SR (1997) Targeting transforming growth factor a expression to discrete loci of the neuroendocrine brain induces female sexual precocity. Proc Natl Acad Sci USA 94: 2735-2740

Rampazzo A, Pivotto F, Occhi G, Tiso N, Bortoluzzi S, Rowen L, Hood L, Nava A, Danieli GA (2000) Characterization of C14orf4, a novel intronless human gene containing a polyglutamine repeat, mapped to the ARVD1 critical region. Biochem Biophys Res Commun 278: 766-774

Tao WA, Aebersold R (2003) Advances in quantitative proteomics via stable isotope tagging and mass spectrometry. Curr Opin Biotechnol 14: 110-118

Terasawa E, Fernandez DL (2001) Neurobiological mechanisms of the onset of puberty in primates. Endocrinol Rev 22: 111-151

Urbanski HF, Ojeda SR (1987) Activation of lutenzing hormone-releasing hormone release advances the onset of female puberty. Neuroendocrinology 46:273-275, 1987

van den Pol AN, Trombley PQ (1993) Glutamate neurons in hypothalamus regulate excitatory transmission. J Neurosci 13: 2829-2836

Watanabe TK, Katagiri T, Suzuki M, Shimizu F, Fujiwara T, Kanemoto N, Nakamura Y, Hirai Y, Maekawa H, Takahashi E (1996) Cloning and characterization of two novel human cDNAs (NELL1 and NELL2) encoding proteins with six EGF-like repeats. Genomics 38: 273-276

Weiner RI, Findell PR, Kordon C (1988) Role of classic and peptide neuromediators in the neuroendocrine regulation of LH and prolactin. In: Knobil E Neill JD (eds) The physiology of reproduction. Vol. 1. Raven Press, New York, pp 1235-1281

# The non-genomic Action of Sex Steroids

*Joe I, Kipp JL, and Ramirez VD*

## Summary

The aim of this paper is to discuss novel and rather recent evidence indicating that estradiol and testosterone have rapid actions by interacting with two different, but physiologically and chemically well-characterized proteins: 1) tubulin, a basic component of microtubules and therefore involved in cellular cytoarchitecture and cellular trafficking; and 2) glyceraldehyde-3-phosphate dehydrogenase (GAPDH), an enzyme involved in glycolysis but also in other important, non-glycolytic functions.

Estradiol and testosterone bind to tubulin at nanomolar concentrations and exert opposite effects on microtubule polymerization in an in vitro assay that uses electron microscopy to visualize the formation of microtubules: estradiol disrupts polymerization whereas testosterone stabilizes microtubules. This finding was confirmed by spectrometric analysis and in vivo cell cultures using image visualization of tubulin. Interestingly, testosterone but not estradiol blocks the colchicine-induced depolymerization effect in both the pure tubulin assay and the cell culture model.

Previously, we reported that estradiol binds with high affinity and selectivity to GAPDH and that a single injection of estradiol (10 µg, s.c.) to ovariectomized rats significantly increased and recovered the reduced catalysis of the enzyme in the plasmalemma-microsomal fraction (P3 fraction) of the hippocampus of these rats to intact levels. Herein, we report that estradiol induces a rapid (within 30 min) translocation of the enzyme to the P3 fraction of primary hippocampus cell cultures as well in the hippocampal cell line (HT-22) that lacks functional alfa and beta estrogen receptors. Importantly, the translocation is accompanied by serine phosphorylation of the GAPDH as shown by Western blot analysis of the P3 fraction. Estradiol treatment (10 nM) of HT-22 cell cultures appears to sequester the GAPDH in membrane organelles visualized by immunocytochemistry, because they become resistant to depletion by the non-ionic detergent Triton-X-100.

Department of Molecular and Integrative Physiology, University of Illinois at Urbana, IL 61801, USA.

Kordon et al.
Hormones and the Brain
© Springer-Verlag Berlin Heidelberg 2005

These results and related reports from other laboratories cited in this paper strongly support the concept that, by interacting with these two proteins and other cellular components, sex steroids are involved in rapid, non-genomic functions in a variety of cells.

## Introduction

The landmark of this evolving and growing field is the rapidity of the steroid-initiated cellular membrane events at multiple target cells involving several signaling pathways. The concept that steroids require a cognate receptor as the only mechanism of action is currently a simplistic view because of the abundance of data indicating that steroids can interact with other type of proteins, particularly enzymes, a major mechanism of action formulated long ago (Tomkins and Maxwell 1963).

In this report, we present novel and rather recent evidence indicating that 17-beta-estradiol (E or E2) and testosterone (T) have rapid actions by interacting with two different but well-known, physiologically and chemically characterized proteins: 1) tubulin, a basic component of microtubules and therefore involved in cellular cytoarchitecture and cellular trafficking; and 2) glyceraldehyde-3-phosphate dehydrogenase (GAPDH), an enzyme involved in glycolysis but also in other non-glycolytic functions.

These novel results and related studies from other laboratories mentioned below strongly suggest that, by rapidly interacting with these two proteins and other cell components, sex steroids are involved in cellular functions such as neuronal plasticity, neuroprotection and exocytosis.

## Estradiol and Testosterone Interact with Tubulin and other Microtubule Proteins

There are several reports indicating that steroid hormones are capable of modifying cell proliferation and neuroplasticity (Ramirez et al. 2001; Wheeler et al. 1987; Wolley and McEwen 1993; McEwen 1999). Early findings showed that E (Szego et al. 1988) and T (Valenti et al. 1979) modify the dynamic of microtubules in the rat endometrium and increase the levels of tubulin in the medial basal hypothalamus and anterior pituitary of castrated rats, respectively. Related to our findings is the report of Szego et al. (1988), who observed a rapid and transient shortening of microtubules in the endometrium of ovariectomized rats after seconds of intravenous administration of E. Others have shown that E binds to the cytoskeleton of erythrocytes (Puca and Sica 1981), modifies the shape of cells (Aizu-Yokota et al. 1994, 1995), is capable of differentiating neuroblasts towards the dopaminergic phenotype (Agrati et al. 1997), induces

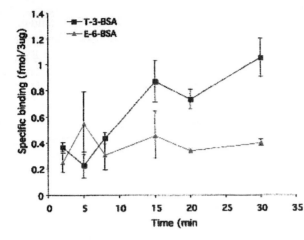

**Fig. 1.** Association binding rate of T-3-[$^{125}$I]-BSA and E-6-[$^{125}$I]-BSA to tubulin (3 µg). Data correspond to several assays with 4-6 values per point, except at 30 min, where the n is equal to 10 for T and 14 for E. Mean+/-SE are shown.

redistribution of GFAP in the rat brain (Tranque et al. 1987), and regulates neurogenesis in vitro and in cell cultures (Blanco et al. 1990) or brain explants (Toran-Allerand 1990) in vivo as well (Woolley and McEwen 1993; Woolley et al. 1990). Interestingly, natural fluctuations during the rat estrous cycle of astrocytes in the dentate gyrus, as well as hormonal regulation, have been reported (Luquin et al. 1993). These examples suggest an effect of steroids on the cytoskeleton organization and function of neurons, glia and other cells, such as tanycytes (Garcia-Segura et al. 1999). In addition, diethylstilbestrol (DES) has been shown to cause microtubule disruption in culture cells (Sakakibara et al. 1991) and to inhibit microtubule formation in vitro (Chaudoreille et al. 1991). In spite of these clear effects of E on the cytoskeleton of different cells, its mechanism is unknown. Our present results indicate that both E and T may have crucial roles in the assembly of microtubules by direct or indirect interactions with tubulin and other stabilizer factors.

Searching for the elusive membrane estradiol receptor in hippocampal membrane fractions, we unexpectedly isolated beta-tubulin and showed that this protein binds E and T at nanomolar concentrations but not other steroids, such as progesterone, the alfa isomer of estradiol, DES, a synthetic estrogen and others (Ramirez et al. 2001). The binding was temperature-sensitive and differentially competed off by colchicine, which has a well-established site in the C-terminal of the beta-subunit of tubulin (Nogales et al. 1998). The E binding was colchicine-resistant whereas the T binding was colchicine-sensitive, suggesting that T may share a similar binding site with colchicine and may differentially affect microtubule functions. The rapid rate of association of the E binding compared to the T binding to tubulin and with different capacities suggests different effects of these two steroids on microtubule dynamics, as demonstrated below (Fig. 1).

It was of interest to study whether microtubule-associated proteins would or not bind the two complexes. As recently reported (Ramirez and Kipp 2002), of the two MAPs tested, MAP2 and tau bound E-6-[$^{125}$I]-BSA and T-3-[$^{125}$I]-BSA with high affinity and using low amounts of proteins. For example, the specific binding of E-6-[$^{125}$I]-BSA to MAP2 in duplicate was 2,515-2,627 at 10 ng, 3,305-3,102 at 20 ng, and around 8,000 cpm at 40 ng. The binding was temperature-resistant and colchicine did not compete off the binding of either of the two ligands, clearly indicating that the binding sites in the MAPs are different from the ones found in the tubulin molecule. These data rule out the possibility that contamination of the tubulin with MAPs was responsible for our binding studies using highly purified tubulin, given the different binding properties of these molecules. On the other hand, the data support the hypothesis that these MAPs, as well as others, can play a role as regulators of the action of E or T on microtubule dynamics in a particular cell or cellular compartment, for instance, different locations between dendrite (where MAP2 locates) and axon (where tau locates), as reported earlier (Jaccioni and Cambiazo 1995).

## Estradiol and Testosterone have Opposite Effects on Microtubule Polymerization

Microtubules are important components of the cytoskeleton and play a role in determining cell shape and facilitating cellular or subcellular movement, such as cilia and flagella activity, meiosis and mitosis, membrane vesicles transport and axonal extension. Microtubules exert these functions through a highly regulated dynamic process of polymerization and depolymerization, which can be demonstrated both in vitro and in vivo. The basic molecule in the formation of microtubule is tubulin. Three well-established subunits, alfa, beta and gamma, appear to be essential in the formation of microtubules. In vivo, the regulation of microtubule dynamics is more complex because a series of stabilizers and destabilizers play specific roles. Examples of the stabilizers with known functions include the MAPs and the destabilizers include katanin, op18/stathmin and XKCM1/XFIF2, among others (Nogales 2000).

Recently, we reported that E and T exerted dramatic opposite effects on the rate of polymerization of tubulin in an in vitro assay (Kipp and Ramirez 2003). It seemed that E tended to modify only the polymerization process without altering the depolymerization. In contrast, T inhibited the microtubule depolymerization without affecting the rate of polymerization, as shown in Figure 2 (taken from Kipp and Ramirez 2003).

The effect of T is remarkably similar to the reported action of a non-hydrolyzable GTP analogue, guanylyl-(alfa,beta)-methylene-diphosphate (GMPCPP). When this analogue was used as the nucleotide to replace the hydrolysable GTP on the exchangeable site in the beta-tubulin, microtubules

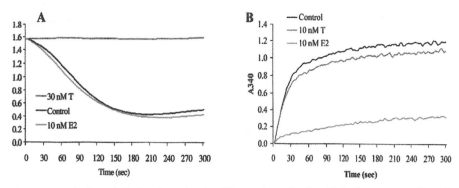

Fig. 2. Rate of microtubule depolymerization (A) or polymerization (B) in the presence of E or T is shown. The spectra shown in both A and B were reconstructed from the mean values of three independent studies. For details, consult Kipp and Ramirez 2003.

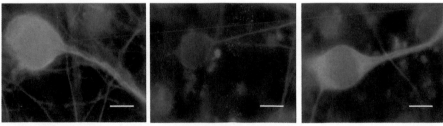

Fig. 3. An example of T blocking the strong effect of colchicine on microtubule density in rat hippocampus primary cell cultures. Cells were incubated with ethanol (control), colchicine or colchicine plus T for 30 min before ICC. Scale bar= 10 mm

were stabilized from depolymerization (Mejillano et al. 1990; Hyman et al. 1992), indicating a critical role of GTP hydrolysis in the depolymerization phenomenon. Hence, reasoning by analogy, we can speculate that T exerts a similar action reinforced by the fact that T seems to bind at the same site that colchicine does in the beta subunit of tubulin, and it is the beta subunit that is responsible for hydrolysis of GTP. Our recent report indicates that the effect of T is not just an in vitro finding, irrelevant to in vivo cells (Kipp and Ramirez 2003); T dramatically blocks the depolymerization action of colchine in hippocampal primary cell culture, as depicted in Figure 3. The fact that colchicine does not block, either in vitro (Ramirez et al. 2001) or in vivo (Kipp and Ramirez 2003), the effect of E on the binding to tubulin or microtubule depolymerization, respectively, is a strong indication that these two steroids have remarkably different mechanisms of action on microtubule functions.

These robust experimental findings – specific binding of T to tubulin at nanomolar concentrations, competition of the binding by colchicine, stabilization of microtubule polymerization in vivo and the increase in number of microtubules in vitro, together with the blocking of the colchicine effect in cell cultures – indicate that T may have a binding site in the beta subunit of tubulin, probably close to or in the same site demonstrated for colchicine. Future studies will be required to clarify these novel findings for T and E and their probable actions on microtubule functions in vivo.

## Rapid Effect of 17-beta-estradiol on GAPDH Translocation in Hippocampal Cells

It is known that GAPDH is involved in vesicle transportation and fusion to cell membrane through interaction with microtubules. For example, endocytosis is impaired in GAPDH mutant cells (Robbins et al. 1995), treatment with anti-GAPDH antibody damages the formation of microtubule network (Tisdale 2002), isoforms of GAPDH from rabbit brain cytosol catalyze membrane fusion activity, and endogenous tubulin inhibits GAPDH's fusogenic activity (Glaser and Gross1995; Glaser et al. 2002), to mention some of the experiments clearly indicating a role of GAPDH in functions other than glycolysis.

Our previous finding indicating that E binds GAPDH with high affinity (Joe and Ramirez 2001) and selectively increases the catalysis of GAPDH in a plasma membrane-microsomal fraction (P3 fraction) of the hippocampus of ovariectomized rats (Ramirez et al. 2001; Joe 2003) – plus the robust effect on microtubule formation discussed above – led us to investigate whether E would modify GAPDH translocation in a cell line, HT-22, that is known to lack both alfa and beta estrogen receptors to eliminate the involvement of these two receptors in the rapid action of E.

Figure 4 shows the total amount of GAPDH detected in Western blot in the P3 fraction from the HT-22 cells incubated with vehicle (control), 10 nM E, 100 nM progesterone or 30 nM T for 30 min before collection for differential centrifugation. It is evident that only E increases the amount of the enzyme in the P3 fraction. A time course indicates that the effect is significant after five minutes, reaching maximal at 30 minutes post-incubation.

Because colchicine is known to disrupt microtubule dynamics and, therefore, movements of intracellular molecules, we tested whether this drug would block the translocation of GAPDH. Figure 5 indicates that this drug indeed reduced the amount of the enzyme in the P3 fraction when the cells were incubated with E and colchicine vs E alone. Colchicine by itself did not significantly change the amount of GAPDH in cells treated with the vehicle as control.

Together these data strongly suggest that E selectively affects the movement of GAPDH from one compartment to another to regulate non-glycolytic functions of GAPDH. In an attempt to further clarify these intriguing results, we decided to visualize by immunocytochemistry the presence of GAPDH in HT-22 cells after E treatment. To accomplish this, it was necessary to reduce

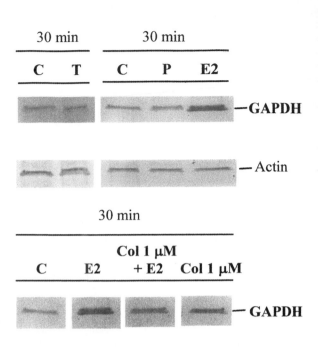

**Fig. 4.** An example of Western blot to identify the amount of GAPDH in the P3 fraction from HT-22 cell cultures in response to steroid treatment is shown. The same amount of protein was loaded (3 µg) in each line with the actin signal to control for loading. After transfer, the blots were incubated with antibodies specific for either GAPDH or Actin. The experiment was repeated at least three times with similar results. For details, see Joe 2003.

**Fig. 5.** An example of the amount of GAPDH detected in Western blot of the P3 fraction from HT-22 cells after E (10 nM) or E plus colchicine (Col), vehicle (control; C) or colchicine alone for 30 min of incubation is shown. For details, see Joe 2003.

the soluble GAPDH with a non-ionic detergent, TritonX-100, to remove non-compartmentalized GAPDH. The results clearly indicate that the treatment removes most of the soluble enzyme. But, when the cells were incubated with E for 30 min and then treated with the detergent, a remarkable amount of GAPDH was still present in what appear to be vesicles or other organelles (Fig. 6).

Therefore, in the presence of E the cells become resistant to TritonX-100 treatment. Further studies will be required to identify precisely in what intracellular organelles this GAPDH is present.

## E-induced Rapid Phosphorylation of GAPDH in Hippocampal Cells

Before addressing this issue, we searched for potential phosphorylation site in the GAPDH molecule using the Prosite Search protocol (Biowork bench). A monomeric GAPDH consists of two domains, a co-factor (NAD+) binding domain (located in the C-termini) and a catalytic domain (N-termini). In the catalytic domain, there are four potential phosphorylation sites: three for protein kinase C and one for caseine kinase 2. Only one potential site was found for tyrosine kinase. These data imply that serine residues in GAPDH are most likely

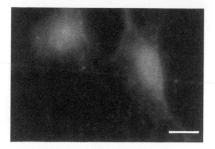 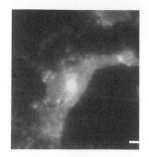

Control                    E 10 nM for 30 r

**Fig. 6.** An example of GAPDH localization in HT-22 cells treated with Triton X-100 is shown. The detergent was used to remove soluble proteins. Cells were prepared for ICC using a specific anti-GAPDH antibody. For details, see Joe 2003.

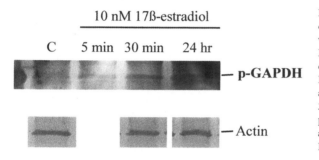

**Fig. 7.** Hippocampal primary cell cultures were incubated with vehicle (control; C) or E for different times. At the end of the experiment, the P3 fraction was prepared and Western blot using 3 μg of protein per lane was performed using a specific anti-phosphoserine antibody. For details, see Joe 2003.

phosphorylated by PKC, an idea that was documented by a study demonstrating phosphorylation of membrane-associated GAPDH by PKC (Tisdale 2002).

First, we studied whether GAPDH would be phosphorylated by E in the P3 fraction of hippocampal cell cultures. The time course indicated that E-induced phosphorylation of serine residues was rapid, reaching maximal level at 30 minutes post-treatment (Fig. 7).

Similar experiments in HT-22 cells showed that only E would phosphorylate the GAPDH present in the P3 fraction at 30 minutes post-incubation, because T and P were ineffective (data not shown).

Next we investigated whether blocking the dephosphorylation rate with a phosphatase inhibitor (okadaic acid at saturating concentrations) would alter the effect of E on the phosphorylation of GAPDH. The rationale for this premise was that E could be affecting either the forward rate of phosphorylation or the backward reaction. As depicted in Figure 8, in the presence of E this inhibitor clearly increased the effect of E alone because the amount of phosphorylated GAPDH was double from the control cell. E or okadaic acid alone increased the level of phosphorylation by only 36 % over controls.

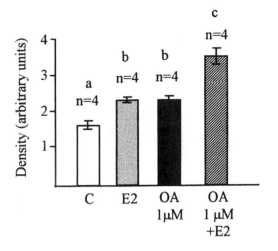

**Fig. 8.** The effect of a phosphatase inhibitor (OA) on the E-induced phosphorylation of GAPDH in the P3 fraction from HT-22 cells is shown. The cells were incubated with vehicle (control; C), E2, OA or OA and E2 together for 30 min. Mean+/- SE are shown for each case. Different letters indicate a p value less than 0.05.

These data indicate that E-induced phosphorylation is probably altering the forward reaction, either directly by affecting the conformation of GAPDH after binding to this protein or indirectly by binding to PKC that would then phosphorylate GAPDH.

## Overview

We have summarized our current findings in Figure 9. This diagram attempts to put into perspective what we have discussed in this paper, considering also the exciting recent, new information about the role of GAPDH in vesicle fusion and exocytosis (Glaser and Gross 1995; Glaser et al. 2002). This new information fits quite well with the known effect of E and the E-BSA complex on rapid release of DA from the striatum (Ramirez and Zheng 1999). Though T has a robust effect in stabilizing microtubule assembly, it is still unclear what the functional role of such a phenomenon is. In contrast, in the case of E, there is prior and current growing evidence indicating that, by affecting microtubule dynamics, E results in changes in movements of vesicles and shape of cells, ending in functional changes of the cells.

In this model, E2 induces translocation of either cytosolic GAPDH or vesicle membrane-associated GAPDH into membrane structures, including the plasma membrane, via changes in microtubule dynamics (Fig. 9, left side). Another effect of E is to activate serine protein kinases located in caveolae-like structures in the plasma membrane, independently of classical estrogen receptors. The activation can be caused either directly by activating PKC (Harvey et al. 2002) or indirectly by interacting with a putative membrane-bound estrogen receptor that binds the PKC. The activated PKC phosphorylates plasma membrane-associated GAPDH that is involved in exocytosis.

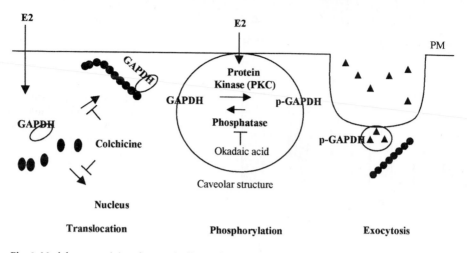

**Fig. 9.** Model summarizing the novel effects of E2 on microtubule dynamics, most likely affecting translocation of GAPDH, phosphorylation of GAPDH and neurotransmitter release by exocytosis. For details, see Robbins et al. 1995; Tisdale 2002; Glaser and Gross 1995; Joe and Ramirez 2001; Joe 2003; Glaser et al. 2002; Ramirez and Zheng 1999; and Harvey et al. 2002. PM, plasma membrane. ● tubulin; ○ vesicles; ●●● microtubule; ▲ neurotransmitter.

Hence, by regulating these three basic cellular functions - translocation, phosphorylation and exocytosis - through GAPDH and other putative proteins, E adds a new avenue of research into understanding the non-genomic action of E and probably other steroids as well.

# References

Agrati P, Ma ZQ, Patrone C, Picotti,GB, Pellicciari C, Bondiolotti G, Bottone MG, Maggi A (1997) Dopaminergic phenotype induced by oestrogens in a human neuroblastoma cell line. Eur Neurosci 9: 1008-1016

Aizu-Yokota E, Ichinoseki K, Sato Y (1994) Microtubule disruption induced by estradiol in estrogen receptor-positive and -negative human breast cancer cell lines. Carcinogenesis 15: 1875-1879

Aizu-Yokota E, Susaki A, Sato Y (1995) Natural estrogens induce modulation of microtubules in Chinese hamster V79 cells in culture. Cancer Res 55: 1863-1868

Blanco G, Diaz H, Carrer HF, Beauge L (1990) Differentiation of rat hippocampal neurons induced by estrogen in vitro: effects on neuritogenesis and Na, K-ATPase activity. J Neurosci Res 27:47-54

Chaudoreille MM, Peyrot V,. Braguer D, Codaccioni F, Crevat A (1991) Qualitative study of the interaction mechanism of estrogenic drugs with tubulin. Biochem Pharmacol 91: 685-693

Garcia-Segura LM, Naftolin F, Hutchison JB, Azcoitia I, Chowen JA (1999) Role of astroglia in estrogen regulation of synaptic plasticity and brain repair. J Neurobiol 40: 574-584

Glaser PE, Gross RW (1995) Rapid plasmenylethanolamine-selective fusion of membrane bilayers catalyzed by an isoform of glyceraldehyde-3-phosphate dehydrogenase:

discrimination between glycolytic and fusogenic roles of individual isoforms. Biochemistry 34:12193-12203

Glaser PE, Han X, Gross RW (2002) Tubulin is the endogenous inhibitor of the glyceraldehyde 3-phosphate dehydrogenase isoform that catalyzes membrane fusion: implications for the coordinated regulation of glycolysis and membrane fusion. Proc Natl Acad Sci USA 99:14104-14109

Harvey BJ, Alzamora R, Healy V, Renard C, Doolan CM (2002) Rapid responses to steroid hormones: from frog skin to human colon. A homage to Hans Ussing. Biochem Biophys Acta 1566: 116-128

Hyman AA, Salser S, Drechsel DN, Unwin N, Mitchison TJ (1992) Role of GTP hydrolysis in microtubule dynamics: Information from a slowly hydrolysable analogue. GMPCPP Mol Biol Cell 3:1155-1167

Jaccioni RB, Cambiazo V (1995) Role of microtubule-associated proteins in the control of microtubule assembly. Physiol Rev 75: 835-64

Joe I (2003) The study of glyceraldehyde-3-phosphate dehydrogenase (GAPDH) function targeted by estrogen and progesterone in the central nervous system and physiological implication. Thesis, Univ. Illinois, Urbana

Joe I, Ramirez VD (2001) Binding of estrogen and progesterone-BSA conjugates to glyceraldehyde-3-phosphate dehydrogenase (GAPDH) and the effects of the free steroids on GAPDH enzyme activity: physiological implications. Steroids 66:529-538

Kipp JL, Ramirez VD (2003) Estradiol and testosterone have opposite effects on microtubule polymerization. Neuroendocrinology 77: 258-272

Luquin S, Naftolin F, Garcia-Segura LM (1993) Natural fluctuation and gonadal hormone regulation of astrocyte immunoreactivity in dentate gyrus. J Neurobiol 2497: 913-924

McEwen BS (1999) Stress and hippocampal plasticity. Ann Rev Neurosci 22:105-22

Mejillano MR, Marton JS, Himes RH (1990) Stabilization of microtubules by GTP analogues. Biochem Biophys Res Commun 166: 653-660

Nogales E (2000) Structural insights into microtubule function. Annu Rev Biochem 69: 277-302

Nogales E, Wolfe SG, Downing KH (1998) Structure of the αβ tubulin dimer by electron crystallography. Nature 391:199-203

Puca GA, Sica V (1981) Identification of specific high affinity sites for the estradiol receptor in the erythrocyte cytoskeleton. Biochem Biophys Res Commun 103: 682-689

Ramirez VD, Kipp JL (2002) A novel non-genomic action of estradiol (E) and (T): regulation of microtubule polymerization. In: Watson CS (ed) The identities of membrane receptors. Kluwer Academic Publishers, Boston, pp 147-156

Ramirez VD, Zheng J (1999) Steroid receptors in brain cell membranes. In: Baulieu EE, Robel P, Schumacher M (eds) Contemporary endocrinology: neurosteroids: a new regulatory function in the nervous system. Humana Press, Totowa, NJ, pp. 269-292

Ramirez VD, Kipp JL, Joe I (2001) Estradiol, in the CNS, targets several physiologically relevant membrane-associated proteins. Brain Res Rev 37: 141-152

Robbins AR, Ward RD, Oliver C (1995) A mutation in glyceraldehydes 3- phosphate dehydrogenase alters endocytosis in CHO cells. J Cell Biol 130:1093-1104

Sakakibara Y, Saito I, Ichinoseki K., Oda T, Kaneko M, Saito H, Kodama M, Sato Y (1991) Effects of diethylstilbestrol and its methyl ethers on aneuploidy induction and microtubule distribution in Chinese hamster V79 cells. Mutat Res 263:269-276

Szego CM, Sjostrand BM, Seeler BJ, Baumer JW, Sjostrand FS (1988) Microtubule and plasmalemmal reorganization: acute response to estrogen. Am J Physiol 254, E775-85

Tisdale EJ (2002) Glyceraldehyde-3-phosphate dehydrogenase is phosphorylated by protein kinase Ciota/lambda and plays a role in microtubule dynamics in the early secretory pathway. J Biol Chem 277: 3334-3341

Tomkins GM, Maxwell ES (1963) Some aspects of steroid hormone action. Ann Rev Biochem 32: 677-708

Toran-Allerand CD (1990) Neurite-like outgrowth from CNS explants may not always be of neuronal origin. Brain Res 513: 353-357

Tranque PA, Suarez I, Olmos G, Fernandez, B, Garcia-Segura LM (1987) Estradiol-induced redistribution of glial fibrillary acidic protein immunoreactivity in the ratbrain. Brain Res 406: 348-351

Valenti C, Vasas M, Cardinalli DP (1979) Effect of castration, estradiol and testosterone on tubulin levels of the medial basal hypothalamus and theadenohypophysis of the rat. Experientia 35: 120-122

Wheeler WJ, Hsu TC, Tousson A, Brinkley BR (1987) Mitotic inhibition and chromosome displacement induced by estradiol in Chinese hamster cells. Cell Motil Cytoskel 7: 235-247

Woolley CS, McEwen BS (1993) Roles of estradiol and progesterone in regulation of hippocampal dendritic spine density during the estrous cycle in the rat. J Comp Neurol 336:293-306

Woolley CS, Gould E, Frankfurt M, McEwen BS (1990) Naturally occurring fluctuation in dendritic spine density on adult hippocampal pyramidal neurons. J Neurosci 10:4035-4039

# Mechanisms of Steroid Hormone Actions on Hypothalamic Nerve Cells: Molecular and Biophysical Studies relevant for Hormone-dependent Behaviors

*Lee-Ming Kow, Nandini Vasudevan[1], Nino Devidze, Andre Ragnauth, and Donald W. Pfaff*

## Summary

Genes turned on by hormones and genes whose products are essential for hormone-controlled behaviors have received intense study during the last 20 years. Now, we see that steroid hormones can also affect nerve cells by rapid membrane actions in addition to slower genomic actions. At the molecular level, in transient transfection studies of neuroblastoma cells using a 2-pulse protocol, we have shown that the rapid effects in the first pulse actually can potentiate the later genomic actions in the facilitation of transcription. Signal transduction from the first, membrane-limited pulse, of the 2-pulse protocol uses multiple signaling pathways. Now, with in vivo behavioral studies on female sex behavior, we have discovered that the logical relations between the two actions are different from the simpler transcription studies in a surprising manner: The rapid membrane action need not be the first hormonal pulse in the 2-pulse experimental protocol. For behavior, the membrane-limited action can be the second pulse. How do these effects on hypothalamic neurons come about? At the neuronal level, estradiol can potentiate the excitatory effects of neurotransmitters such as histamine or NMDA. Using patch clamp studies (now followed up with calcium imaging studies), we see that estradiol can excite electrical activity in two ways, by increasing an inward current and by decreasing an outward current. The inward-going current is a sodium current; the outward-going current is a potassium current.

Tremendous progress has been made in discovering and conceptualizing hormone actions on gene expression in the CNS. Genes induced by estrogens in the mammalian forebrain influence a variety of neural functions. Among them, reproductive behavior mechanisms are very well understood. Their functional genomics provide a solid theoretical paradigm for linking genes to neural circuits to behavior. We propose that estrogen-induced genes are organized in modules: Growth of hypothalamic neurons; Amplification of the

The Laboratory of Neurobiology and Behavior, Rockefeller University, New York, N.Y. 10021
[1] Present address: Penn State University, State College, PA.

Kordon et al.
Hormones and the Brain
© Springer-Verlag Berlin Heidelberg 2005

estrogen effect by progesterone; Preparative behaviors; Permissive actions on sex behavior circuitry; and Synchronization of mating behavior with ovulation (GAPPS). These modules represent mechanistic routes for CNS management of successful reproduction. The gene networks involved have been reviewed by Mong and Pfaff (2003); our paper develops the ideas and references presented there. Moreover, new microarray results add estrogen-dependent genes to our list for further study.

## Genomic routes activating functional modules (GAPPS)

Causal routes from hormone to gene to behavior include direct effects, from gene induction to neural circuit to behavioral change. These would include hormone effects on neurotransmitter receptors in ventromedial hypothalamic neurons, which directly trigger the rest of the lordosis circuit. Noradrenergic $\alpha_{1b}$ receptors are induced by estrogen treatment in ventromedial hypothalamic (VMH) cells (Etgen et al. 2001), which govern the rest of the lordosis behavior circuit. Muscarinic receptors responding to the neurotransmitter acetylcholine are also found on VMH neurons. Estrogen treatment increases their activities as well (Kow et al. 1995).

Causal routes also include indirect effects, from gene induction to downstream genes to behavioral change. Some hormone effects occur early, long before the onset of reproductive behaviors, and set the stage for later developments:

**Neuronal growth:** Growth promotion by estrogens in VMH neurons follows from the stimulation of synthesis of ribosomal RNA, which precedes the elaboration of dendrites and synapses on VMH neurons observed after hormonal treatment.

**Amplification by progesterone:** Administration of progesterone 24 or 48 hours after estrogen (E) priming greatly amplifies the effect of E on mating behavior. This effect requires the nuclear progesterone receptor (PR), as it disappears after antisense DNA against PR mRNA has been administered in the VMH.

**GnRH:** The physiological importance of estrogenic elevation of gonadotropin releasing hormone (GnRH, LHRH) mRNA levels under positive feedback conditions – as well as elevation of the receptor mRNA for GnRH – must be to synchronize reproductive behavior with the ovulatory surge of luteinizing hormone (LH).

Finally, hormone/gene/behavior causal routes include indirect effects, from gene induction to intermediate behaviors. Some of the genes affected by estrogens work by altering other behaviors, which then prepare the animal for the behavior in question, in this case mating:

**Analgesia:** The enkephalin gene is turned on rapidly, within about 30 min, by estrogens, and this is proven to represent a hormone-facilitated transcriptional facilitation. The route of action upon lordosis of the enkephalin gene product is indirect, through other behaviors. That is, we propose that, through the reduction of pain, enkephalins help to allow the female to engage in mating behavior despite the mauling she receives from the male.

**Anxiety reduction:** The oxytocin gene and the gene for its receptor are both expressed by hypothalamic neurons at higher levels in the presence of estrogens. The indirect route of action of this multiplicative set of gene inductions on mating behavior is likely through a behavioral link: anxiety reduction allows courtship and mating.

Emerging from 1) this series of individual gene inductions by estrogens acting in the basal forebrain, and 2) a recounting of downstream genes and their physiological routes of action, comes 3) a systematic molecular "formula" (GAPPS) that appears to account for the causal relations between sex hormones and female mating behaviors. First, there is a hormone-dependent growth response, which permits hormone-facilitated, behavior-directing hypothalamic neurons a greater range of input/output connections and, thus, physiological power. Secondly, progesterone can amplify the estrogen effect, in part through the downstream genes listed above. Then, through indirect behavioral means – the reduction of anxiety and a partial analgesia – the female as an organism is prepared for engaging in reproductive behavior sequences. Here the genes for oxytocin (and its receptor) as well as the genes for the opioid peptide enkephalin (and its receptors) are important. Next, neurotransmitter receptor induction by estradiol permits the neural circuit for lordosis behavior to be activated. The noradrenaline a1 receptor and the muscarinic acetylcholine receptors are key here, in the ventromedial nucleus of the hypothalamus. Finally, induction of the decapeptide that triggers ovulation, GnRH, as well as its cognate receptor acts to synchronize mating behavior with ovulation in a biologically adaptive fashion.

## Fast, membrane-initiated actions

For more than 40 years, interpretations of steroid hormone actions as nuclear, transcriptional events have been seen as "competing" against inferences of rapid membrane actions. We (Vasudevan et al. 2001) have discovered conditions where membrane-limited effects potentiate later transcriptional actions in a nerve cell line. Making use of a 2-pulse hormonal schedule in a transfection system, early and brief administration of conjugated, membrane-limited estradiol was necessary but not sufficient for full transcriptional potency of the second estrogen pulse. The efficacy of the first pulse depended on intact signal transduction pathways, including PKC, PKA and calcium-signaling pathways. Surprisingly, the efficacy of both the first and second pulses was blocked by a classical nuclear estrogen receptor (ER) antagonist. Thus, two different modes of steroid hormone action can synergize.

We have followed up the initial transient transfection experiments with a series of biophysical and behavioral studies (Kow et al. 2002, 2003, 2004). Using electrophysiological recording techniques from nerve cells *in vitro* in slices of hypothalamic tissue, it is clear that brief applications of estradiol can potentiate excitatory responses to a transmitter such as histamine, crucial for the initiation of sexual arousal, and increase inward and decrease outward membrane currents, both in favor of increasing neuronal excitability. The behavioral results are more surprising. It appears that under the experimental conditions of 2-pulse administration, the application of membrane-limited estradiol to the hypothalamus does not have to be in the first pulse, as found in cell line studies (Vasudevan et al. 2001), but can also be in the second pulse of hormone administration.

Current initiatives add two innovations, one technical and the other strategic. Identification of cells with the same completeness and precision as in the visceral and buccal ganglia of Aplysia, for example, is a goal that has long eluded students of the mammalian CNS. Now, using patch clamp and RT/PCR technology, we can suck the cytoplasmic messenger RNA out of the recorded cell after the recording is finished and thereby identify that cell with respect to 1) genes expressed, 2) cell body shape, 3) cell body size, 4) neuronal location, and, therefore, 5) behavioral importance.

In terms of experimental strategy, we can continue to direct our analyses toward the complete explanation of simple sex behaviors such as lordosis (building on previous work reviewed in Pfaff 1999) and the locomotion of courtship behavior in the female mouse (Garey et al. 2002). However, similar sex hormonal mechanisms also elevate sexual arousal, a specific manifestation of the global arousal of the CNS (Pfaff et al. 2001; Pfaff 2004). In this sense the discoveries for a simple concrete behavior pattern like lordosis can be used as a "stepping stone," strategically, to attack the mechanisms for broader underlying concepts.

## References

Etgen AM, Ansonoff MA, Quesada A (2001) Mechanisms of ovarian steroid regulation of norepinephrine receptor-mediated signal transduction in the hypothalamus: implications for female reproductive physiology. Horm Behav 40:169-77

Garey J, Kow L-M, Huynh W, Ogawa S, Pfaff DW (2002) Temporal and spatial quantitation of nesting and mating behaviors among mice housed in a semi-natural environment. Horm Behav 42:294-306

Kow L-M, Pfaff DW (2002) Acute estrogen effects on rat ventromedial hypothalamus: Potentiating neuronal excitation and facilitating lordosis-inducing genomic action. Society for Neuroscience Abstr. # 482.16

Kow L-M, Pfaff DW (2004) The membrane actions of estrogens can potentiate their lordosis behaviorfacilitating genomic actions. PNAS, in press

Kow L-M, Tsai Y-F, Weiland NG, McEwen BS, Pfaff DW (1995) In vitro electro-pharmacological and autoradiographic analyses of muscarinic receptor subtypes in rat hypothalamic ventromedial nucleus: implications for cholinergic regulation of lordosis. Brain Res 694: 29-39

Kow L-M, Devidze N, Shibuya I, Pfaff D (2003) Acute estradiol application increases inward and decrease outward whole-cell currents of neurons in rat hypothalamic ventromedial nucleus (VMN). Society for Neuroscience Abstr. # 610.7

Mong J, Pfaff D (2004) Hormonal symphony; genetic network serving estrogenic effects on reproductive behaviors. Mol Psychiat, 9:550-556

Pfaff D (1999) Drive. Cambridge: The MIT Press

Pfaff D (2004) Brain Arousal and Information Theory. Cambridge, Harvard University Press, in press

Pfaff D, Frohlich J, Morgan M (2002) Hormonal and genetic influences on arousal–sexual and otherwise. Trends Neurosci 25:45-50

Vasudevan N, Kow, L-M, Pfaff DW (2001) Early membrane estrogenic effects required for full expression of slower genomic actions in a nerve cell line. Proc Natl Acad Sci USA 98: 12267-12271.

# Biological Effects and Markers of Exposure to Xenosteroids and Selective Estrogen Receptor Modulators (SERMs) at the Hypothalamic-Pituitary Unit

*M. Tena-Sempere[1] and E. Aguilar[1]*

## Summary

Estrogen is a pivotal factor in the regulation of a wide array of biological systems, in both the male and the female, which include not only the reproductive axis but also bone, the cardiovascular system, adipose tissue and the brain. In recent years, the biological effects and mechanisms of action of estrogen have been deeply revisited, and extensive efforts have been made to better understand both the physiology and pathophysiology of estrogen actions in different target tissues. In this context, a major concern has recently emerged about the potential deleterious effects on human and wildlife health of a wide array of natural and synthetic compounds with sex steroid-like (mostly estrogenic) bioactivities; these compounds are globally termed xenosteroids. In addition, synthetic drugs have been developed with combined estrogenic and anti-estrogenic actions, depending on the cellular context. These molecules, collectively named selective estrogen receptor modulators (SERMs), are provided with obvious pharmacological applications, but they may also serve in the characterization of the complex mode of action of estrogen in different physiological systems. Similarly, estrogen receptor (ER)-selective ligands have been recently identified or engineered, thus providing an experimental tool to dissect out the contribution of each of the two major ER isoforms (ERα and ERβ) in signaling the plethora of estrogen effects in multiple target tissues. The hypothalamic-pituitary (HP) unit is highly sensitive to the actions of estrogen, although several aspects of estrogen effects upon the development and regulation of the HP unit remain partially unknown. The aim of this review is to provide a comprehensive overview of our recent work in the identification of molecular mechanisms and markers of exposure to xenoestrogens, as well as in the analysis of the biological effects of SERMs and ER-selective ligands at the HP unit.

[1] Department of Cell Biology, Physiology and Immunology, University of Córdoba, 14004 Córdoba, Spain

Kordon et al.
Hormones and the Brain
© Springer-Verlag Berlin Heidelberg 2005

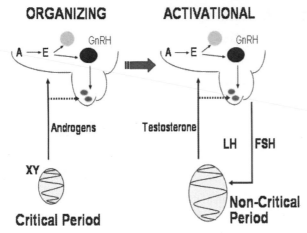

**Fig. 1.** Organizing and activational effects of estrogen upon the HP unit and the paradigm of brain sex differentiation in the male. During the *critical period* of hypothalamic differentiation, estrogen (E), produced locally after aromatization of testosterone (A) secreted by the embryonic testis, imprints the plastic development of the neuronal networks involved in the neuroendocrine control of reproductive function, thus promoting a characteristic male-pattern of morphological and functional differentiation of the brain (left side). Outside this period, testosterone, together with other testicular factors, participates in the regulation of gonadotropin secretion through feedback mechanisms (right side). However, at this stage, sex steroids are devoid of organizing effects. Taken from Tena-Sempere et al. 2000b, with minor modifications.

## Introduction

Despite the classical contention that estrogen is the female reproductive hormone, an enormous body of data has now firmly established that estrogen is a key regulator of multiple physiological events in both males and females, including not only fertility and reproduction but also bone homeostasis, adipose and immune functions, cardiovascular physiology and different aspects of central nervous system function (Clark and Mani 1994; Sharpe 1998). Moreover, in multiple target tissues, estrogen, produced locally through aromatization of testosterone, is the molecular signal responsible for conducting the biological actions of androgens (Sharpe 1998). Such a plethora of biological actions is mostly conducted through the so-called genomic pathway, where estrogen interacts with specific nuclear receptors that operate as ligand-activated transcriptional factors. So far, two different subtypes of estrogen receptor (ER) have been identified: the classical ER (renamed ERα) and the newly cloned ERβ (White and Parker 1998; Kuiper et al. 1998). Although they possess a similar domain structure, the α and β forms of ER have partially different functional properties and show distinct patterns of tissue distribution and gene regulation (for examples, see Kuiper et al. 1998; Paech et al. 1997; Osterlund et al. 1998; Tena-Sempere et al. 2000a; Schreihofer et al. 2000), which may contribute to the complexity and plasticity of the biological actions of estrogen. An additional source of diversity in estrogen signaling may derive from the generation of multiple variants of ERα and ERβ, detected both in normal tissues and tumor cells, whose functional role in conducting the biological effects of estrogen remains to be fully elucidated (Shupnik 2002).

Among other target systems, the hypothalamic-pituitary (HP) unit is highly sensitive to both the developmental and regulatory effects of estrogen. Notably, depending on the stage of development, the actions of estrogen on the HP system can be considered as organizing or activational effects (Fig. 1). The former involve biological actions during sensitive periods of development (conventionally termed "critical periods") that result in permanent effects in the functional programming of the HP unit. Within such a critical period, changes in the sex steroid input upon differentiating brain induce a permanent reprogramming of its pattern of development. Outside this organizing period, the HP unit remains sensitive to the regulatory effects of estrogen. However, at this stage, changes in estrogen input result in transient regulatory events (i.e., activational), such as modulation of gonadotropin-releasing hormone (GnRH), luteinizing hormone (LH), follicle-stimulating hormone (FSH) and prolactin (PRL) secretion (for a review, see Tena-Sempere et al. 2000b). Both organizing and activational effects of estrogen contribute to the normal function of the HP unit throughout the life span. Conversely, disruption of estrogen effects at different stages of development may be detrimental to the organization and function of this system.

## Mechanisms and Markers of Exposure to Xenosteroids at the HP Unit

Among other physiological systems, the HP unit plays a central role in the integrated control of reproductive function. As indicated above, during critical periods of development the functional organization of the hypothalamus is driven by sex steroids, and changes in the steroid input are able to induce permanent effects in terms of programming of the function of the reproductive axis. In rodents, sex differentiation of brain structures related to the neuroendocrine control of reproductive function and sex behavior takes place perinatally (E17.5-postnatal day 10) and involves androgen and estrogen (Tena-Sempere et al. 2000b). Interestingly, the signals ultimately responsible for masculinization or feminization of the developing HP unit are similar, because estrogen, in a dose-dependent manner, is able to promote female (low levels) or male (high levels) patterns of brain sex differentiation (Tena-Sempere et al. 2000b; MacLusky and Naftolin 1981; Dohler and Hancke 1978; see Fig. 2).

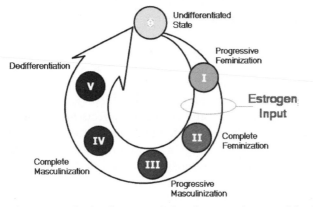

**Fig. 2.** Hypothesis of estrogen-induced progressive sexual brain differentiation. Estrogen is the molecular signal responsible for either feminization or masculinization of the developing hypothalamus, depending on the level of exposure (represented by the circular arrow). Low estrogenic input promotes a female pattern of differentiation. However, increased estrogen interaction induces a male pattern of sex differentiation. Finally, supra-maximal estrogenic exposure disrupts the normal differentiation process, thus resulting in the absence of either female or male development. This stage of dedifferentiation resembles, but is not analogous to, the original undifferentiated state of brain sex development. This hypothesis may explain why the administration of supra-physiological doses of estrogenic compounds is deleterious to male reproductive function. Taken from Tena-Sempere et al. 2000b, with minor modifications.

## Endocrine Disruption of Reproductive Function Direct Actions at the HP unit?

In recent years, a major concern has been raised as to the potential deleterious effects on human and wildlife health of a wide array of natural and synthetic compounds with sex steroid-like bioactivities, termed xenosteroids. These belong to the large family of endocrine disrupters (EDC), i.e., factors with the ability to interact with and disturb different endocrine systems which in turn results in adverse health effects that may appear later in life. Indeed, plant compounds and manmade chemicals and by-products, whose levels of exposure have increased steadily in Western countries, have been proven to be estrogenic (xenoestrogens), androgenic or anti-androgenic. Moreover, many epidemiological studies have revealed significant trends of deterioration in reproductive health in different species. In humans, increasing incidences of testicular cancer and genital malformations, together with decreased sperm counts and fertility, have been reported. This plethora of disorders has been recently grouped under the so-called Testicular Dysgenesis Syndrome (Boisen et al. 2001). The etiology of such a syndrome is not completely elucidated, but the potential involvement of environmental EDCs (such as xenoestrogens) has been proposed. Whether endocrine disruption takes place at other levels of the reproductive axis has received less attention. However, on the basis of physiological data on the sensitivity of the HP unit to estrogen, it is possible that the impact of xenoestrogens upon the reproductive axis may derive, at least partially, from primary actions in the pituitary and/or hypothalamus.

When considering the potential endocrine-disrupting activity of xenoestrogens, it has been argued that most of the synthetic EDCs in the environment have very weak estrogenic activity, thus casting doubts on the possibility that, at the conventional range of exposure, they would elicit significant biological effects. However, in addition to their ability to bioaccumulate, two relevant phenomena have to be considered. First, exposure to synthetic EDCs usually takes place from mixtures of similarly acting or dissimilarly acting compounds, and experimental evidence obtained using in vitro systems indicates that exposure to complex mixtures of xenoestrogens at individual doses below their no-observed-effect level (NOEL) is able to induce robust estrogenic responses (Silva et al. 2002). Second, complex mixtures of weak xenoestrogens are able to modulate the effects of potent steroid hormones, such as endogenous estradiol (Rajapakse et al. 2002). Thus, it becomes possible that, although single exposure to individual weak xenoestrogens may not pose a significant risk in terms of endocrine disruption, exposure to complex mixtures of similarly or dissimilarly acting EDCs may evoke adverse responses, either through concentration addition among the different xenoestrogens or by modulation of the effects of endogenous steroids. In the latter case, and considering the mode of action of estrogen in promoting sex differentiation of the hypothalamus, it is tempting to speculate that exposure to xenoestrogens may enhance the estrogenic input upon the developing HP unit, which in turn may result in altered patterns of sex differentiation (Fig. 2).

## Neonatal Estrogenization as an Experimental Model of Disruption at the HP unit

Most of the efforts toward characterization of the deleterious effects of xenoestrogens on the reproductive system have so far focused on the analysis of their direct actions upon genitalia and gonads. However, considering that the developing HP unit is highly sensitive to endogenous estrogen, and that estrogen is able to induce permanent organizing effects, it is conceivable that early exposure to exogenous estrogens (xenoestrogens) may have an impact on the function of this system later in life. Indeed, most of the effects attributed to EDCs are characterized by a delayed onset, and some of them (advanced or delayed puberty, infertility) may have a central origin at the HP unit. Moreover, based on physiological data, the sensitivity of the developing HP unit is expected to be much higher than that of the reproductive tract. However, scientific evidence for the potential disruption of the reproductive axis at the HP level is still pending, mostly due to our very limited knowledge about the sensitivity

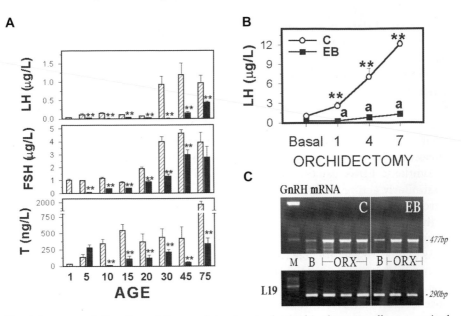

**Fig. 3.** Summary of alterations of the gonadotropic axis observed in the neonatally estrogenized male rat. In panel **A**, serum LH, FSH and testosterone (T) levels are presented in control and neonatally estrogenized males, at different time points between day 1 and 75 of age. In addition, in panels **B** and **C**, the patterns of serum LH response and hypothalamic GnRH gene expression after orchidectomy in control (C) and neonatally estrogenized  male rats are shown. When relevant, values are given as means ± SEM. ** $P < 0.01$ vs values from corresponding controls (ANOVA followed by Turkey's test). EB, estradiol benzoate. Taken from Tena-Sempere et al. 2000a, with modifications.

of this system to EDCs and their mechanism(s) of actions, as well as novel endpoints and biomarkers of exposure.

To extend our knowledge about the mechanisms of action and novel endpoints of xenoestrogens at the HP unit, appropriate experimental animal models need to be used. In our laboratory, we have used rats treated with high doses of the synthetic estrogen estradiol benzoate during the critical neonatal period of hypothalamic sex differentiation (Tena-Sempere et al. 2000b). Given the specific timing of sex differentiation of the brain, this model is especially suitable to specifically target key events in the organization of the HP system controlling reproductive function. However, disruption of reproductive function in rodents by neonatal exposure to high doses of estrogenic compounds is probably a multi-faceted phenomenon that involves direct effects at different levels of the hypothalamic-pituitary-gonadal axis (Tena-Sempere et al. 2000b).

In terms of the function of the HP unit, a striking effect of neonatal estrogenization in the rat is the persistent decrease in plasma LH and FSH levels (Fig. 3A). Moreover, LH response to gonadectomy is reduced in neonatally estrogenized animals (Fig. 3B), thus proving the impairment of the feedback mechanisms responsible for the control of gonadotropin secretion (Tena-Sempere et al. 2000b). Such a suppression of gonadotropin levels is likely related to a decrease in the release of hypothalamic GnRH. In fact, a primary defect at the level of gonadotropes can be ruled out, as pituitary responsiveness to GnRH, both in vivo and in vitro, was maintained, and even enhanced, by neonatal estrogenization (Tena-Sempere et al. 2000b). Furthermore, impaired release of GnRH is not attributable to the inherent damage of GnRH neurons, as basal and depolarization-induced release of hypothalamic GnRH in vitro was higher in estrogenized male rats (Tena-Sempere et al. 2000b) and basal and gonadectomy-induced expression of GnRH gene was similar in control and estrogenized animals (Fig. 3C). In contrast, a constitutive lack of activation of excitatory systems governing GnRH release seems to be involved. In this sense, activation of aminoacidergic pathways, by means of administration of specific agonists for N-methyl-D-aspartic acid (NMDA) and kainic acid (KA) receptors, restored the defective LH response to orchidectomy and selectively elicited LH secretion in adult, neonatally estrogenized male rats (Tena-Sempere et al. 2000b). The latter finding points out that the neural circuitry governing hypothalamic GnRH release is a target for the actions of both endogenous and exogenous estrogens.

## Identification of Novel Mechanisms and Markers of Exposure to Xenoestrogens

Using the neonatally estrogenized rat as an experimental model, we have recently initiated a search for novel mechanisms of action and new endpoints and biomarkers of exposure to estrogenic compounds during critical periods of development at the HP unit. To this end, we have undertaken two complementary strategies. First, based on the scientific literature, we have chosen a panel of genes that are either acutely regulated by estrogen or encode relevant factors in estrogen actions. Second, in the context of FP-5 EU project EDEN QLK4-CT-2002-00603, we have started an analysis of differentially expressed genes in the hypothalamus and pituitary following neonatal exposure to estrogen.

For the first approach, expression profiling by RT-PCR of selected gene candidates has included ERα and β and progesterone receptor (PR) in the hypothalamus as well as ERα, ERβ, the truncated ER product TERP-1 and PR in the pituitary. The data so far obtained may have mechanistic implications. For instance, neonatal exposure to high doses of estrogen results in a persistent decrease of expression of ERα and ERβ genes in the pituitary, which is associated with an increase in relative expression levels of the mRNAs encoding the truncated ER product TERP-1 (Tena-Sempere et al. 2001a,b; Fig. 4). Considering that ERα and ERβ are the functionally active forms and that TERP-1 may function as dominant negative of full-length ERs, it is tempting to propose that disruption of pituitary function following neonatal estrogenization

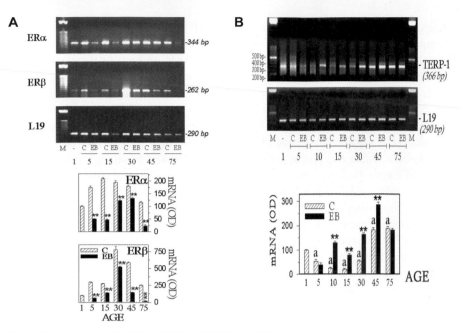

**Fig. 4.** Expression profile of ERα, ERβ and TERP-1 mRNAs in male rat pituitary during postnatal development and effects of neonatal exposure to estrogen. In panel **A**, pituitary relative mRNA levels of ERα and ERβ are presented in control and neonatally estrogenized males, at different time points between day 1 and 75 of age. Similarly, in panel **B**, expression mRNA levels of the truncated variant TERP-1 in pituitaries from estrogenized males are shown. Neonatal exposure to estrogen induces two complementary responses for decreasing pituitary estrogen sensitivity: decreased expression of the mRNA encoding the fully functional forms of ER, and increased expression of the dominant negative isoform TERP-1. Semi-quantitative data are expressed as mean ± SEM (four independent determinations per group). ** P ≤ 0.01 vs. control samples; a P ≤ 0.01 vs. day 1 samples (ANOVA followed by Turkey's test). Taken from Tena-Sempere et al. 2001a,b.

might involve homologous down-regulation of the ER system by at least two complementary pathways: 1) decreased expression of the mRNAs encoding the fully functional forms of ER, and 2) increased expression of TERP-1 mRNA, a dominant negative isoform of ERα and ERβ when expressed at ratios of 1:1 or greater (Shupnik 2002; Tena-Sempere et al. 2001b). In the hypothalamus, our results demonstrate that neonatal exposure to estrogen induces a persistent increase in relative mRNA levels of ERα and ERβ, which might contribute to the altered function of the GnRH system in this model (Tena-Sempere et al. 2001a). In addition, neonatal exposure to estrogen resulted in increased expression of the PR gene in the hypothalamus in both male and female rats. Given the recently proposed role of PR in hypothalamic sex differentiation (Quadros et al. 2002), the involvement of such a phenomenon in the plethora of reproductive defects of the neonatally estrogenized rat is presently under investigation.

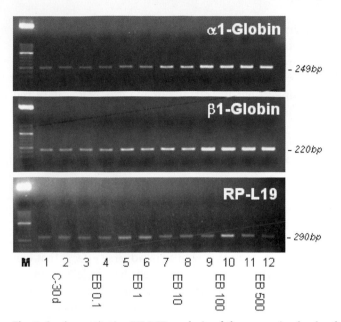

**Fig. 5.** Semi-quantitative RT-PCR analysis of the expression levels of α- and β-globin mRNAs in male rat pituitary following neonatal exposure to estrogen. Upon initial identification of the phenomenon by means of differential display RT-PCR, characterization of dose responsiveness for the induction of globin mRNA expression in male rat pituitary was conducted. Groups of males were exposed on day 1 post-partum to increasing doses of estradiol benzoate (ranging from 0.1-500 µg/rat), and samples of pituitary tissue were collected on day 30 post-partum. A clear-cut dose-response pattern was demonstrated for both targets. These results have been fully confirmed by real-time RT-PCR assays (data not shown).

For the second strategy, a degenerated oligoprimer (DOP)-based PCR approach has been implemented in collaboration with Dr. H. Leffers at the Department of Growth and Reproduction of Rigshospitalet (University Hospital, Copenhagen, Denmark), to identify differentially expressed genes in the pituitary and hypothalamus of rats exposed neonatally to high doses of estrogen. Although analysis of DOP-PCR differential display assays is still underway, several estrogen-induced genes have already been identified. For example, seven different primer combinations identified selective up-regulation of β-globin gene in the pituitary of 30-day-old male and female rats treated on Day 1 post-partum with high doses of estradiol benzoate. Similarly, induction of expression of α-globin gene in the pituitary has also been demonstrated in neonatally estrogenized animals. These DOP-PCR assays have been followed by detailed expression profiling by means of semi-quantitative and real-time RT-PCR analyses. These analyses fully confirmed our initial observations, indicating that persistently increased expression of α- and β-globin mRNA levels in the pituitary takes place in a dose-dependent manner (Fig. 5).

Moreover, such a persistent induction appears to be selectively detected in the pituitary, as no increase was observed in an array of additional tissues such as the hypothalamus, cortex, cerebellum, liver and testis. Thus, globin genes may constitute suitable continuous biomarkers of exposure to estrogenic compounds in the pituitary. We plan to employ such markers in our analyses of low-dose and mixture effects of xenosteroids in the HP unit.

## Effects of SERMs Upon Sex Differentiation of the HP Unit

As reviewed in previous sections, inappropriate estrogen input (e.g., after exposure to xenoestrogens) at different levels of the hypothalamic-pituitary-gonadal axis may result in detrimental reproductive effects. In addition, as estrogen is playing multiple roles in different physiological systems, deprivation of endogenous estrogen (e.g., at menopause) results in adverse effects that can be prevented by hormonal replacement therapy. Indeed, beneficial actions of estrogen have been reported in bone, cardiovascular system and central nervous system (CNS). However, estrogen also conducts  potent tropic actions in breast and uterus that are associated with an increased risk of estrogen-dependent cancer. Thus, pure estrogen replacement is undesirable. Alternatively, tissue-specific estrogens, with agonistic activity in the skeleton and the cardiovascular system but antagonistic effects in breast and endometrium, would be optimal for replacement protocols. Different compounds with this pharmacological profile have been developed in recent years. Given their combined activities at the ER, they have been globally termed selective ER modulators (SERMs; McDonnell 1999; Jordan and Morrow 1999).

## SERMs: Tamoxifen and Raloxifene

Development of tissue-specific estrogens was founded in structural and clinical studies seeking  nonsteroidal antiestrogens. The first antiestrogen reported in the literature was MER25, which presented serious side effects in clinical trials (Jordan and Morrow 1999). However, analysis of the structure of this compound led to the generation of triphenylethylene derivatives that resulted in the generation of tamoxifen (TX; Fig. 6). Initially, TX was considered as a pure anti-estrogen in the management of estrogen-responsive breast cancer. Accordingly, given its proposed antiestrogenic activity, adverse effects in terms of bone density were anticipated. Clinical trials, however, demonstrated that TX behaved as estrogen in the skeleton, increasing bone mineral density. This observation raised the possibility of combined tissue-specific estrogenic/antiestrogenic actions of TX, and ultimately proved the existence of a novel family of compounds: the SERMs. These compounds have obvious therapeutical

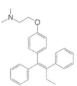

### Tamoxifen

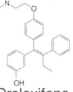

### Droloxifene

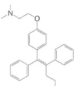

### Toremifene

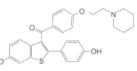

### Raloxifene

**Fig. 6.** Chemical structure of several selective estrogen receptor modulators (SERMs). Tamoxifen and other triphenylethylene derivatives, as well as the benzothiophene derivative raloxifene, are shown. In addition, structures of ER-selective ligands, propyl-pyrazole-triol (PPT; selective ERα ligand) and diarylpropionitrile (DPN; potency-selective ERβ agonist) are presented. Taken from McDonnell 1999, Jordan and Morrow 1999, Stauffer et al. 2000, Meyers et al. 2001, with minor modifications.

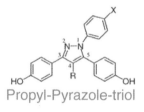

Propyl-Pyrazole-triol        Diarylpropionitrile

applications (e.g., estrogen-dependent cancer, prevention of osteoporosis). In addition, they have interesting physiological implications. Indeed, discovery of the mode of action of SERMs has helped to enlarge our present understanding of the molecular mechanisms for the wide variety of effects of estrogen in multiple target tissues. Moreover, the generation of synthetic molecules with tissue-specific effects at the ER raises the possibility that SERMs are actually mimicking a physiological system wherein different endogenous estrogens are playing different roles, depending on the cell and tissue context. This question remains to be fully answered (McDonnell 1999).

Despite the potential beneficial effects of TX in estrogen replacement, in terms of prevention of osteoporosis (estrogenic effects) without increasing the incidence of breast cancer (antiestrogenic action), clinical and experimental studies demonstrated that TX possesses estrogenic activity in the uterus and increases the risk of endometrial cancer. The latter finding precludes the use of TX in conventional management and prevention of osteoporosis at menopause. Indeed, recently developed derivatives of TX, such as toremifene and, more recently, droloxifene and idoxifen (see Fig. 6), are anticipated to have SERM activities similar to TX in clinical studies. Thus, development of novel SERMs with improved pharmacological and clinical profiles was required. In this context, a non-steroidal benzothiophene derivative, termed Raloxifene (RX), was generated (Fig. 6). This compound mimicked the effects of estrogen and TX in bone, but unlike them it was devoid of significant uterotropic activity (McDonnell 1999; Avioli 1999). Moreover, RX decreases circulating cholesterol levels and is antiestrogenic in the breast. On this basis, RX was approved by the USA FDA for the prevention of postmenopausal osteoporosis.

## Actions of SERMs in different target tissues. Actions at CNS?

On the basis of their mechanism of action, SERMs may target all estrogen-responsive tissues and, depending on the cell context, elicit estrogenic or antiestrogenic responses. Most of these effects have been evaluated in great detail and were reviewed in the previous section. However, the actions of SERMs upon the CNS remain partially undefined. In principle, most SERMs, such as TX and RX, are able to cross the blood-brain barrier (Somjen et al. 1996), and some adverse side effects of TX upon the CNS have been described in clinical trials. Conversely, some estrogenic effects of SERMs upon the CNS might be beneficial. Recent studies have demonstrated that synaptic plasticity and neuroprotection are estrogen-mediated events, and potential disease-modifying or neuroprotective effects of estrogen in the elderly have been proposed (Schneider and Finch 1997; Reibel et al. 2000). Given the optimal pharmacological profile of RX in postmenopausal patients, the possibility that RX may conduct estrogenic effects in the CNS merits further investigation.

## Effects of Raloxifene upon sex differentiation of the HP unit

Concerning the central effects of RX, little attention has been paid to the effects of this SERM on the circuitry controlling neuroendocrine function and reproduction, and it remains to be fully elucidated whether RX is conducting predominantly estrogenic or antiestrogenic actions in this context. Taking advantage of the fact that the developing HP unit is highly sensitive to endogenous and exogenous estrogens, we have recently undertaken a series of studies to characterize the potential actions of RX upon the HP unit at critical stages of sex differentiation. Our aim was two-fold: 1) to provide further evidence for the effects of RX upon the reproductive axis at certain stages development, and 2) to evaluate whether RX is conducting central estrogenic and/or antiestrogen effects in a highly estrogen-sensitive system.

Data so far obtained indicate that RX is mostly estrogenic at the HP unit. Indeed, administration of different doses of RX to male and female rats on day 1 post-partum evoked an array of reproductive defects that resembled those of neonatal estrogenization. These included decreased gonadotropin secretion, hyperprolactinaemia, advanced vaginal opening, persistent vaginal estrus,

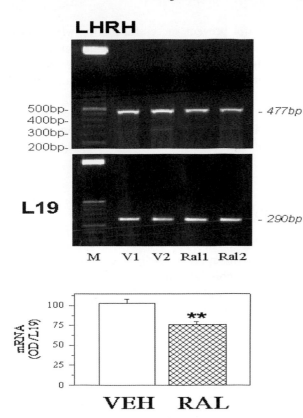

**Fig. 7.** Hypothalamic expression of GnRH mRNA in 23-day-old female rats injected neonatally with Raloxifene (500 μg/rat/day) or vehicle. A representative ethidium bromide-stained gel electrophoresis of GnRH mRNA levels in hypothalamic samples from control (V) and raloxifene-treated animals is presented. In addition, semi-quantitative data of GnRH mRNA steady-state levels in control (VEH) and raloxifene-treated (RAL) groups are shown. Semi-quantitative data are expressed as mean ± SEM. * P ≤ 0.05 vs. control samples (ANOVA followed by Turkey's test).

inhibition of positive and negative feedback between estrogen and LH, and anovulation and infertility in females, whereas in males, neonatal RX treatment resulted in delayed puberty onset and hyperprolactinaemia (Pinilla et al. 2001a, 2002a). Further demonstration that neonatal RX is acting as an estrogen upon the developing HP unit comes from co-administration experiments where RX was injected together with estradiol benzoate. In this setting, RX was unable to prevent the plethora of reproductive defects associated with neonatal estrogenization, thus suggesting that RX is not an anti-estrogen at this level (Pinilla et al. 2002b). The mechanisms for altered function of the gonadotrope axis following neonatal exposure to RX may involve decreased GnRH expression at the hypothalamus (Tena-Sempere et al. 2003a; see Fig. 7), although reduced pituitary LH content and/or decreased pituitary responsiveness to hypothalamic GnRH might also be involved. Additional evidence for an estrogen-like action at the HP unit was obtained after acute administration of RX to ovariectomized female rats, which inhibited LH secretion and stimulated PRL secretion (Pinilla et al. 2001b). Interestingly, however, RX is apparently not acting as an estrogen upon the organization of the neuronal system involved in the control of sexual receptivity in female rats, as it did not prevent successful mating with males of proven fertility. Moreover, RX carried out an antiestrogenic action in adult ovariectomized (OVX) estrogen-primed female rats, as it blocked the ability of estrogen to promote successful mating in OVX females (Pinilla et al. 2002b). Overall, our data on the central actions of RX strongly suggest a high degree of cell specificity within the hypothalamus for the estrogenic/antiestrogenic effects of RX. The physiological implications of this phenomenon for the complete elucidation of the mode of estrogen action in the developing HP unit remain to be analyzed.

## ER-Selective Ligands and Analysis of HP Unit Functions

As indicated in previous sections, the biological actions of estrogen are mostly conducted through interaction with the specific nuclear receptors ERα and ERβ, whose activity may be partially modulated by several ER variants. The existence of such heterogeneity in ER expression has been considered as a major contributing factor to the diversity of effects of estrogen in different target tissues. In fact, this phenomenon has been linked to the tissue specificity of the actions of endogenous estrogens as well as SERMs, although conclusive evidence on this point is still missing. However, the specific contribution of each of the two major ER subtypes in signaling the plethora of biological actions of estrogen is not yet fully elucidated. This problem has been recently approached by the use of knockout mouse models, where either the α or β form of ER is selectively eliminated throughout development. These models are tremendously instrumental but have some physiological limitations, related to potential developmental defects and activation of compensatory mechanisms in the absence of one receptor that partially hamper interpretation of results. As a complementary approach, novel ER isoform-selective ligands have been recently developed, thus allowing specific activation of one ER subtype in the physiological presence of the other subtype and ER variants (Harris et al. 2002; Frasor et al. 2003). This is especially relevant for the ER pathway, given the proposed role of several ER isoforms, including ERβ, as regulators of ERα signaling in target tissues.

Although several studies have attempted to identify ERα- and ERβ-selective ligands, the most conclusive work in the area has been conducted by the Katzenellenbogens' group at the University of Illinois (USA). Extensive structural and biological studies have allowed them to identify several ER ligands with interesting agonistic or antagonistic properties at the ER. Thus, pyrazole derivatives, such as propyl-pyrazole-triol (PPT), have been identified as selective ERα agonists, whereas diarylpropionitriles as DPN have been characterized as ERβ potency-selective agonists (Stauffer et al. 2000; Meyers et al. 2001). Moreover, additional compounds with combined agonistic/

antagonistic activities have been generated, such as R,R-tetrahydrochrysene (R,R-THC), which acts as an agonist at ERα but as an antagonist at ERβ (Harrington et al. 2003). These newly developed ER-selective ligands provide an optimal experimental approach for in vivo analysis of the respective roles of ERα and ERβ in signaling the biological actions of estrogen in different target tissues.

## Regulation of ER isoforms by ER-selective ligands in female rat pituitary

We have recently undertaken the analysis of the effects of ER-selective ligands in terms of regulation of several ER isoform expressions in female rat pituitary. Specifically, both PPT (as ERα agonist) and DPN (as ERβ ligand) were used initially. PPT displays a 400-fold higher affinity binding for ERα and it is virtually unable to activate ERβ (Stauffer et al. 2000 e). In contrast, DPN is a potency-selective agonist for ERβ, with a 70-fold higher binding affinity for ERβ and over a 170-fold higher biopotency in ERβ than in ERα (Meyers et al. 2001). In our setting, the ability of these compounds to modulate the expression of the transcripts encoding ERα and ERβ isoforms, as well as those for the truncated ERα product (TERP) and the variant ERβ2, in pituitaries from OVX rats was evaluated. Notably, as observed for estradiol, the selective ERα agonist PPT fully reversed the responses to OVX, whereas the ERβ ligand DPN failed to induce any significant effect except for a partial stimulation of TERP-1 and –2 mRNA expression levels. Furthermore, the ERβ-agonist was ineffective in altering pituitary expression of progesterone receptor-B mRNA, i.e., a major estrogen-responsive target (Tena-Sempere et al. 2003b; see Fig. 8). These data indicate that endogenous estrogen differentially regulates pituitary expression of the mRNAs encoding several ER isoforms with distinct functional properties, by a mechanism that is mostly conducted through ERα. Moreover, it is proposed that interaction of ERα protein with its own ligands not only activates signaling but also turns on different mechanisms for fine-tuning the pituitary responsiveness to estrogen. These mechanisms would include repression of inhibitory ERβ forms, which may be essential for the full expression of estrogen effects at the ERα, as well as induction of dominant negative isoforms, such as TERP-1, which may participate in the auto-limitation of estrogen effects. In addition, although activation of ERβ failed to modify its own expression levels, it did induce a significant stimulation of TERP-1 and TERP-2 mRNA levels. This may constitute an additional, novel mechanism whereby ERβ is able to repress ERα signaling activity in the pituitary (see Fig. 9). The molecular mechanisms for such regulatory cross-talk between ERα and ERβ isoforms remain to be elucidated.

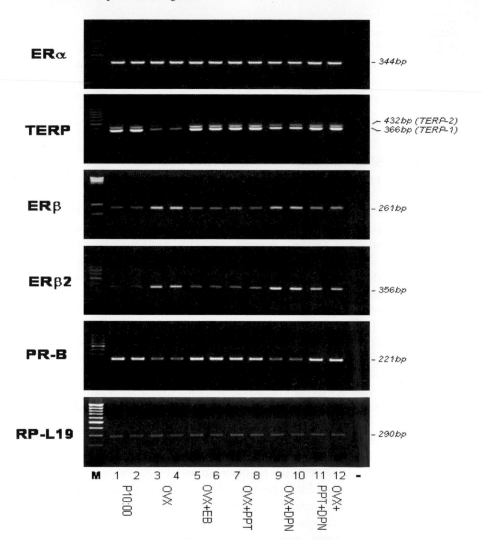

**Fig. 8.** Expression of ERα, TERP-1 and -2, ERβ, ERβ2, and PR-B mRNAs in pituitaries from two-week-old OVX rats treated with estradiol benzoate (EB), the ERα-selective ligand PPT, the potency-selective ERβ-agonist DPN, or combination of PPT+DPN. Pituitary mRNA levels of the targets in two-week-old OVX rats and control females on the morning of proestrus (P10:00) are also presented. Representative RT-PCR assays of the expression levels of ER-isoform and PR-B mRNAs in the different experimental groups are shown. In each gel, representative –RT negative controls (from OVX RNA samples) are presented (-). Parallel amplification of RP-L19 served as internal control. Assays from two independent RNA samples per experimental group are presented. Taken from Tena-Sempere et al. 2003b.

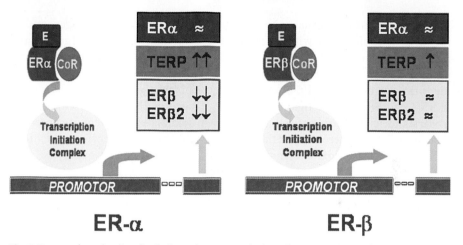

**Fig. 9.** Proposed mechanism for the homologous regulation of ER expression in the pituitary based on the use of ER-selective ligands. Estrogen differentially regulates mRNAs levels of several ER isoforms by a mechanism that is mostly conducted through ERα. These regulatory responses would include repression of inhibitory ERβ forms, as well as induction of dominant negative isoforms, such as TERP-1. In addition, although activation of ERβ failed to modify its own expression levels, it did induce a significant stimulation of TERP-1 and TERP-2 mRNA levels.

## Future Perspectives and Conclusions

As reviewed above, research on estrogen effects and mechanisms of action in different target tissues has attracted considerable attention over the last decades. Indeed, this area represents a good example of how basic and applied science can cooperate effectively, with mutual benefits. For instance, the emergence of major concerns about the possibly deleterious health effects of environmental xenoestrogens has allowed us to revisit some aspects of estrogen action during development and its implication in normal sex differentiation. Conversely, basic knowledge about the physiological role of estrogen in brain sex differentiation and reproductive tract maturation has paved the way for better prediction and/or understanding of the adverse effects of xenoestrogen in reproduction. Similarly, the development of SERMs has resulted not only in safer hormone replacement protocols but also in a significant advance towards the characterization of the mechanism(s) whereby estrogen conducts quite diverse biological effects in different target tissues. Additional extensive research efforts on the physiology and pathophysiology of estrogen actions are foreseen. In this sense, future perspectives in the area will certainly involve the exhaustive analysis of the biological effects of xenosteroids, with special attention to the characterization of low-dose and mixture effects, identification of novel mechanisms of action and endpoints, and risk assessment in terms of wildlife and human health. In addition, the generation and use of novel selective ER modulators and ligands will help to further delineate the complex mode of action of estrogen and to identify, in conjunction with different experimental approaches (genetically modified organisms with null mutations of ERα and ERβ, genomics and proteomics), isoform-specific ER responses. In this context, our studies on the identification of molecular markers and mechanisms of action of xenoestrogens, SERMs and ER-selective ligands upon the HP unit will help us to enlarge our understanding of the role of estrogen in brain sexual development, its potential disruption by xenosteroids, and the mode of action and therapeutic implications of SERMs, such as raloxifene, in the CNS.

## Acknowledgments

M.T.-S. is indebted to Dr. Henrik Leffers and Dr. Niels E. Skakkebaek (Department of Growth and Reproduction, Rigshospitalet, Copenhagen, Denmark) for providing data from differential display analyses and for helpful collaboration at different stages of the EDEN project. In addition, the friendly collaboration of Dr. Jose E. Sanchez-Criado (Physiology Section, University of Cordoba) in studies involving ER-selective ligands is cordially appreciated. The authors acknowledge also the contribution of Dr. Leonor Pinilla and other members of our research group at the University of Cordoba, for outstanding assistance in conducting the experimental studies. This work was supported by grants BFI 2000-0419-CO3-03 and BFI 2002-00176 from DGESIC (Ministerio de Ciencia y Tecnología, Spain), and European Union Research Contract EDEN QLK4-CT-2002-00603.

## References

Avioli LV (1999) SERM drugs for the prevention of osteoporosis. Trends Endocrinol Metab 10:317-319.

Boisen KA, Main KM, Rajpert-De Meyts E, Skakkebaek NE (2001) Are male reproductive disorders a common entity? The testicular dysgenesis syndrome. Ann NY Acad Sci 948: 90-99.

Clark JH, Mani SK (1994) Actions of ovarian steroids. In: Knobil E, Neill JD (eds) The physiology of reproduction. Raven Press, New York, pp 1011-1062.Döhler KD, Hancke JL (1978) Thoughts on the mechanisms of sexual brain differentiation. In: Dorner G, Kawakami M (eds) Hormones and brain development. Elsevier, Amsterdam, pp 153-158.

Frasor J, Barnett DH, Danes JM, Hess R, Parlow AF, Katzenellengogen BS (2003) Response-specific and ligand dose-dependent modulation of estrogen receptor (ER) α activity by ERβ in the uterus. Endocrinology 144:3159-3166

Harrington WR, Sheng S, Barnett DH, Petz LN, Katzenellenbogen JA, Katzenellenbogen BS (2003) Activities of estrogen receptor alpha- and beta-selective ligands at diverse estrogen responsive gene sites mediating transactivation or transrepression. Mol Cell Endocrinol 206:13-22.

Harris HA, Katzenellenbogen JA, Katzenellenbogen BS (2002) Characterization of the biological roles of estrogen receptors, ERα and ERβ, in estrogen target tissues in vivo through the use of an ERα-selective ligand. Endocrinology 143:4172-4177.

Jordan VC, Morrow M (1999) Tamoxifen, raloxifene and the prevention of breast cancer. Endocrinol Rev 20:253-278.

Kuiper GGJM, Shughrue PJ, Merchenthaler I, Gustafsson J-A (1998) The estrogen receptor β subtype: A novel mediator of estrogen actions in neuroendocrine systems. Frontiers Neuroendocrinol 19:253-286.

MacLusky NJ, Naftolin F (1981) Sexual differentiation of the central nervous system. Science 211:1294-1302.

McDonnell DP (1999) The molecular pharmacology of SERMs. Trends Endocrinol Metab 10: 301-311.

Meyers MJ, Sun J, Carlson KE, Marriner GA, Katzenellenbogen BS, Katzenellenbogen JA (2001) Estrogen receptor-β potency-selective ligands: structure-activity relationship studies of diarylpropionitriles and their acetylene and polar analogues. J Med Chem 44: 4230-4251.

Österlund M, Kuiper GGJM, Gustafsson J-A, Hurd YL (1998) Differential distribution of estrogen receptor-α and -β mRNA within the female rat brain. Brain Res Mol Brain Res 54:175-180.

Paech K, Webb P, Kuiper GGJM, Nilsson S, Gustafsson J-A, Kushner PJ, Scanlan TS (1997) Differential ligand activation of estrogen receptors ERα and ERβ at AP1 sites. Science 277:1508-1510.

Pinilla L, Gonzalez LC, Gaytan F, Tena-Sempere M, Aguilar E (2001a) Oestrogenic effects of neonatal administration of raloxifene on hypothalamic-pituitary-gonadal axis in male and female rats. Reproduction 121:915-924.

Pinilla L, Gonzalez LC, Tena-Sempere M, Aguilar E (2001b) Evidence for an estrogen-like action of raloxifene upon the hypothalamic-pituitary unit: raloxifene inhibits luteinizing hormone secretion and stimulates prolactin secretion in ovariectomized female rats. Neurosci Lett 311:149-152.

Pinilla L, Barreiro ML, Gonzalez LC, Tena-Sempere M, Aguilar E (2002a) Comparative effects of testosterone propionate, oestradiol benzoate, ICI 182,780, tamoxifen and raloxifene on hypothalamic differentiation in the female rat. J Endocrinol 172:441-448.

Pinilla L, Barreiro ML, Tena-Sempere M, Aguilar E (2002b) Raloxifene effects upon the neuronal system controlling sexual receptivity in female rats. Neurosci Lett 329:285-288.

Quadros PS, Pfau JL, Goldstein AY, De Vries GJ, Wagner CK (2002) Sex differences in progesterone receptor expression: a potential mechanism for estradiol-mediated sexual differentiation. Endocrinology 14310:3727-3739.

Rajapakse N, Silva E, Kortenkamp A (2002) Combining xenoestrogens at levels below individual no-observed-effect concentrations dramatically enhances steroid hormone action Environ Health Perspect 110:917-921.

Reibel S, Andre V, Chassagnon S, Andre G, Marescaux C, Nehlig A, Depaulis A (2000) Neuroprotective effects of chronic estradiol benzoate treatment on hippocampal cell loss induced by status epilepticus in the female rat. Neurosci Lett 281:79-82.

Schneider LS, Finch CE (1997) Can estrogens prevent neurodegeneration. Drugs Aging 11: 87-95.

Schreihofer DA, Stoler MH, Shupnik MA (2000) Differential expression and regulation of estrogen receptors (ERs) in rat pituitary and cell lines: Estrogen decreases ERa protein and estrogen responsiveness. Endocrinology 141:2174-2184.

Sharpe RM (1998) The roles of oestrogen in the male. Trends Endocrinol Metab 9:371-377.

Shupnik MA (2002) Oestrogen receptors, receptor variants and oestrogen actions in the hypothalamic-pituitary axis. J Neuroendocrinol 14:85-94.

Silva E, Rajapakse N, Kortenkamp A (2002) Something from "nothing": eight weak estrogenic chemicals combined at concentrations below NOECs produce significant mixture effects. Environ Sci Technol 36:1751-1756.

Somjen D, Waisman A, Kaye AM (1996) Tissue selective action of tamoxifen methiodide, raloxifene and tamoxifen on creatine kinase B activity in vitro and in vivo. J Steroid Biochem Mol Biol 59:389-396

Stauffer SR, Coletta CJ, Tedesco R, Nishiguchi G, Carlson K, Sun J, Katzenellenbogen BS, Katzenellenbogen JA (2000) Pyrazole ligands: structure-affinity/activity relationships and estrogen receptor-a-selective agonists. J Med Chem 43:4934-4947.

Tena-Sempere M, Navarro J, Pinilla L, Gonzalez LC, Huhtaniemi I, Aguilar E (2000a) Neonatal exposure to estrogen differentially alters estrogen receptor α and β messenger ribonucleic acid expression in rat testis during postnatal development. J Endocrinol 165:345-357.

Tena-Sempere M, Pinilla L, Gonzalez LC, Aguilar E (2000b) Reproductive disruption by exposure to exogenous estrogenic compounds during sex differentiation: lessons from the neonatally estrogenized male rat. Curr Topics Steroid Res 3:23-37.

Tena-Sempere M, Gonzalez LC, Pinilla L, Huhtaniemi I, Aguilar E (2001a) Neonatal imprinting and regulation of estrogen receptor alpha and beta mRNA expression by estrogen in the pituitary and hypothalamus of the male rat. Neuroendocrinology 73:12-25.

Tena-Sempere M, Barreiro ML, Gonzalez LC, Pinilla L, Aguilar E (2001b) Differential neonatal imprinting and regulation by estrogen of estrogen receptor subtypes α and β and of the truncated estrogen receptor product (TERP-1) mRNA eexpression in the male rat pituitary. Neuroendocrinology 74:347-358.

Tena-Sempere M, Barreiro ML, Aguilar E, Pinilla L (2003a) Mechanisms for altered reproductive function in female rats following neonatal administration of raloxifene. Eur J Endocrinol, 150:397-403.

Tena-Sempere M, Navarro VM, Mayen A, Bellido C, Sanchez-Criado JE (2003b) Regulation of estrogen receptor (ER) isoform messenger RNA expression by different ER ligands in female rat pituitary. Biol Reprod 2004; 70:671-678.

White R, Parker MG (1998) Molecular mechanisms of steroid hormone action. Endocr Relat Cancer 5:1-14.

# Regulation of Neurosteroid Biosynthesis by Neurotransmitters and Neuropeptides

H. Vaudry[1], J.L. Do Rego[1], D. Beaujean-Burel[1], J. Leprince[1], L. Galus[1],
D. Larhammar[2], R. Fredriksson[2], V. Luu-The[3], G. Pelletier[3],
M.C. Tonon[1], and C. Delarue[1]

## Summary

It is now established that the brain has the capability of synthesizing biologically
active steroids, termed neurosteroids, that participate in the regulation of
various neurophysiological and behavioral processes. However, the neuronal
mechanisms regulating the activity of neurosteroid-producing cells have not
yet been elucidated. We recently found that, in the frog brain, three enzymes
involved in steroid biosynthesis are actively expressed in hypothalamic neurons:
3β-hydroxysteroid dehydrogenase/$\Delta^5$-$\Delta^4$ isomerase (3β-HSD), cytochrome P450
17α-hydroxylase/C17,20-lyase (P450$_{C17}$) and hydroxysteroid sulfotransferase
(HST). Concurrently, we showed that frog hypothalamic explants can convert
tritiated pregnenolone ([$^3$H]$\Delta^5$P) into various bioactive steroids, including 17-
hydroxypregnenolone (17OH-$\Delta^5$P), progesterone (P), 17-hydroxyprogesterone
(17OH-P), dehydroepiandrosterone (DHEA), $\Delta^5$P sulfate ($\Delta^5$PS) and DHEA
sulfate (DHEAS). The hypothalamic nuclei, where the 3β-HSD-, P450$_{C17}$- and
HST-expressing neurons are located, receive afferent fibers containing a variety
of neurotransmitters and neuropeptides. Here, we show that GABA, endozepines
and neuropeptide Y (NPY) regulate neurosteroid biosynthesis.

Double immunohistochemical labeling of hypothalamic slices with antisera
against 3β-HSD and various subunits of the GABA$_A$ receptor revealed that most
3β-HSD-positive neurons also express the α3 and β2/β3 subunits of the GABA$_A$
receptor. Incubation of hypothalamic explants with graded concentrations of
GABA induced a dose-dependent inhibition of the conversion of [$^3$H]$\Delta^5$P into
radioactive metabolites. The effect of GABA on neurosteroid biosynthesis was
mimicked by the GABA$_A$ receptor agonist muscimol and was blocked by the
selective GABA$_A$ receptor antagonists bicuculline and SR95531. The GABA$_A$

[1] European Institute for Peptide Research, Laboratory of Cellular and Molecular
Neuroendocrinology, INSERM U413, UA CNRS, University of Rouen, 76821 Mont-
Saint-Aignan, France
[2] Department of Neuroscience, Unit of Pharmacology, Uppsala University, 75124
Uppsala, Sweden
[3] Laboratory of Molecular Endocrinology and Oncology, Laval University Medical
Center, Québec, Canada G1V 4G2.

Kordon et al.
Hormones and the Brain
© Springer-Verlag Berlin Heidelberg 2005

receptor complex encompasses a central-type benzodiazepine receptor (CBR). Thus, we investigated the effect of the endozepine octadecaneuropeptide (ODN), an endogenous ligand of CBR, on neurosteroid biosynthesis. Using an antiserum against human ODN, we observed that ODN-positive glial cells send thick processes in the close vicinity of 3β-HSD-containing neurons. Incubation of hypothalamic explants with synthetic ODN induced a dose-dependent stimulation of the conversion of $[^3H]\Delta^5P$ into various neurosteroids. The β-carbolines β-CCM and DMCM, two inverse agonists of CBR, mimicked the stimulatory effect of ODN on neurosteroid biosynthesis, whereas the CBR antagonist flumazenil significantly reduced the stimulatory responses induced by ODN, β-CCM and DMCM. These data indicate that GABA, acting through $GABA_A$ receptors, inhibits 3β-HSD activity and that ODN, acting as an inverse agonist on the $GABA_A$/CBR complex, stimulates neurosteroid biosynthesis.

Labeling of brain sections revealed the existence of NPY-immunoreactive varicosities in close proximity to HST-containing perikarya. In situ hybridization studies showed that $Y_1$ and $Y_5$ receptor mRNAs are expressed in the anterior preoptic area and the dorsal magnocellular nucleus. Pulse-chase experiments with $^{35}S$-labeled 3'-phosphoadenosine 5'-phosphosulfate as a sulfate donor, and $[^3H]\Delta^5P$ or $[^3H]DHEA$ as a steroid precursor, demonstrated that NPY inhibits the conversion of $\Delta^5P$ into $\Delta^5PS$ and DHEA into DHEAS by hypothalamic explants. The inhibitory effect of NPY on the formation of sulfated neurosteroids was mimicked by PYY, a non-selective NPY receptor agonist, and by $[Leu^{31},Pro^{34}]NPY$, an agonist for non-$Y_2$ receptors, and was completely suppressed by the $Y_1$ receptor antagonist BIBP3226. Conversely, the $Y_2$ receptor agonist NPY(13-36) and the $Y_5$ receptor agonist $[D-Trp^{32}]NPY$ did not affect the biosynthesis of $\Delta^5PS$ and DHEAS. These data indicate that NPY, acting through $Y_1$ receptors, exerts an inhibitory influence on the biosynthesis of sulfated neurosteroids. The present study provides evidence that, in the brain, neurotransmitters and neuropeptides regulate the activity of neurosteroid-producing neurons. Since neurosteroids have been implicated in the control of a number of behavioral and metabolic activities, these data strongly suggest that some of the neurophysiological effects of neurotransmitters and neuropeptides can be mediated through modulation of neurosteroid biosynthesis.

## Introduction

Biologically active steroids play an essential role in the development, growth and differentiation of the central nervous system (for review, see McEwen 1994). Owing to their lipophilic nature, steroid hormones secreted by the adrenal gland, testis, ovary and placenta can easily cross the blood-brain barrier. Thus, it has long been assumed that steroids acting on nerve cells in the brain were exclusively produced by endocrine glands. However, pioneering studies conducted by Baulieu and Robel showed that the concentrations of pregnenolone ($\Delta^5$P) and dehydroepiandrosterone (DHEA) in the central nervous system (CNS) remained elevated long after adrenalectomy and gonadectomy (Corpéchot et al. 1981, 1983) and that the circadian variations of the levels of these steroids in brain tissue are not synchronized with those of circulating steroids (Robel et al. 1986), suggesting that the brain may be a source of biologically active steroids. Subsequently, immunohistochemical localization of cytochrome P450 side-chain cleavage (P450scc) in the rat brain and the observation that this brain enzyme was capable of converting cholesterol into $\Delta^5$P (Le Goascogne et al. 1987) confirmed that the brain was a steroidogenic organ. The presence of most of the enzymes involved in the biosynthetic pathways of steroids has now been demonstrated, either in neurons or in glial cells, by immunohistochemical or in situ hybridization approaches. These include: P450scc, a desmolase that cleaves the $C_{20}$-$C_{22}$ bond of cholesterol; 3β-hydroxysteroid dehydrogenase/$\Delta^5$-$\Delta^4$ isomerase (3β-HSD), which catalyzes the formation of $\Delta^4$-3-ketosteroids; cytochrome P450 17α-hydroxylase/C17,20-lyase (P450$_{C17}$), which catalyzes the production of $\Delta^5$-3β-hydroxysteroids; 17β-hydroxysteroid dehydrogenase (17β-HSD), which catalyzes the interconversion of 17-ketosteroids (androstenedione, estrone) and 17β-hydroxysteroids (testosterone, 17β-estradiol); 5α-reductase, which causes the reduction of the $C_4$-$C_5$ double bond to produce 5α-reduced metabolites including dihydrotestosterone (5α-DHT) and dihydroprogesterone (5α-DHP); cytochrome P450aromatase, which converts androgens into estrogens; hydroxysteroid sulfotransferase (HST), which is responsible for the synthesis of sulfated steroids such as $\Delta^5$P sulfate ($\Delta^5$PS) and DHEA sulfate (DHEAS); and sulfatase, which hydrolyzes sulfated steroids to produce unconjugated steroids (Mensah-Nyagan et al. 1999; Mellon and Vaudry 2001). The term neurosteroids has been coined to designate all biologically active steroids synthesized from cholesterol or other, early precursors in the CNS (Robel and Baulieu 1994).

There is now clear evidence that neurosteroids are involved in the regulation of various neurophysiological and behavioral processes, including cognition, stress, anxiety, sleep, and sexual and feeding behaviors (Majewska 1992; Robel and Baulieu 1994). However, the neuronal mechanisms regulating the activity of neurosteroid-producing cells remain poorly understood. We recently found that, in the frog brain, three enzymes involved in the synthesis of neuroactive steroids - 3β-HSD, P450$_{C17}$, and HST - are intensely expressed in hypothalamic neurons, and we showed that frog hypothalamic explants can very actively convert tritiated $\Delta^5$P ($[^3H]\Delta^5$P) into various bioactive steroids, including 17-hydroxypregnenolone (17OH-$\Delta^5$P), progesterone (P), 17-hydroxyprogesterone (17OH-P), DHEA, $\Delta^5$PS and DHEAS. The hypothalamic nuclei where 3β-HSD-, P450$_{C17}$- and HST-expressing neurons are located receive afferent fibers containing a variety of neurotransmitters and neuropeptides. The frog hypothalamus is thus a very suitable model in which to investigate the neuronal control of neurosteroid biosynthesis.

## Regulation of neurosteroid synthesis by GABA

In the frog brain, the neurons expressing 3β-HSD and/or P450$_{C17}$ are exclusively located in the anterior preoptic area and in a few hypothalamic nuclei, including the suprachiasmatic nucleus, the ventral part of the magnocellular preoptic nucleus, the posterior tuberculum, the nucleus of the periventricular organ, the dorsal hypothalamic nucleus and the ventral hypothalamic nucleus (Mensah-Nyagan et al. 1994). Since these diencephalic nuclei are richly innervated by GABAergic fibers (Franzoni and Morino 1989), we investigated the possible effect of GABA in the control of neurosteroid biosynthesis. Double immunohistochemical labeling of hypothalamic slices with antisera against 3β-HSD and various subunits of the GABA$_A$ receptor revealed that many 3β-HSD-positive neurons also express the α3 and the β2/β3 subunits of the GABA$_A$ receptor (Do Rego et al. 2000). Incubation of hypothalamic explants with graded concentrations of GABA induced a dose-dependent inhibition of the conversion of [$^3$H]Δ$^5$P into radioactive metabolites, e.g., 17OH-Δ$^5$P, P, 17OH-P and DHEA (Do Rego et al. 2000). The inhibitory effect of GABA on neurosteroid biosynthesis was mimicked by the GABA$_A$ receptor agonist muscimol and was

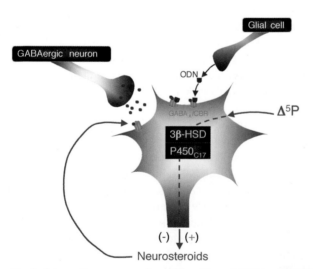

**Fig. 1.** Schematic representation of the effect of GABA and ODN on neurosteroid biosynthesis. GABA, acting through GABA$_A$ receptors, inhibits the biosynthesis of 17-hydroxypregnenolone, progesterone, 17-hydroxyprogesterone and dehydroepiandrosterone. Concurrently, the endozepine octadecaneuropeptide (ODN), released by glial cell processes ending in the vicinity of 3β-hydroxysteroid dehydrogenase (3β-HSD)- /cytochrome P450$_{C17}$ (P450$_{C17}$)-immunoreactive neurons, stimulates the biosynthesis of neurosteroids by acting as an inverse agonist on central-type benzodiazepine receptors (CBR) that are associated with the GABA$_A$ receptor complex. Neurosteroids, released by these neurons, may in turn modulate allosterically the activity of the GABA$_A$ receptor and thus control their own biosynthesis. Δ$^5$P, pregnenolone.

blocked by the selective $GABA_A$ receptor antagonists bicuculline and SR95531. In contrast, the $GABA_B$ receptor agonist baclofen did not affect neurosteroid synthesis. Interestingly, bicuculline and SR95531, when administered alone, induced a significant increase in steroid biosynthesis, suggesting that neurosteroid-producing neurons are under the inhibitory control of endogenous GABA (Do Rego et al. 2000). Since neurosteroids are potent allosteric regulators of $GABA_A$ receptor function (Covey et al. 2001), these data suggest the existence of an ultrashort regulatory feedback loop by which neurosteroids may regulate their own production through modulation of $GABA_A$ receptor activity (Fig. 1).

## Regulation of neurosteroid synthesis by endozepines

The activity of the $GABA_A$ receptor can be allosterically regulated by various compounds, including neuroactive steroids, barbiturates, ethanol, zinc and benzodiazepines (Hevers and Luddens 1998). The existence of specific binding sites for benzodiazepines in the brain has led to the characterization of endogenous ligands for benzodiazepine receptors, a family of molecules termed endozepines. All endozepines identified so far derive from an 86-amino acid polypeptide called diazepam-binding inhibitor (DBI; Guidotti et al. 1983). Proteolytic cleavage of DBI has the potential to generate several biologically active fragments, including the triakontatetraneuropeptide (TTN) and the octadecaneuropeptide (ODN; Fig. 2). While ODN is a preferential ligand for the central-type benzodiazepine receptor (CBR) that belongs to the $GABA_A$ receptor complex (Ferrero et al. 1986), TTN is a specific ligand for the peripheral-type benzodiazepine receptor (Slobodyansky et al. 1989).

Immunohistochemical labeling of consecutive frog brain slices with antibodies against $3\beta$-HSD and human ODN (Duparc et al. 2003) revealed that ODN-positive periventricular glial cells send thick immunoreactive processes in the close vicinity of $3\beta$-HSD-containing neurons in various hypothalamic nuclei (Do Rego et al 2001). Incubation of hypothalamic explants with synthetic rat or human ODN stimulated, in a dose-dependent manner, the conversion of $[^3H]\Delta^5P$ into various neurosteroids. The $\beta$-carbolines $\beta$-CCM and DMCM, two inverse agonists of CBRs, mimicked the effect of ODN on neurosteroid biosynthesis, whereas flumazenil, a CBR antagonist, significantly reduced the stimulatory response induced by ODN, $\beta$-CCM and DMCM. In fact, flumazenil induced a significant reduction of neurosteroid production on its own, indicating that endogenous ODN exerts a stimulatory influence on steroidogenic neurons (Do Rego et al. 2001). In addition, the ODN-evoked stimulation of steroid synthesis was markedly attenuated by GABA. These data indicate that the inhibitory effect of GABA on neurosteroid biosynthesis can be modulated by ODN, acting as an inverse agonist on the $GABA_A$/central-type benzodiazepine receptor complex (Fig. 1).

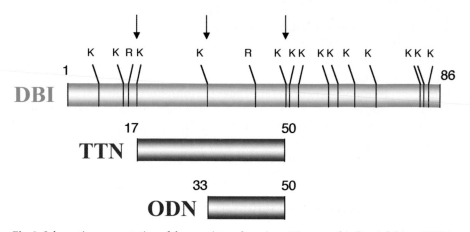

**Fig. 2.** Schematic representation of three major endozepines. Diazepam-binding inhibitor (DBI) is an 86-amino acid polypeptide that encompasses a high proportion of basic residues, i.e., Lys (K) or Arg (R). Proteolytic cleavage of DBI at some of these basic amino acids (arrows) can generate several processing products, including the triakontatetraneuropeptide (TTN; $DBI_{17-50}$) and the octadecaneuropeptide (ODN; $DBI_{33-50}$). DBI and ODN act as preferential ligands for central-type benzodiazepine receptors (CBRs) that are part of the $GABA_A$ receptor complex, whereas TTN is a specific ligand for peripheral-type benzodiazepine receptors that are primarily located at the outer surface of mitochondria.

The occurrence of peripheral-type benzodiazepine receptors in the frog diencephalon and telencephalon has been demonstrated by immunohistochemistry using antibodies against the 18-kDa subunit of peripheral-type benzodiazepine receptors (Do Rego et al. 1998). Double labeling of brain slices with antisera against 3β-HSD and the 18-kDa subunit of peripheral-type benzodiazepine receptors revealed that most hypothalamic neurons expressing 3β-HSD also contained peripheral-type benzodiazepine receptor-like immunoreactivity. Exposure of hypothalamic explants to TTN induced a dose-related increase in the production of 17OH-$\Delta^5$P, 17OH-P and a novel neurosteroid that has not yet been identified (Do Rego et al. 1998). The stimulatory effect of TTN on the formation of neurosteroids was mimicked by the peripheral-type benzodiazepine receptor agonist Ro5-4864 and was markedly reduced by the peripheral-type benzodiazepine receptor antagonist PK11195. In contrast, the CBR antagonist flumazenil did not affect the activation of neurosteroid biosynthesis induced by TTN (Do Rego et al. 1998). These data indicate that TTN, acting via peripheral-type benzodiazepine receptors, stimulates the activity of several key steroidogenic enzymes, including 3β-HSD and P450$_{C17}$.

## Regulation of neurosteroid synthesis by neuropeptide Y

In the frog brain, HST-positive neurons are located in the anterior preoptic area and the dorsal magnocellular nucleus (Bcaujean et al. 1999), two diencephalic nuclei that are richly innervated by neuropeptide Y (NPY)-containing fibers (Danger et al. 1985; Caillez et al. 1987; Lázár et al. 1993). Concurrently, there is evidence that sulfated neurosteroids and NPY are involved in the regulation of similar behavioral activities. For instance, $\Delta^5$PS and DHEAS, like NPY, are implicated in the control of food intake in rodents (Reddy and Kulkarni 1998; Schwartz et al. 2000). Similarly, $\Delta^5$PS and NPY are known to regulate reproductive behavior (Wehrenberg et al. 1989; Kavaliers and Kinsella 1995). These observations prompted us to investigate the possible effects of NPY on the biosynthesis of sulfated neurosteroids.

Double labeling of frog brain sections revealed the existence of NPY-immunoreactive varicosities in close proximity to HST-containing perikarya (Beaujean et al. 2002). Partial sequences of frog (Rana esculenta) $Y_1$, $Y_2$, $Y_5$ and $y_6$ receptor cDNAs have been cloned, and riboprobes have been used to localize the NPY receptor mRNAs in the frog brain. Expression of $Y_1$ and $Y_5$ receptor mRNAs was visualized in the anterior preoptic area and the dorsal magnocellular nucleus, i.e., in the two diencephalic nuclei where HST-immunoreactive neurons are located. Neither $Y_2$ nor $y_6$ receptor transcripts were found in the frog diencephalon, suggesting that NPY might regulate the activity of HST neurons through activation of $Y_1$ and/or $Y_5$ receptors (Beaujean et al. 2002).

The effect of NPY on the biosynthesis of sulfated steroids has been studied by means of a pulse-chase technique using either $[^3H]\Delta^5P$ or $[^3H]DHEA$ as a steroid precursor and $^{35}S$-labeled 3'-phosphoadenosine 5'-phosphosulfate as a sulfate donor. Incubation of diencephalic explants with graded concentrations of frog NPY (Chartrel et al. 1991) induced a dose-dependent inhibiton of $[^3H]\Delta^5PS$ and $[^3H]DHEAS$ formation (Beaujean et al. 2002). The inhibitory effect of NPY on the biosynthesis of sulfated neurosteroids was mimicked by peptide YY (PYY), a nonselective NPY receptor agonist, and by $[Leu^{31},Pro^{34}]NPY$, an agonist for non-$Y_2$ receptors. In contrast, the N-terminally truncated NPY analogue NPY(13-36), a selective $Y_2$ receptor agonist, and $[D-Trp^{32}]NPY$, a specific $Y_5$ receptor agonist, did not significantly affect the production of $\Delta^5PS$ and DHEAS. Moreover, compound BIBP3226, a selective $Y_1$ receptor antagonist, abolished the effect of NPY on neurosteroid formation. These observations indicate that NPY-induced inhibition of $\Delta^5PS$ and DHEAS production is mediated through the $Y_1$ receptor subtype. The fact that the $Y_1$ receptor gene is actively expressed in the anterior preoptic area and dorsal magnocellular nuclei, which contain HST-immunoreactive cell bodies (Beaujean et al. 1999), provides additional support for the involvement of $Y_1$ receptors in the inhibitory effect of NPY on HST activity in the diencephalon. Concurrently, we observed that the $Y_1$ receptor antagonist BIBP3226 alone provoked a modest increase in the biosynthesis of

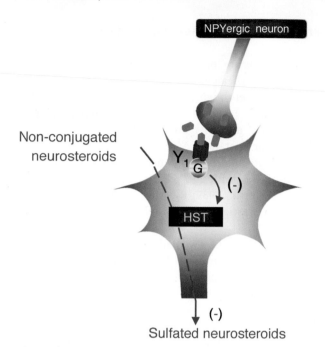

**Fig. 3.** Schematic representation of the effect of neuropeptide Y (NPY) on neurosteroid biosynthesis. NPY-producing neurons send fibers in the vicinity of hydroxysteroid sulfotransferase (HST)-immunoreactive neurons located in the anterior preoptic area and the dorsal magnocellular nucleus. NPY, acting through $Y_1$ receptors negatively coupled to adenylyl cyclase, inhibits the biosynthesis of pregnenolone sulfate and dehydroepiandrosterone sulfate.

$\Delta^5$PS and DHEAS, suggesting that endogenous NPY may actually exert a tonic inhibitory action on sulfated neurosteroid biosynthesis (Beaujean et al. 2002), (Fig. 3).

## Conclusion

The present report provides evidence that, in the brain, various neurotransmitters and neuropeptides regulate the activity of neurosteroid-producing neurons (Fig. 4). Since neurosteroids have been implicated in the control of a number of behavioral and metabolic activities, such as response to novelty, food consumption, sexual activity, aggressiveness, anxiety, depression, body temperature and blood pressure, these data strongly suggest that some of the neurophysiological effects of GABA, endozepines and NPY (and possibly those of many other neurotransmitters and neuropeptides) can be mediated through modulation of neurosteroid biosynthesis.

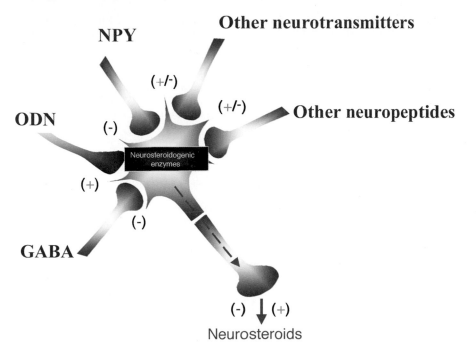

**Fig. 4.** Schematic representation of the control of neurosteroid-producing neurons by neurotransmitters and neuropeptides. Fibers containing various stimulatory or inhibitory factors innervate neurosteroid-producing neurons. Several of these factors have been shown to modulate the biosynthesis of neurosteroids. It is thus conceivable that some of the neurophysiological effects of neurotransmitters and neuropeptides can be mediated through modulation of neurosteroid biosynthesis. GABA, γ-amino-butyric acid; NPY, neuropeptide Y; ODN, octadecaneuropeptide.

## Acknowledgments

This work was supported by grants from INSERM (U413), a FRSQ-INSERM exchange program (to G.P. and H.V.), and the Conseil Régional de Haute-Normandie.

## References

Beaujean D, Mensah-Nyagan AG, Do Rego JL, Luu-The V, Pelletier G, Vaudry H (1999) Immunocytochemical localization and biological activity of hydroxysteroid sulfotransferase in the frog brain. J Neurochem 72: 848-857

Beaujean D, Do Rego JL, Galas L, Mensah-Nyagan AG, Fredriksson R, Larhammar D, Fournier A, Luu-The V, Pelletier G, Vaudry H (2002) Neuropeptide Y inhibits the biosynthesis of sulfated neurosteroids in the hypothalamus through activation of $Y_1$ receptors. Endocrinology 143: 1950-1963

Cailliez D, Danger JM, Andersen AC, Polak JM, Pelletier G, Kawamura K, Kikuyama S, Vaudry H (1987) Neuropeptide Y (NPY)-like immunoreactive neurons in the brain and pituitary of the amphibian *Rana catesbeiana*. Zool Sci 4: 123-134

Chartrel N, Conlon JM, Danger JM, Fournier A, Tonon MC, Vaudry H (1991) Characterization of melanotropin release-inhibiting factor (melanostatin) from frog brain: homology with human neuropeptide Y. Proc Natl Acad Sci USA 88: 3862-33866

Corpéchot C, Robel P, Axelsön M, Sjövall J, Baulieu EE (1981) Characterization and measurement of dehydroepiandrosterone sulfate in the rat brain. Proc Natl Acad Sci USA 78: 4704-4707

Corpéchot C, Synguelakis M, Talha S, Axelson M, Sjovall J, Vihko R, Baulieu EE, Robel P (1983) Pregnenolone and its sulfate ester in the rat brain. Brain Res 270:119-125

Covey DF, Evers AS, Mennerick S, Zorumski CF, Purdy RH (2001) Recent development in structure-activity relationships for steroid modulators of GABA$_A$ receptors. Brain Res Rev 37: 91-97

Danger JM, Guy J, Benyamina M, Jégou S, Leboulenger F, Coté J, Tonon MC, Pelletier G, Vaudry H (1985) Localization and identification of neuropeptide Y (NPY)-like immunoreactivity in the frog brain. Peptides 6: 1225-1236

Do Rego JL, Mensah-Nyagan AG, Feuilloley M, Ferrara P, Pelletier G, Vaudry H (1998) The endozepine triakontatetraneuropeptide diazepam-binding inhibitor [17-50] stimulates neurosteroid biosynthesis in the frog hypothalamus. Neuroscience 83: 555-570

Do Rego JL, Mensah-Nyagan AG, Beaujean D, Vaudry D, Sieghart W, Luu-The V, Pelletier G, Vaudry H (2000) γ-Aminobutyric acid, acting through γ-aminobutyric acid type A receptors, inhibits the biosynthesis of neurosteroids in the frog hypothalamus. Proc Natl Acad Sci USA 97: 13925-13930

Do Rego JL, Mensah-Nyagan AG, Beaujean D, Leprince J, Tonon MC, Luu-The V, Pelletier G, Vaudry H (2001) The octadecaneuropeptide ODN stimulates neurosteroid biosynthesis through activation of central-type benzodiazepine receptors. J Neurochem 76: 128-138

Duparc C, Lefebvre H, Tonon MC, Vaudry H, Kuhn JM (2003) Characterization of endozepines in the human testicular tissue: effect of triakontatetraneuropeptide on testosterone secretion. J Clin Endocrinol Metab 88: 5521-5528

Ferrero P, Santi MR, Conti-Tronconi B, Costa E, Guidotti A (1986) Study of an octadecaneuropeptide derived from diazepam binding inhibitor (DBI): biological activity and presence in rat brain. Proc Natl Acad Sci USA 83: 827-831

Franzoni MF, Morino P (1989) The distribution of GABA-like-immunoreactive neurons in the brain of the newt, *Triturus cristatus carnifex*, and the green frog *Rana esculenta*. Cell Tissue Res 255: 155-166

Guidotti A, Forchetti CM, Corda MG, Konkel D, Bennett CD, Costa E (1983) Isolation, characterization, and purification to homogeneity of an endogenous polypeptide with agonistic action on benzodiazepine receptors. Proc Natl Acad Sci USA 80: 3531-3535

Hevers W, Luddens H (1998) The diversity of GABA$_A$ receptors. Pharmacological and electrophysiological properties of GABA$_A$ channel subtypes. Mol Neurobiol 18: 35-86

Kavaliers M, Kinsella DM (1995) Male preference for the odors of estrous female mice is reduced by the neurosteroid pregnenolone sulfate. Brain Res 682: 222-226

Lázár G, Maderdrut JL, Trasti SL, Liposits Z, Toth P, Kovicz T, Merchenthaler I (1993) Distribution of proneuropeptide Y-derivated peptides in the brain of *Rana esculenta* and *Xenopus laevis*. J Comp Neurol 327: 551-571

Le Goascogne C, Robel P, Gouézou M, Sananès N, Baulieu EE, Waterman M (1987) Neurosteroids: cytochrome P450scc in rat brain. Science 237: 1212-1215

Majewska MD (1992) Neurosteroids: endogenous bimodal modulators of the GABAA receptor. Mechanism of action and physiological significance. Prog Neurobiol 38: 379-385

McEwen BS (1994) Endocrine effects on the brain and their relationship to behavior. In: Siegel GJ, Agranoff BW, Albers RW, Molinoff B (eds) Basic neurochemistry. Raven Press, New York, pp 1003-1023

Mellon S, Vaudry H (2001) Biosynthesis of neurosteroids and regulation of their synthesis. Int Rev Neurobiol 46: 33-78

Mensah-Nyagan AG, Feuilloley M, Dupont E, Do Rego JL, Leboulenger F, Pelletier G, Vaudry H (1994) Immunocytochemical localization and biological activity of 3β-hydroxysteroid dehydrogenase in the central nervous system of the frog. J Neurosci 14: 7306-7318

Mensah-Nyagan AG, Do-Rego JL, Beaujean D, Luu-The V, Pelletier G, Vaudry H (1999) Neurosteroid: expression of steroidogenic enzymes and regulation of steroid biosynthesis in the central nervous system. Pharmacol Rev 51: 63-82

Reddy DS, Kulkarni SK (1998) The role of the GABA-A and mitochondrial diazepam-binding inhibitor receptors on the effects of neurosteroids on food intake in mice. Psychopharmacology 137: 391-400

Robel P, Baulieu EE (1994) Neurosteroids. Biosynthesis and function. Trends Endocrinol Metab 5: 1-8

Robel P, Corpéchot C, Clarke C, Groyer A, Synguelakis M, Vourc'h C, Baulieu EE (1986) Neurosteroids: 3β-hydroxy-$\Delta^5$-derivatives in the rat brain. In: Fink AJ, Harmar AJ, McKerns KW (eds) Neuroendocrine molecular biology. Plenum Press, New York, pp 367-377

Schwartz MW, Woods SC, Porte Jr D, Seeley RJ, Baskin DG (2000) Central nervous system control of food intake. Nature 404: 661-671

Slobodyansky E, Guidotti A, Wambebe C, Berkovich A, Costa E (1989) Isolation and characterization of a rat brain triakontatetraneuropeptide, a posttranslational product of diazepam binding inhibitor: specific action at the Ro5-4864 recognition site. J Neurochem 53: 1276-1284

Wehrenberg WB, Corder R, Gaillard RC (1989) A physiological role for neuropeptide Y in regulating the estrogen/progesterone induced luteinizing hormone surge in ovariectomized rats. Neuroendocrinology 49: 680-682

# Progestins and antiprogestins: mechanisms of action, neuroprotection and myelination

*M. Schumacher[1], A. Ghoumari[1], R. Guennoun[1], F. Labombarda[2], S.L. Gonzalez[2], M.C. Gonzalez Deniselle[2], C. Massaad[1], J. Grenier[1], K.M. Rajkowski[1], F. Robert[1], E.E. Baulieu[1], and A.F. De Nicola[2]*

## Summary

Progesterone, originally considered as a hormone involved only in reproductive functions, exerts pleiotropic effects throughout the central and peripheral nervous systems. As early as 10 years ago, its role in myelination had been demonstrated in the regenerating peripheral nerve and in cocultures of neurons and Schwann cells. More recently, it has been shown that progesterone also accelerates myelin formation by oligodendrocytes in cerebellar organotypic cultures. Attention to the neuroprotective effects of progesterone was attracted at the end of the 1980s by the observation that female rats with high endogenous levels of progesterone recover better from traumatic brain injury and have less edema and secondary neuron loss than males. The protective effects of progesterone have been mainly studied in lesion models. However, progesterone also protects neurons from neurodegeneration, as has been documented in the Wobbler mouse, a murine model of spinal cord motoneuron degeneration. These findings have significant clinical implications, but an efficient therapeutic use of progestins for treating lesions or diseases of the nervous system would require a better understanding of their mechanisms of action in neurons and glial cells. We have indeed only a rudimentary understanding of the molecular mechanisms by which progestins exert their pleiotropic effects in the brain. Their study should provide a substantial basis for the design of progesterone analogs with much safer and selective actions. This review will summarize our current knowledge of the multiple mechanisms of progesterone action: the role of different progesterone receptor isoforms, the importance of coregulator proteins in modulating their transcriptional activities, and novel progesterone actions mediated by membrane receptors. The detailed account of the multiple mechanisms of progesterone action is followed by a discussion of recent studies, documenting the promyelinating and neuroprotective effects of progestins and of mifepristone (RU486), known as an antiprogestin or selective progesterone

[1] INSERM U488, 80, rue du Général Leclerc, 94276 Kremlin-Bicêtre, France;
[2] Laboratory of Neuroendocrine Biochemistry, Instituto de Biologia y Medicina Experimental, University of Buenos Aires, Argentina.

Kordon et al.
Hormones and the Brain
© Springer-Verlag Berlin Heidelberg 2005

receptor modulator (SPRM). Their actions involve both classical and novel mechanisms.

## Introduction

Progesterone is an important female reproductive hormone that, together with estradiol, regulates functions of reproductive organs, sexual behavior and the release of gonadotropins (Schumacher et al. 1999). It is particularly well known as a hormone necessary for the initiation and maintenance of pregnancy. First produced by the mother's corpus luteum, progesterone is synthesized by the placenta as pregnancy progresses. However, progesterone is not only present in females, and significant amounts of the steroid, produced by the adrenal glands, also circulate in males (Kalra and Kalra 1977; Gutai et al. 1977). The circulating progesterone easily crosses the blood-brain barrier and diffuses throughout the nervous tissues because of its lipid solubility, and elevated levels of progesterone have been measured in different brain regions of men and women (Hammond et al. 1983; Weill-Engerer et al. 2002).

In addition to the steroidogenic endocrine glands, progesterone is also synthesized locally within the brain, spinal cord and peripheral nerves by neurons and glial cells, either de novo from cholesterol or from blood-derived pregnenolone (Robel et al. 1999; Baulieu et al. 2001). Within these three compartments of the nervous system, the 3β-hydroxysteroid dehydrogenase (3β-HSD), which catalyzes the conversion of pregnenolone to progesterone, is widely distributed (Guennoun et al. 1995, 1997; Coirini et al. 2002, 2003a, b). The regulation of progesterone synthesis within the nervous system has so far not been explored in detail, but involves neurotransmitters, neuropeptides and cellular interactions (Beaujean et al. 2002; Mellon and Vaudry 2001). For example, Schwann cells, the myelinating glial cells in the peripheral nervous system (PNS), synthesize progesterone in response to a diffusible neuronal signal (Robert et al. 2001).

Progesterone mediates part of its effects on target cells via intracellular receptors, which also show a widespread distribution within the nervous system (MacLusky and McEwen 1980; Hagihara et al. 1992; Lauber et al. 1991; Labombarda et al. 2000b). In addition, progesterone and its metabolites exert some of their effects through progesterone receptor (PR)-independent mechanisms. For example, they are potent modulators of neurotransmitter receptors and they bind to specific membrane receptors. All these observations are congruent with the pleiotropic effects of progestins in the nervous system. It is indeed now well established that the functions of progesterone are not restricted to reproduction but that it is also concerned with  vital neuronal and glial functions. Thus, progesterone has been shown to play an important role in myelination and in neuron viability (Stein 2001; Schumacher et al. 2001;

Schumacher and Robert 2002; De Nicola et al. 2004). Although these findings open the way for interesting therapeutic possibilities, their development is seriously hampered due to a serious lack of knowledge concerning the mechanisms of action of progestins within the nervous system. Understanding these mechanisms is required for the development of more efficient and selective progesterone analogs for the treatment of disorders and lesions of the nervous system.

Now that the important trophic functions of progesterone in the nervous system have been recognized, the time has come to elucidate the underlying mechanisms and to identify the target genes. It is the right time, because the multiple novel mechanisms of progesterone action have recently been discovered in different experimental systems and because a variety of synthetic progestins have become available for therapeutic applications. This review summarizes our current knowledge of the mechanisms of action of progestins, followed by some specific examples of their promyelinating and neuroprotective effects. The aim is to encourage further mechanistic explorations of the trophic effects of progestins and of SPRMs in the nervous system.

## Mechanisms of progesterone action

### Transcriptional regulation by progesterone receptor isoforms

*The PR-A and PR-B isoforms of the progesterone receptor*

The genomic actions of progesterone are mediated by two different-sized receptor isoforms, PR-A (94 kDa) and PR-B (114 kDa), which are generated from a single  gene by differential promoter utilization (Kastner et al. 1990; Conneely and Lydon 2000). Binding of the hormone to either PR isoform causes conformational changes, resulting in the dissociation of a chaperone protein complex, receptor dimerization, increased receptor phosphorylation, binding of the receptor dimer to specific hormone-responsive DNA elements (HRE) located on target genes and interactions of the receptor complex with nuclear coactivators (Tsai and O'Malley 1994; Li and O'Malley 2003; Conneely et al. 2003). The PR-A and PR-B isoforms have been shown to form either homodimers (A:A and B:B) or heterodimers (A:B; DeMarzo et al. 1991, 1992).

Both PR-A and PR-B have a modular structure with distinct functional domains, including the N-terminal domain (A/B-domain), a centrally located DNA binding domain (DBD = C-domain) with two highly conserved zinc fingers, a hinge-domain (H = D-domain) and a hydrophobic ligand-binding domain (LBD = E-domain) in the C-terminal region (Fig. 1). The hinge region contains the nuclear localization signal (NLS), a large region of 61 amino acids that extends over the second zinc finger (Tyagi et al. 1998; Guiochon-Mantel

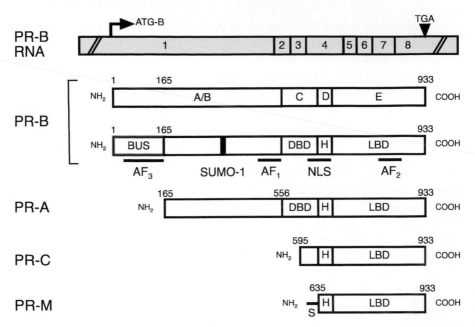

**Fig. 1.** Schematic representation of the four different human PR isoforms (PR-B, PR-A, PR-C, PR-M) resulting from the use of different transcription or translation start sites. The cDNA of PR-B is represented on top and shows the eight exons that encode the different functional domains (A-E) of the PR-B protein (933 amino acids) presented just below. Exon 1 encodes the A/B domain (N-terminal domain), exons 2 and 3 the C-domain (DNA binding-domain, DBD), exons 4-8 the D-domain (hinge region, H) and the E-domain (ligand binding-domain, LBD). AF 1-3 correspond to distinct activation domains. A consensus binding site for SUMO-1 is located within an inhibitory domain (IF). The nuclear localization signals (NLS) extend over the hinge region and the second zinc finger of the DBD. The PR-B and PR-A isoforms, which differ by an N-terminal 164-amino-acid segment called BUS (B-receptor upstream segment), result from two distinct transcription start sites within exon 1. The transcription start site of PR-C, which lacks the N-terminal region and one of the two zinc fingers, is located within exon 2. Initiation of transcription of the recently cloned PR-M occurs within intron 3. PR-M corresponds to the hinge region and the LBD, preceded by a hydrophobic signal peptide of 16 aminoacids (S).

2000). The NLS can be functionally divided into two regions: the constitutively active C-terminal region and the N-terminal region (second zinc finger), which is only active in the presence of ligand (Guiochon-Mantel et al. 1989). It is indeed now well established that the PR undergoes a continuous nucleo-cytoplasmic shuttling, resulting from its continuous active transport into the nucleus and its diffusion out into the cytoplasm (Guiochon-Mantel and Milgrom 1993). The different functional domains of the human PR are encoded by the eight exons of the open reading frame of the PR gene: exon 1 encodes the N-terminal domain, exons 2 and 3 encode the DBD (each exon coding for one of the two zinc fingers) and exons 4-8 encode the hinge-domain and the LBD (Misrahi et al. 1993; Rousseau-Merck et al. 1987). PR-B differs from PR-A only by an additional 164-

amino acid segment in its N-terminal region, called BUS (B-receptor Upstream Segment; Takimoto et al. 2003).

The transcriptional activities of the two PR isoforms are regulated by nuclear coregulator proteins, which bind to distinct activation functions (domains; AF): the constitutive AF-1 located just upstream of the DBD, the ligand-dependent AF-2 located within the LBD and AF-3 in the PR-B-specific BUS segment (Sartorius et al. 1994; Fig. 1). In addition to the AF, two inhibitory functions (IF) have been described: one located within the BUS segment has been linked to the regulation of AF-3 function and one located N-terminally to AF1 is common to both PR isoforms (Hovland et al. 1998). Within the latter, a consensus binding site for the small ubiquitin-like modifier protein SUMO-1 has been identified. Sumoylation plays an important role in the targeting, stability and transcriptional activity of nuclear proteins and has also been shown to regulate the actions of steroid receptors (Poukka et al. 2000; Muller et al. 2001). For instance, binding of SUMO-1 to the PR decreases its transcriptional activity by inhibiting the synergistic interactions between the AFs, a phenomenon known as "autoinhibition" (Abdel-Hafiz et al. 2002; Takimoto et al. 2003). However, overexpression of SUMO-1 has recently been shown to enhance PR-mediated gene transcription (Chauchereau et al. 2003).

Both in vitro and in vivo experiments have provided evidence that PR-A and PR-B have different functions. Their different cell- and promoter-specific transactivation properties have been related to the additional AF3 in the BUS segment and to the recruitment of different coregulators, which may explain the stronger transactivation properties of PR-B (Horwitz et al. 1995; Giangrande et al. 1997, 2000). In addition, the activity of inhibitory domains can be masked in PR-B. Thus, the corepressor SMRT (*silencing mediator of retinoid and thyroid receptors*) has been reported to interact more strongly with PR-A than with PR-B (Giangrande and Mcdonnell 1999).

PR-B is indeed a more active transactivator than PR-A, as has been shown by transfecting various cell lines lacking endogenous steroid receptors with PR-B or PR-A expression vectors and progesterone-responsive reporter gene constructs. Moreover, only the B-isoform can mediate activation of gene transcription by antiprogestins such as mifepristone (Horwitz et al. 1995; Dijkema et al. 1998). In well-defined cell and promoter contexts, the PR-A can even act as a repressor of PR-B-mediated gene transcription. This inhibitory function of PR-A may involve direct protein-protein interactions with PR-B, as a PR-A mutant lacking the DBD still showed the same inhibitory effects (Vegeto et al. 1993; Wen et al. 1994). Furthermore, PR-A has been shown to inhibit the transcriptional activity of other steroid receptors, including androgen, estrogen, glucocorticoid and mineralocorticoid receptors (Vegeto et al. 1993; Wen et al. 1994; Mcdonnell et al. 1994; Mcdonnell and Goldman 1994; Kraus et al. 1995). The term "transrepression" has been coined to refer to the suppression of the transcriptional activities of steroid receptors by PR-A. Interestingly, the "transrepressor activity" of PR-A involves the same domains of the PR as the above described "autoinhibitory activity" to the SUMO-1-binding motif (Abdel-Hafiz et al. 2002). The mechanisms of transrepression are still not understood. Engineered cells and transgenic mice have allowed the demonstration that PR-A and PR-B regulate the expression of different subsets of genes in vivo. Thus, microarray analysis of breast cancer cell lines expressing either PR isoform or different isoform ratios has demonstrated that PR-A and PR-B activate the transcription of different genes (Jacobsen et al. 2002; Richer et al. 2002). Regulated expression of both isoforms in vivo is required for normal mammary gland development, as shown by transgenic mice overexpressing either the A or the B form of the PR (Shyamala et al. 1998, 2000). Subsequently, the creation of mice selectively lacking either PR-A or PR-B has allowed the unequivocal demonstration that the two PR isoforms function as distinct transcription factors and mediate different physiological responses to progesterone. Their generation was achieved by introducing a point mutation into the PR gene at the PR-B or PR-A translation start sites (Conneely et al. 2002). Inactivation of PR-B resulted in reduced mammary ductal morphogenesis but did not affect ovarian and uterine development. In contrast, mice lacking PR-A had normal mammary glands but displayed severe ovarian and uterine anomalies. In these mice, the antiproliferative effect of progesterone in uterine epithelium is absent and progesterone potentiates the mitogenic effect of estradiol (Mulac-Jericevic et al. 2000; Conneely et al. 2002).

As PR-B and PR-A have different transactivation functions, differently influence the actions of other steroid receptors and also activate the transcription of different progesterone-responsive genes, their relative expression within a cell is important for determining the effects of progestins and also of other steroids (Mote et al. 1999; Fang et al. 2002). In human breast cells, the coordinated expression of the two PR isoforms can be lost (Mote et al. 2002).

The respective functions of PR-A and PR-B have so far only been explored with respect to reproduction. Their presence throughout the gestational period in a wide range of fetal tissues also suggests an important role of progesterone in the development of fetal organs (Inoue et al. 2001). In the nervous system, their biological properties and their role in the cell-specific actions of progestins are not well defined. Many studies performed over the past decade have documented that regulation of PR-A and PR-B expression varies between different brain regions according to sex, hormonal status and age (Kato et al. 1993; Camacho-Arroyo et al. 1994; Szabo et al. 2000; Guerra-Araiza et al. 2002, 2003; Beyer et al. 2002; Inoue et al. 2002)

### Novel isoforms of the progesterone receptor

A third N-terminally truncated PR isoform, named PR-C (60 kDa), has been identified in T47D human breast cancer cells (Fig. 1). PR-C arises from the initiation of translation at a methionine located C-terminally to the start sites that generate the larger A- and B-isoforms. It lacks the first zinc finger of the DBD but contains the second one and a complete LBD with the sequences necessary for receptor dimerization and nuclear localization. Although PR-C binds progestins and antiprogestins with similar affinity to PR-A and PR-B, it is transcriptionally silent because it does not possess the two zinc fingers required for DNA binding. However, PR-C can form heterodimers with the A- and B-isoforms and modulate their transcriptional activities (Wei et al. 1996). The functional role of PR-C in progesterone action is not well understood and its tissue distribution has not been well defined. In addition to breast cells, abundant expression of PR-C has also been described for decidual cells of the rat uterus, where its levels are significantly increased during late pregnancy (Ogle et al. 1998; Ogle 2002)

Recently, a novel truncated PR, named PR-M, has been cloned from human adipose and aortic cDNA libraries. The PR-M mRNA is the product of an alternative transcription start site located within intron 3 just prior to exon 4, and the corresponding protein (38 kDa) is only composed of the hinge region and the LBD (Saner et al. 2003). The potential functions of the PR-M isoform, which has so far been located in human aortic cells and T47D breast cancer cells, remain to be determined. PR-M may correspond to a novel membrane receptor of progesterone, because it lacks the DBD and portion of the NLS, and hydropathy analysis indicates a hydrophobic N-terminal signal sequence (Saner et al. 2003).

In addition to the four PR isoforms generated by the alternative use of different transcription or translation start sites (PR-A, PR-B, PR-C and PR-M), various PR transcripts resulting from the deletion of one or more exons have been identified in normal and malignant cells of human breast, endometrium, ovary and vascular smooth muscles (Richer et al. 1998; Misao et al. 1998; Hodges et al. 1999; Balleine et al. 1999). Analysis of the exon-deleted PR mRNA variants has revealed perfect junctions between the exons surrounding the deletion area, strongly suggesting that they may be generated by alternative splicing of wild-type PR transcripts (Misao et al. 2000). The possibility that the exon-deleted PR mRNA variants may be expressed as proteins is supported by the detection by immunoblotting of multiple PR bands in many tumor cells (Richer et al. 1998; Yeates et al. 1998). At least some of these PR variants may be functional and may influence the transcriptional activities of the other isoforms. For example, it has been proposed that the putative exon 6-deleted PR variant may function as a dominant-negative transcription inhibitor (Richer et al. 1998).

Recent structural studies indicate that the structure of the PR gene may be more complex than initially thought. They have revealed the presence of additional exons located in regions previously specified as introns. Four such "intronic" exons have been identified: exons T and S located between exons 3 and 4, and exons i45a and i45b, located between exons 4 and 5 (Hirata et al. 2003a, b;

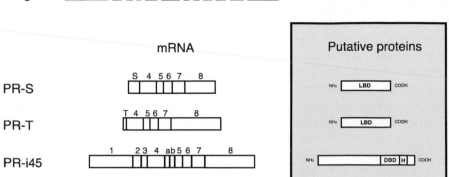

**Fig. 2.** Schematic presentation of the human PR gene. The coding region encompasses the previously described exons 1-8 as well as four recently described exons located in regions previously specified as introns: exons T and S between exons 3 and 4 and exons i45a (a) and i45b (b) between exons 4 and 5. In frame stop, codons are located within the new exons S, T, i45a and i45b. Thus, the longest putative PR protein encoded by PR mRNA variants S and T would correspond to almost the entire part of the ligand- binding domain (LBD). The longest putative PR protein encoded by PR mRNA variants i45 would correspond to the N-terminal A/B domain, the DNA-binding domain (DBD), the hinge region (H) and a small part of the LBD (adapted from Hirata et al. 2003a, b).

Fig. 2). The use of these new exons, when linked to exons 4-8, generates many variants of PR mRNA in human tissues and cell lines. The structures of the proteins encoded by these mRNAs are still unclear. As in frame stop codons are located within the new exons, the T and S isoforms would encode a protein that contains almost the entire LBD, but lacks the DBD and the N-terminal domain, and may thus be involved in non-genomic actions of progesterone (Hirata et al. 2003b).The presence and biological significance of these novel PR isoforms are still unknown.

### Coregulators of the progesterone receptor

The transcriptional activity of liganded PR isoforms is determined by nuclear coregulatory proteins, which form complexes with the AF or IF through protein-protein interactions. They are either coactivators, which enhance transcription, or corepressors, which suppress it. Limiting amounts of coregulators have been proposed to result in "transcriptional interference" or "squelching" between steroid receptors (McKenna et al. 1999; Rowan and O'Malley 2000).

The first coactivator for the steroid receptor family, steroid receptor coactivator-1 (SRC-1), was cloned and characterized by the O'Malley group (Onate et al. 1995). It was identified by using a yeast two-hybrid screen of a human lymphocyte cDNA library, with the hormone-bound PR-LBD as bait. SRC-1 increases the transcriptional activity of the PR by interacting predominantly with AF-2 of the LBD but also with AF-1 of the N-terminal domain. Interactions between the PR and SRC-1 have recently been shown to be increased by sumoylation (Chauchereau et al. 2003). SRC-1 possesses a weak intrinsic histone acetyltransferase (HAT) activity and recruits more general coactivators with strong histone-modifying enzyme activities such as the CREB-binding protein (CBP) or the arginine-specific histone methyltransferase (CARM-1) to the DNA-bound PR transcription complex (Spencer et al. 1997; Onate et al. 1998). Its biological role has been demonstrated in SRC-1 knockout mice, which exhibit partial progesterone resistance in mammary gland and uterus (Xu et al. 1998). Subsequent to SRC-1, other coactivators of the PR have been identified, including two other p160 family members with intrinsic HAT activity, namely SRC-2 (NCoA-2, GRIP1, TIF-2) and SRC-3 (p/CIP, ACTR, TRAM-1,RAC-3) (Leo and Chen, 2000; Rowan and O'Malley 2000; Robyr et al., 2000; Glass and Rosenfeld, 2000; Gehin et al., 2002).

Whereas the interactions between p160 coactivators and AF-2 have been well characterized, less is known about AF-1. The yeast two-hybrid screening strategy has recently allowed the identification of several proteins that selectively interact with the N-terminal domain of PR-A, such as the jun dimerization protein-2 (JDP-2), previously known as a natural repressor of jun and other leucine zipper transcription factors (Edwards et al. 2003). Chromatin immunoprecipitation (ChIP) showed that JDP-2 and PR are indeed recruited to the promoter of a progesterone-responsive target gene in vivo (Wardell et al. 2002).

As already mentioned, coregulatory proteins control several aspects of the activities of steroid receptors, such as their efficacy and determine specificity. Thus, elevated levels of p160 coactivators decrease the EC50 values of agonist complexes with the PR, defined as the concentration of agonist required for half-maximal induction of gene expression (Giannoukos et al. 2001; Simons 2003). The opposing actions of coactivators and corepressors also determine the effects of PR antagonists such as mifepristone. In fact, mifepristone can display both agonist and antagonist activities with the PR, depending on the cellular context or the phosphorylation status of the receptor. It thus qualifies as a "selective progesterone receptor modulator" (SPRM) with mixed antagonist/ agonist properties (Katzenellenbogen and Katzenellenbogen 2002; Leonhardt et al. 2003). However, mifepristone can act as a partial agonist only with PR-B and not with PR-A (Meyer et al. 1990; Leonhardt et al. 2003). Its binding to PR-B induces conformational changes that are distinct from those induced by agonists. As a result, the antagonist-bound PR-B has a reduced affinity for coactivators and an increased affinity for corepressors such as the nuclear receptor corepressor (NCoR) and the silencing mediator for retinoic acid and thyroid hormone receptor (SMRT Jackson et al. 1997; Wagner et al. 1998; Zhang et al. 1998). In nuclear extracts of T47D human breast cancer cells and of HeLa cells, mifepristone-dependent activity, ranging from transcriptional activation to repression, was found to be dependent on the relative levels of SRC-1 and

SMRT (Liu et al. 2002). AF-1 has also been shown to be involved in the partial agonist activity of mifepristone. Thus, overexpression of the coactivator JDP-2, which binds to AF-1 as already mentioned, strongly potentiated the partial agonist activity of mifepristone when cotransfected into Cos-1 cells with a PR-B expression vector and a progesterone-sensitive reporter gene (Edwards et al. 2003; Wardell et al. 2002). The small leucine zipper-containing protein L7/SPA, which binds to the hinge region, also increases the partial agonist activity of mifepristone. In contrast, binding of the corepressors N-CoR or SMRT to AF-2 suppresses mifepristone-mediated partial agonist activity (Jackson et al. 1997). There is now experimental evidence that the recruitment of coregulators is dependent on the physiological context. Expression of nuclear coactivators and corepressors is regulated in different reproductive tissues by steroid and thyroid hormones (Misiti et al. 1998), and it varies during the estrous cycle (Shiozawa et al. 2003).

### Coregulators of steroid receptors in the brain

The biological functions of steroid receptor coactivators or corepressors in the nervous system and their interactions with steroid receptors have so far not been explored in detail. There is some evidence that the regulation of coregulator expression may play an important role in the control of steroid hormone actions in the brain and may contribute to the cell-specific actions of steroids within the nervous system. Several recent studies have thus documented the selective expression and regulation of steroid receptor coactivators within different compartments of the nervous system. For example, SRC-1 is broadly expressed in the adult rat brain, whereas SRC-2 is mainly present in the anterior pituitary gland. The two splice variants of SRC-1, SRC-la and SRC-le, are differentially expressed within distinct brain regions (Misiti et al. 1998; Meijer et al. 2000). Within the rat hippocampus, SRC-1 was mainly found in neurons and only in some astrocytes (Ogawa et al. 2001).

SRC-1 mRNA and protein levels are also influenced by gender and by environmental conditions in a brain region-specific manner. Thus, SRC-1 is expressed at higher levels in the hippocampus of males under basal conditions, but stress increases hippocampal SRC-1 levels only in females (Bousios et al. 2001). An in situ hybridization study of SRC-1 mRNA expression in the female rat brain demonstrated its presence in discrete brain regions throughout development, and its expression is positively regulated by estrogen in the ventromedial nuclei of the hypothalamus but not in the cerebral cortex. In the brains of canaries, SRC-1 transcripts are strongly expressed within steroid-sensitive nuclei of the song system (Charlier et al. 2003). Both SRC-1 and CBP are down-regulated in spinal motoneurons innervating the bulbocavernosus in aged rats, and reduced coactivator levels have been proposed to contribute to the reduced steroid sensitivity observed in aged animals (Jezierski and Sohrabji

2001; Matsumoto 2002). Together, these still fragmentary findings strongly suggest that SRC-1 may be involved in the amplification of hormone actions within the brain in a temporally and spatially coordinated manner (Mitev et al. 2003).

The use of SRC-1 antisense oligodeoxynucleotides and the generation of null mutants for SRC-1 (SRC-1$^{-/-}$) have indeed provided evidence that this coactivator may play an important role in hormone-dependent brain processes. Thus, infusion of SRC-1 antisense oligodeoxynucleotides into the rat brain impaired the process of sexual differentiation during development and inhibited progesterone-facilitated sexual receptivity in adult females (Auger et al. 2000; Molenda et al. 2002). The process of sexual differentiation of the brain and of behavior could also be disturbed by using CBP antisense oligodeoxynucleotides (Auger et al. 2002). Antisense oligonucleotides to SRC-1 and SRC-2, but not to SRC-3, inhibited lordosis behavior and the induction of the PR by estrogen within the ventromedial hypothalamus in rats and mice. This observation is consistent with the presence of SRC-1 and SRC-2 and the absence of SRC-3 within this brain region (Apostolakis et al. 2002). SRC-1$^{-/-}$ mice are viable and only show partial hormone resistance and slight loss in reproductive functions, due to compensation by SRC-2 (Xu et al. 1998). During early postnatal development, disruption of SRC-1 delays the development of cerebellar Purkinje cells, leading to moderate motor dysfunctions in adulthood. However, at later postnatal stages, when SRC-2 starts to be expressed, both morphology and number of Purkinje cells recover, in agreement with the compensation by SRC-2 (Nishihara et al. 2003).

### Interactions of the progesterone receptor with other transcription factors

Classical nuclear PRs not only regulate gene expression by their direct binding to DNA but also through protein-protein interactions with other nuclear transcription factors. Such cross-talk generally concerns negative gene regulation. Examples are PR-mediated repression of the transcriptional activities of NF-κB, Stat-5 and AP-1 (fos/jun) (Kalkhoven et al. 1996; Leonhardt et al. 2003). Interestingly, the SPRM mifepristone and the pure PR antagonist onapristone (ZK98299) can both mimic the effects of PR agonists on target genes via PR interactions with other transcription factors (Edwards et al. 2000; Leonhardt et al. 2003).

### Progesterone receptor phosphorylation and ligand-independent activation

The PR is a phosphoprotein whose transcriptional activity is regulated by phosphorylation (Weigel 1996). This process appears highly complex, as the receptor bears at least 15 phosphorylation sites (Knotts et al. 2001). There is now ample evidence that several intracellular phosphorylation cascades are involved in the phosphorylation of the PR and also of its associated proteins. Of note is the phosphorylation of the PR by mitogen-activated protein kinases (MAPKs), which affects ligand-dependent PR downregulation and the transcriptional synergy between peptide growth factors and progestins on several gene promoters (Qiu and Lange 2003). In addition, phosphorylation also affects the ligand specificity of the PR. For example, mifepristone can behave like an agonist and activate gene transcription when intracellular phosphorylation pathways are activated (Beck et al. 1993; Nordeen et al. 1993; Sartorius et al. 1993).

A number of studies have reported that the phosphorylated PR may regulate gene transcription even in the absence of progesterone. This phenomenon, named "ligand-independent receptor activation," has been observed for PRs and other steroid receptors in transient transfection experiments (Power et al. 1992). However, the molecular mechanisms of the ligand-independent activation of steroid receptors are not well understood. During ligand-independent activation of the chicken PR-A with the 8-bromo-cAMP, no alteration in receptor phosphorylation was observed (Bai et al., 1997). This finding raised the possibility that ligand-independent activation of the PR may be mediated through changes in the phosphorylation of coregulators or other protein factors interacting with the receptors. In fact, SRC-1 was later found to be a target of cAMP-dependent signalling, indicating that cross-talk between a signalling pathway and a nuclear receptor coactivator may be involved in the regulation of PR activity (Rowan et al., 2000).

The biological relevance of this mechanism was suggested by the observation that it may play a role in the activation of sexual receptivity (lordosis behavior) in female rodents (Mani et al. 1994, 1996; Apostolakis et al. 1996). The significance of ligand-independent PR activation has been further substantiated by a recent microarray study that has allowed the identification of several brain target genes for the unliganded PR (Jacobsen et al. 2002). Two of these genes, coding for Ectodermal-Neural Cortex 1 (ENC-1) and Down Syndrome Cell Adhesion Molecule (DSCAM), are expressed at significant levels in the nervous system and are likely to play an important role in the development and maintenance of neuronal networks (Hernandez et al. 1998; Barlow et al. 2001; Agarwala et al. 2001).

## Novel mechanisms of progesterone action

*Novel mechanisms of action involving the classical progesterone receptors*

The classical PR not only interacts with specific DNA sequences or other transcription factors in the nucleus but also with cytoplasmic proteins implicated in intracellular signalling pathways. The N-terminal domain common to PR-A and PR-B indeed contains a "SH3 domain interaction motif," which was shown by pull-down assays to selectively interact with Src tyrosine kinase family members. Interactions of the PR with the SH3 domain of these signalling molecules were found to be transient and ligand-dependent and correspond to a unique feature of the PR (Edwards et al. 2003; Boonyaratanakornkit et al. 2001). Both PR-A and PR-B can activate Src kinases, in vitro and in cultured cells, and they can both influence cell proliferation via this mechanism of action (Edwards et al. 2003). The effect of progesterone on Src kinase activities could be mimicked by the selective PR agonist R5020 and prevented by mifepristone. A functional consequence of PR interaction with the SH3 domain of Src kinase is the activation of the Src/Ras/MAPK signalling pathway, as has been documented in MCF-7 breast cancer cells (Migliaccio et al. 1998; Leonhardt et al. 2003).

A model is emerging that suggests that intracellular steroid receptors may be targeted both to the nucleus, where they regulate gene transcription, and to the cell membrane, where they may mediate rapid membrane effects. How a subpopulation of steroid receptors translocates to the cell membrane is an important question that remains to be elucidated. This model has been documented for the PR in *Xenopus laevis* oocytes. Reinitiation of oocyte meiosis was the first well-documented rapid action of progesterone at the level of the cell membrane and does not require gene transcription (Baulieu et al. 1978; Godeau et al. 1978). The effect of progesterone involved an increase in intracellular $Ca^{2+}$ and the regulation of intracellular signalling pathways, in particular the inactivation of the adenylate cyclase/protein kinase A (PKA) system and the activation of mitogen-activated protein kinase (MAPK; Finidori-Lepicard et al. 1981; Ferrell 1999). Twenty years later, the nongenomic signalling of progesterone in Xenopus oocytes has been shown to involve the amphibian homolog of the mammalian PR, named the Xenopus PR (XPR), which shows both cytoplasmic localization and membrane association (Bayaa et al. 2000; Maller 2001; Bagowski et al. 2001). XPR was shown to associate with active phosphatidylinositol 3-kinase (PI3-K) and MAPK in a progesterone-specific manner (Bagowski et al. 2001). In heterologous cotransfection experiments using COS cells, XPR was shown to activate transcription in response to progesterone and R5020 and this effect was blocked by mifepristone (Bayaa et al. 2000). However, it is not certain whether XPR mediates all the effects of progesterone on oocyte maturation. Membrane receptors of progesterone, such as those recently identified in fish oocytes, could also play an important role (see below).

### Pregnane X receptor

The nuclear pregnane X receptor (PXR) plays a key role in drug metabolism and efflux by activating the expression of cytochrome P450 enzymes and of transporters involved in multidrug resistance (Kliewer et al. 2002). PXR is a promiscuous xenobiotic receptor that is also activated by naturally occuring steroids, including pregnenolone, progesterone, its metabolite 5β-pregnane-

3,20-dione, mifepristone and glucocorticoids (Kliewer et al. 1998; Moore et al. 2002). During pregnancy, PXR shows a progesterone-mediated 50-fold induction (Masuyama et al., 2001). This novel steroid signalling pathway could thus play an important role in steroid homeostasis.

The capacity of PXR to bind many structurally diverse ligands has been explained by solving the crystal structure of its LBD, revealing an enlarged, highly flexible and hydrophobic ligand binding pocket with 5 polar residues (Watkins et al. 2001; Ekins and Schuetz, 2002). PXR binds as a heterodimer with 9-cis retinoic acid receptors (RXRs) to a HRE on target genes (Kliewer et al. 1998) and interacts with nuclear coactivator proteins such as SRC-1 (Masuyama et al. 2001). Binding of SRC-1 has been shown to stabilize the LBD of PXR and to have marked effects on the manner in which the receptor interacts with ligands (Watkins et al. 2003).

PXR is highly expressed in the hepatogastrointestinal tract and also in the kidney, stomach, lung, uterus, ovary and placenta (Masuyama et al. 2001; Kliewer et al. 2002). An immunohistochemical study has revealed the presence of PXR in neurons of the basal ganglia, thalamus and cerebellum of human fetuses (Suzuki et al. 1996). The functions of PXR in the nervous system remain to be explored.

### Membrane receptors of progesterone

There is now compelling evidence for rapid membrane actions of progesterone in reproductive tissues and in the nervous system, which have been related in numerous cases to the regulation of $Ca^{2+}$ flux. In addition to the classical PR, which may associate with the cell membrane, specific membrane receptors of progesterone (mPR) may be involved in the rapid non-genomic effects of the steroid. However, the identity and properties of mPRs, as is the case for steroid membrane receptors in general, are still not well defined (Schmidt et al. 2000; Lösel et al. 2003; Lösel and Wehling 2003; Bramley 2003).

The characterization of membrane binding sites for progesterone has always been tentative and has usually been limited to immunostaining and molecular weight determination. Another common approach was the use of progestins coupled to a protein or a polymer, which presumably do not enter cells. Thus, progesterone conjugated to radiolabeledBSA has been used to identify and characterize putative receptors in brain cell membranes. Progesterone linked to [125I]BSA at carbon 11 (PROG-11-[125I]-BSA) was shown to bind to specific membrane sites in different regions of the rat brain, such as the hypothalamus, cerebellum and brainstem (Ke and Ramirez 1990). In the hypothalamus of female rats, binding of PROG-11-[125I]-BSA was found to be inducible by estrogen and was higher in females than in males. An attempt to affinity purify the membrane receptor showed a band of 40-50 kDa that also bound [3H]progesterone (Tischkau and Ramirez 1993).

A progesterone membrane-binding protein was then isolated and cloned from porcine liver. This putative membrane receptor of progesterone comprises 194 amino acids with a single membrane-spanning domain (Falkenstein et al. 1996; Meyer et al. 1996). Binding of [$^3$H]progesterone to the porcine membrane protein was reversible, saturable and showed steroid selectivity : moderate affinity for corticosterone, cortisol, and testosterone and no affinity for aldosterone, dexamethasone and estradiol (Meyer et al. 1996). Subsequently, homologous proteins were cloned in rat (25-Dx), cattle and humans (Selmin et al. 1996; Cenedella et al. 1999; Gerdes et al. 1998). The native proteins are likely to form oligomeric complexes of about 200 kDa, composed of 28 kDa monomers and 56 kDa dimers (Meyer et al. 1998).

Although progesterone exerts rapid effects on the cell membrane of pig hepatocytes, progesterone binding was found to be associated with endomembranes rather than with plasma membranes. Moreover, expression of the cDNA of the progesterone-binding protein in CHO cells (Chinese Hamster Ovary Cells) resulted in increased microsomal progesterone binding (Falkenstein et al. 1999). Based on these observations, the membrane-binding protein of progesterone would rather qualify as an "endomembrane-binding protein." Whether this protein corresponds to an authentic receptor of progesterone or whether it has other functions remains to be established. Thus, based on sequence homology with a protein of the inner zone of the rat adrenal cortex involved in steroid hydroxylation, this protein has been proposed to play a role in steroid metabolism (Raza et al. 2001). Nevertheless, the human progesterone membrane-binding protein was found to be exposed on the cell surface of spermatozoa (Buddhikot et al. 1999; Falkenstein et al. 1999) and the rat 25-Dx protein on the cell surface of neuronal GT1-7 cells after the transfection of a green fluorescent protein (GFP) fusion construct (Krebs et al. 2000).

The distribution of 25-DX protein transcripts has been examined in the female rat brain by in situ hybridization. The highest levels of 25-Dx protein mRNA were found in the ventromedial nucleus of the hypothalamus, the paraventricular nucleus, the amygdala, the supraoptic nucleus, hippocampus and the zona incerta. Lower expression was observed throughout the cortex and striatum and no expression was seen in the ventral tegmental area and in the cerebellum. In the ventromedial nucleus, expression 25-Dx protein was increased by estrogen treatment. Interestingly, 25-Dx protein expression was found to be higher in the hypothalamus of female PRKO mice than in wild-type littermates, suggesting that the classical PR may repress its expression (Krebs et al. 2000).

An important recent event was the cloning of an authentic membrane receptor of progesterone (mPR) of 40 kDa from fish oocytes. The fish mPR is unrelated to known nuclear steroid receptors and, for the first time, it met all the criteria of a membrane receptor: structure of a membrane-spanning protein, plasma membrane localization, expression in steroid target tissues, selective steroid binding, regulation of intracellular signalling pathways, regulation by hormones and biological functions (Zhu et al. 2003). In the spotted seatrout, the mPR is selectively expressed in reproductive endocrine tissues and in the brain. Computer modeling predicted a protein with seven transmembrane domains, characteristic of G protein-coupled receptors. In fact, the fish mPR was shown to activate a pertussis toxin-sensitive inhibitory G protein, consistent with the inhibition of adenylate cyclase activity. Progesterone also activated the MAPK pathway in a mammalian cell line transfected with the fish mPR. The recombinant protein bound progesterone in a saturable manner with high affinity. The role of the fish mPR in mediating progestin induction of oocyte meiotic maturation was demonstrated by injecting antisense oligonucleotides into oocytes (Zhu et al. 2003).

Subsequently, 13 new genes closely related to the fish mPR were cloned from several vertebrate species, including human, mouse and pig (Zhu and Thomas 2003). They all encode proteins with seven transmembrane domains with the characteristics of G protein-coupled receptors and they have been classified into three subtypes: mPRα, mPRβ and mPRγ. Three mammalian genes, each representative of one of the three mPR subtypes, were shown to encode proteins (Kd = 30-40 kDa) with high affinity and saturable binding for progesterone, but not for synthetic progestins and antiprogestins The human α, β and γ transcripts showed distinct tissue localization : the α form localized in reproductive tissues (ovary, testis, adrenal glands and placenta), the β form exclusively localized to neural tissues (brain and spinal cord) and the γ form was present in kidney, lung and colon (Zhu and Thomas 2003).

The mPRα may also be involved in mediating the rapid effects of progesterone on human sperm (Zhu and Thomas 2003), which has become one of the most studied models of the rapid non-genomic actions of steroids. That is, progesterone and 5α-dihydroprogesterone induce $Ca^{2+}$ influx and the acrosome reaction in human sperm within seconds (Osman et al. 1989). In contrast, testosterone, estradiol, corticosterone, androstenedione, pregnenolone and dehydroepiandrosterone were found to be inactive (Blackmore et al. 1990). The action of progesterone on $Ca^{2+}$ influx and the acrosome reaction could also be mimicked by the synthetic progestin R5020 and could be partially inhibited by mifepristone. When administered alone, mifepristone induced an immediate and dose-dependent decrease of intracellular free $Ca^{2+}$ by itself, thus behaving as an inverse agonist (Yang et al. 1994). However, although very much studied, the mechanisms by which progesterone activates the acrosome reaction are still poorly understood and controversial. Although mPRα is a candidate for the receptor involved in the rapid actions of progesterone on human sperm, it is most likely that multiple membrane receptors and signalling pathways are involved. Thus, the potential membrane receptor of progesterone that has been cloned from porcine liver is also present at the surface of human sperm, and antibodies raised against this protein allowed the inhibition of the progesterone-initiated

$Ca^{2+}$ increase and acrosome reaction (Buddhikot et al. 1999; Falkenstein et al. 1999). Alternative transcripts of the classical PR, such as the above described PR-S, may also be expressed in sperm (Hirata et al. 2000; Luconi et al. 2002). In addition, there are indications of the presence of novel membrane receptors of progesterone that still need to be characterized (Luconi et al. 2002). Finally, there is also evidence that steroid-sensitive $GABA_A$ receptors linked to $Ca^{2+}$ channels as well as voltage-operated $Ca^{2+}$ channels may play a role in the effects of progesterone on human sperm (Shi et al. 1997; Kirkman-Brown et al. 2003).

## Modulation of membrane neurotransmitter receptors by progestins

Progesterone and its metabolites have been shown to rapidly modulate the activities of several neurotransmitter receptors, including sigma-1 (σ1) receptors, nicotinic acetylcholine receptors and $GABA_A$ receptors. However, despite intensive research efforts in many laboratories over the past decades, the mechanisms by which progestins and other steroids modulate the activity of neurotransmitter receptors remain elusive.

Sigma receptors were first defined by their ability to bind a variety of pharmacologically active drugs, named "sigma ligands," with high affinity, and drug discrimination studies have allowed σ1 and σ2 receptor subtypes to be identified (Quirion et al. 1992; Bastianetto et al. 1999). The molecular nature of the σ receptors remained enigmatic until the purification and cloning of a σ1 receptor (25 kDa) from guinea pig liver microsomes (Hanner et al. 1996). Subsequently, the cDNA for the human homolog of this receptor was cloned from a placental cell line and the exon-intron structure of its gene was established (Kekuda et al. 1996; Prasad et al. 1998). The same group also cloned a σ 1 receptor from mouse kidney and from rat brain cDNA libraries (Seth et al. 1998).

It has been proposed that progesterone may be one of the endogenous ligands of σ1 receptors, because it acts as competitive inhibitor of the σ1 agonist (SKF-10,047) binding (Su et al. 1988; McCann et al. 1994). Progesterone also inhibits the binding of haloperidol to cloned rat σ1 receptor (Hanner et al. 1996). The physiological relevance of the interactions between progesterone and σ1 receptors has been documented by several observations. Thus, the potentiation of the N-methyl-D-aspartate (NMDA) response of hippocampal neurons and the NMDA-evoked norepinephrine release from preloaded hippocampal slices by σ1 ligands were strongly reduced in the presence of progesterone (Monnet et al. 1995; Debonnel et al. 1996; Bergeron et al. 1999). Furthermore, progesterone has been shown to influence the behavioral efficacy of σ1-receptor ligands in mice (Phan et al. 2002).

Another neurotransmitter receptor that has been shown to be sensitive to high concentrations of progesterone is the nicotinic acetylcholine receptor (nAChR). The activity of native and reconstituted neuronal nAChRs was inhibited by micromolar concentrations of progesterone (Léna and Changeux 1993; Valera et al. 1992). Results from several studies are compatible with the negative allosteric modulation of nAChR by progesterone (Buisson and Bertrand 1999).

One of the best studied steroid effects on a membrane neurotransmitter receptor is the modulation of γ-aminobutyric acid type A (GABA$_A$) receptors by allopregnanolone (3α,5α-tetrahydroprogesterone). At physiological concentrations, allopregnanolone is a potent positive modulator of GABA$_A$ receptors, which explains some of its psychopharmacological actions, in particular its anesthetic, analgesic and anxiolytic effects as well as its role in stress, depression, memory, seizure susceptibility and alcohol dependence (Morrow et al. 2001; Schumacher and Robert 2002; Lambert et al. 2003). The enantioselectivity of allopregnanolone interactions with GABA$_A$ receptors strongly suggested the presence of specific binding sites (Covey et al. 2001). However, recombinant GABA$_A$ receptor subunit expression coupled with site directed mutagenesis have so far not allowed identification of a steroid binding pocket on the GABA$_A$ receptor oligomer (Lambert et al. 2003). A recent study has investigated the photoaffinity labeling of rat brain membrane preparations with an azide derivative of the GABA$_A$ receptor-active neurosteroid 3α,5β-tetrahydroprogesterone. Although this compound enhanced GABA-evoked currents, it did not directly label GABA$_A$ receptor subunits but was incorporated into a membrane protein identified as the voltage-dependent anion channel-1 (VDAC-1; Darbandi-Tonkabon et al. 2003). These data suggested that the effects of progestins on GABA$_A$ receptors may be mediated by an accessory membrane protein, the VDAC-1. However, this conclusion has been brought into question by a subsequent study by the same group showing that the azide derivative of 3α,5β-tetrahydroprogesterone is still able to modulate GABA$_A$ receptor functions in VDAC-1-deficient mice (Darbandi-Tonkabon et al. 2004).

Whatever the mechanisms by which pregnane steroids interact with GABA$_A$ receptors, their GABA-modulatory effects are neuron- and brain region-specific and are dynamically regulated by phosphorylation (Lambert et al. 2003). Recent studies have also highlighted the important role of glial GABA$_A$ receptors and their modulation by allopregnanolone in myelin formation. In peripheral nerves, Schwann cells indeed express functional GABA$_A$ receptors and allopregnanolone, via these receptors, increases the expression of the peripheral myelin protein PMP22 and affects the morphology of the myelinated fibers in peripheral nerves (Magnaghi et al. 2001; Azcoitia et al. 2003).

## The effects of progestins and antiprogestins on myelination and neuronal survival

There is now ample evidence that progesterone and its metabolites, either derived from the circulation or locally synthesized within the nervous system, play an important role in the process of myelination and in the viability of neurons. However, the molecular mechanisms involved in the promyelinating and neuroprotective effects of progestins are only poorly understood, contrasting with the extensive study of their actions in reproductive tissues. Fragmentary data indicate that multiple signalling mechanisms underlie the actions of progestins in the central nervous system (CNS) and in peripheral nerves.

## Promyelinating effects of progestins

### Promyelinating effects of progesterone in the peripheral nervous system

The promyelinating effects of progestins are not well understood and involve nuclear PR-mediated actions and, surprisingly, also membrane GABA$_A$ receptors. A role for progesterone in myelination was first demonstrated in the regenerating mouse sciatic nerve after lesion and in cocultures of rat dorsal root ganglia (DRG) sensory neurons and Schwann cells, the myelinating glial cells of the PNS (Koenig et al. 1995). Prolonged treatment with progestins was also shown to reverse the age-related decrease in myelin protein expression and the age-dependent structural abnormalities of peripheral myelin sheaths. These effects of progesterone and its metabolites were specific, as androgens were inactive (Melcangi et al. 1998; Azcoitia et al. 2003).

In neuron-Schwann cell cocultures, progesterone works by enhancing the rate of myelin formation. This was shown by measuring the incorporation of a fluorescent ceramide analog into myelin lipids (Chan et al. 1998). In the same study, levels of transcripts coding for the enzymes involved in the synthesis of progesterone were reported to be markedly increased during peak myelin formation, congruent with an important role of locally formed progesterone. That is, Schwann cells express the cytochrome P450scc, which converts cholesterol to pregnenolone, and the 3β-hydroxysteroid dehydrogenase (3β-HSD), which converts pregnenolone to progesterone, and these cells have the capacity to synthesize progesterone in response to a neuronal signal (Chan et al. 2000; Robert et al. 2001).

How does progesterone promote the formation of new myelin sheaths by Schwann cells? In myelinating cocultures of neurons and Schwann cells, Chan and collaborators (2000) found PR-immunoreactivity mainly located in the neurons. Based on this observation, they proposed that progesterone may indirectly regulate Schwann cell myelination by activating the transcription of neuronal genes. In favor of this interpretation was the finding that progesterone induced the expression of neuronal genes in the cocultures (Chan et al. 2000).

However, although it is conceivable that progesterone may influence Schwann cell myelination indirectly by acting on adjacent neurons, there is strong evidence that Schwann cells are also targets for the direct actions of progestins (Schumacher et al. 2001; Magnaghi et al. 2001). PR mRNA and protein have been detected in Schwann cells by RT-PCR and immunocytochemistry and specific and saturable binding of the selective PR ligand [$^3$H]ORG 2058 has been measured in cytosols prepared from rat sciatic nerves and in cultured Schwann cells (Jung-Testas et al. 1996; Magnaghi et al. 1999). The inhibition of myelin sheath formation in the regenerating mouse sciatic nerve by mifepristone also pointed to a PR-mediated action of progesterone (Koenig et al. 1995). However, the genomic effects of progesterone in Schwann cells remain poorly defined. It is not known whether they involve different PR isoforms and the target genes of progesterone still need to be identified. Transient transfection experiments have shown that progesterone increases the promoter activity of genes encoding the peripheral myelin proteins P0 and PMP22 (Désarnaud et al. 1998). However, it is not known whether these genes are direct targets of the PR. Results of a recent study have provided proof of principle that the PR of myelin-forming Schwann cells is a pharmacological target for the therapy of Charcot-Marie-Tooth disease (CMT-1A), characterized by the overexpression of PMP22. In an animal model of the disease, transgenic rats moderately overexpressing the myelin protein, administration of progesterone further increased PMP22 expression, resulting in enhanced Schwann cell pathology. In contrast, administration of the pure PR antagonist onapristone (ZK98299) reduced the overexpression of PMP22 and improved the disease phenotype (Sereda et al. 2003).

It should, however, be mentioned that not all the effects of progestins on Schwann cells necessarily involve the intracellular PR. Thus, allopregnanolone has recently been shown to activate the expression of the PMP22 gene via Schwann cell GABA$_A$ receptors (Melcangi et al. 2003). The importance of such alternative pathways of progesterone signalling is further supported by the observation that the structure of peripheral nerves appears normal in PR knockout (PRKO) mice (Jung-Testas et al. 1999).

### Promyelinating effects of progesterone in the central nervous system

That progesterone also promotes myelination in the CNS, where axons are myelinated by oligodendrocytes, has been demonstrated in explant cultures of cerebellar slices taken from seven-day-old (P7) rats and mice (Ghoumari et al. 2003b). These organotypic cultures closely reproduce developmental events and provide a unique model for examining neuronal survival and maturation and the myelination of axons. P7 rats were used for these experiments because Purkinje cells die by apoptosis if explants are prepared between P1 and P5 (Dusart et al. 1997; Ghoumari et al. 2002). Moreover, during the second postnatal week, myelination is very intense, levels of progesterone are elevated and expression of the 3β-HSD is high in the cerebellum (Notterpek et al. 1993; Ukena et al. 1999). Myelination was evaluated by immunofluorescence analysis of the myelin basic protein (MBP). The quantification of MBP immunostaining indeed provides a

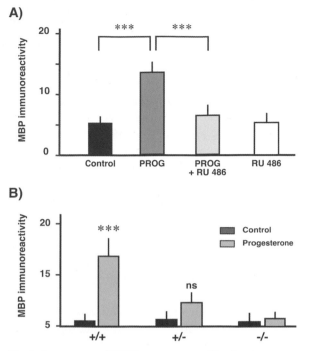

**Fig. 3.** Progesterone (PROG) promotes myelination in organotypic cerebellar slice cultures via the classical intracellular PR. (**A**) Cerebellar slices from P7 rats were treated for seven days with progesterone (20 μM) and/or the PR antagonist mifepristone (RU486; 10 μM). Control cultures were exposed to vehicle (DMSO) alone. Myelination was evaluated by myelin basic protein (MBP) immunostaining using NIH image software (expressed as percentage of an arbitrary staining level). (**B**) Cerebellar slices prepared from P7 wild-type (+/+) or PR knockout (PRKO) mice (+/-, heterozygous; -/-, homozygous) were cultured for seven days in the presence or absence of PROG (20 μM). *** p ≤ 0.001 when compared to the respective controls or as indicated by Newman–Keuls tests after one-way ANOVA (adapted from Ghoumari et al. 2003b).

reliable method for assessing the process of myelination in the brain (Hamano et al. 1996; Muse et al. 2001).

In these cerebellar explant cultures, progesterone and, although to a lesser extent, allopregnanolone accelerated myelination (Ghoumari et al. 2003b). The stimulatory effect of progesterone on myelination, which was observed in cerebellar slices of both sexes, was mediated by the classical PR:1) it could be mimicked by the PR agonist R5020; 2) it was completely abolished by mifepristone; and 3) it was not observed in P7-cerebellar slice cultures from PRKO mice (Fig. 3). In addition, the increase in myelination by allopregnanolone involved membrane GABA$_A$ receptors, as it could be inhibited by the GABA$_A$ receptor antagonist bicuculline and mimicked by the agonist muscimol. Progesterone was indeed converted to allopregnanolone within the cerebellar slices, and this metabolic pathway was involved in the pro-myelination effect of the steroid:

the 5α-reductase inhibitor L685-273 partly inhibited the stimulatory effect of progesterone on MBP expression and this inhibitory effect could be reversed by the simultaneous administration of allopregnanolone (Ghoumari et al. 2003b). How the nuclear and membrane progesterone signalling systems interact during the process of myelination, and whether they are operational in the same or in distinct cell types, remains to be elucidated. Whatever the mechanisms of their concerted actions, binding of progesterone to its intracellular receptor is a prerequisite, as progesterone did not promote myelination either in the presence of mifepristone or in slices from PRKO mice. Once the PR signalling is activated, allopregnanolone may exert additional stimulatory effects via membrane GABA$_A$ receptors (Ghoumari et al. 2003b). In the cerebellar peduncle of older male rats, the systematic administration of progesterone to some extent promoted the remyelination of axons by oligodendrocytes after toxin-induced demyelination (Ibanez et al. 2004).

## Neuroprotective effects of progestins and antiprogestins

Since the observation that females have more favorable outcomes following brain injury, increasing attention has been focused on the neuroprotective and neuroregenerative effects of progesterone (Roof et al. 1993; Stein 2001). They have been mainly examined in lesion models, including traumatic brain injury (TBI), cerebral ischemia and nerve transection. Thus, females with high endogenous levels of progesterone and males treated with progesterone showed improved recovery from TBI (Roof et al. 1993; Roof et al. 1994). Progesterone dramatically reduced cerebral edema, prevented secondary neuronal degeneration and reduced the behavioral impairments resulting from contusion of the medial frontal cortex (Roof et al. 1994). Most importantly, progesterone was still effective in reducing brain damage when treatment was delayed until 24 hours after TBI (Roof et al. 1996).

Progesterone has also been shown to promote the survival of nerve cells in other models of injury. Thus, treatment with progesterone prevented the death of facial motoneurons following nerve transection (Yu 1989) and promoted both neurological and functional recovery after cerebral ischemia and contusion injury of the spinal cord (Jiang et al. 1996; Thomas et al. 1999). In cats, progesterone treatment completely prevented neuron loss after acute global cerebral ischemia in the hippocampus and in the caudate nucleus, which both belong to the brain areas most vulnerable to ischemia (Cervantes et al. 2002; Gonzalez-Vidal et al. 1998). In humans, women have recently been shown to have smaller oxidative damage loads than men, as measured by cerebral spinal fluid (CSF) markers of excitotoxicity, ischemia and oxidative damage (Wagner et al., 2004). Although the neuroprotective effects of progesterone have mostly been examined in models of injury, models of neurodegeneration have largely been neglected. These neuroprotective effects have recently been observed in a murine model of spinal cord motoneuron degeneration, the Wobbler mouse (Gonzalez Deniselle et al. 2002, 2003).

The mechanisms by which progesterone exerts its protective effects in the brain and spinal cord are not well understood. Progestins may have beneficial effects after injury because they decrease the excitability of neurons. As early at the 1940s, progesterone had been reported to reduce the excitability of nerve cells and to protect the brain from seizures (Seyle 1942). In the cerebellum, progesterone was shown to suppress the excitatory responses of Purkinje cells to glutamate and to increase their inhibitory responses to GABA (Smith 1991). Progesterone can also protect cultured spinal cord neurons from glutamate toxicity (Ogata et al. 1993). As mentioned earlier, progesterone is indeed a negative modulator of excitatory neurotransmitter receptors such as the nAChR and, indirectly, via its binding to $\sigma 1$-receptors, of NMDA receptors (Bergeron et al. 1996; Valera et al. 1992). On the other hand, its metabolite allopregnanolone is a positive modulator of inhibitory $GABA_A$ receptors and has been shown to decrease the excitability of hippocampal neurons and to diminish hippocampal damage after seizures (Landgren et al. 1998; Frye 1995; Lambert et al. 2003). After injury to the medial frontal cortex, allopregnanolone was found to be more potent than progesterone in facilitating repair. This observation suggests that at least part of the neuroprotective effects of progesterone after TBI may be mediated by its metabolite, possibly via potentiating $GABA_A$ receptor activity (Djebaili et al. 2004).

Other actions of progesterone may be involved in its neuroprotective effects. For example, progesterone has antioxidant effects and reduces peroxidation of membrane lipids, which may explain its sparing effects on the blood-brain barrier after injury (Roof et al. 1997). Lipid peroxidation also shows gender differences after clinical TBI in humans, as assessed by CSF levels of F(2)-isoprostane (a marker of lipid peroxidation after TBI; Bayir et al. 2004). Progesterone has also been shown to scavenge free radicals (Betz and Coester 1990), to stabilize cell membranes by associating with phospholipids (Carlson et al. 1983), to down-regulate reactive gliosis and astrocyte proliferation (Garcia-Estrada et al. 1993), to increase microtubule associated protein 2 (MAP2) protein in the hippocampus (Reyna-Neyra et al. 2002) and to regulate the expression of specific glial and neuronal genes after injury (see below).

## Neuroprotective effects of progesterone after spinal cord injury

Progesterone has been shown to promote the survival of neurons in the spinal cord after contusion injury and to protect cultured spinal neurons against glutamate toxicity (Ogata et al. 1993; Thomas et al. 1999). After transection of the spinal cord in adult male rats, progesterone prevented motoneuron degeneration and regulated the expression of specific neuronal and glial genes (Labombarda

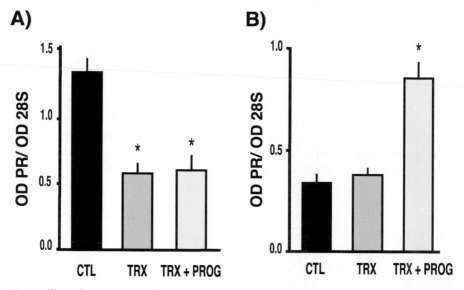

**Fig. 4.** Effects of progesterone (PROG) treatment of rats with spinal cord transection (TRX) on PR (A) and 25-Dx protein mRNA expression (B). mRNA levels were measured by semi-quantitative RT-PCR and were normalized with 28s rRNA. CTL = control animals. * $p \le 0.05$ when compared to the control group (A) or to the control and TRX groups (B) by Newman–Keuls tests after one-way ANOVA (adapted from Labombarda et al. 2003).

et al. 2002; Gonzalez et al. 2004). The regulation of different motoneuron and astrocyte markers by progesterone was examined by in situ hybridization and immunocytochemistry. NADPH-diaphorase is a histochemical marker for nitric oxide synthase, which can be either detrimental or beneficial for nerve cells (Choi 1993). In the intact spinal cord, repeated injections of progesterone did not affect NADPH-diaphorase expression in astrocytes. However, following transection of the spinal cord, expression of NADPH-diaphorase was significantly increased by progesterone in the astrocytes reacting to trauma (Labombarda et al. 2000a).

Likewise, several markers of spinal motoneurons were upregulated by progesterone only after spinal cord transection, namely, the acetylcholine acetyltransferase (ChAT), GAP-43 and the α3 and β1 subunits of the $Na^+/K^+$-ATPase (Labombarda et al. 2002). In the case of ChAT and the $Na^+/K^+$-ATPase subunits, progesterone treatment restored their reduced expression levels after injury. A particularly important observation was the increase of brain-derived neurotrophic factor (BDNF) mRNA and protein by progesterone treatment in motoneurons of rats with spinal cord injury (Gonzalez et al. 2004). This growth factor may mediate some of the neuroprotective effects of progesterone, as BDNF has been shown to be neuroprotective for motoneurons undergoing degeneration and to rescue motoneurons from axotomy-induced cell death (Koliatsos et al. 1993; Sendtner et al. 1992; Yan et al. 1992; Ikeda et al. 1995; Tsuzaka et al. 2001).

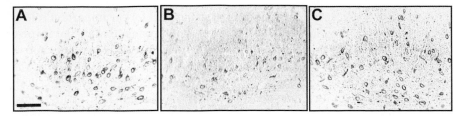

**Fig. 5.** Effect of transection (TRX) and progesterone treatment on 25-DX protein immunostaining in the male rat spinal cord. (**A**) Control spinal cord, (**B**) TRX spinal cord, (**C**) TRX + progesterone. After TRX, progesterone restored the number of immunolabeled cells to a level similar to control. Scale bar = 50 μm (adapted from Labombarda et al. 2003).

Of course, whether genes encoding BDNF and the other markers are direct targets of progesterone remains to be determined.

The neuroprotective effects of progesterone in the spinal cord may involve the B-isoform of the PR, which has been detected by immunocytochemistry in motoneurons of the ventral horn, in glial cells of gray and white matter and in ependymal cells of the male and female rat spinal cord (Labombarda et al. 2000b, 2003). Whether other PR isoforms are expressed and functional in the spinal cord remains to be determined. As shown by semi-quantitative RT-PCR, spinal cord PR mRNA was very abundant as it amounted to a third of that measured in the estrogen-stimulated uterus. After complete spinal cord transection, levels of PR mRNA were significantly decreased and remained low after treatment of the lesioned rats with progesterone (Fig. 4A; Labombarda et al. 2003).

In addition to the nuclear PR, the neuroprotective effects of progesterone are likely to involve other signalling mechanisms. Thus, the rat homologue of the putative progesterone membrane receptor cloned from porcine liver, 25-Dx protein, is also expressed in the rat spinal cord (Labombarda et al. 2003). In contrast to the widespread localization of PR-B, present in neurons and glial cells, immunostaining of 25-Dx protein was exclusively neuronal, showing a preferential staining of neurons in the dorsal horns and around the central canal. As expected for a putative membrane receptor of progesterone, 25-Dx protein localized to the cell membrane. Therefore, both the cellular and subcellular distributions of PR-B and 25-Dx protein in the spinal cord are very different. Moreover, the regulation of their expression is dissimilar: whereas PR mRNA levels were reduced after spinal cord injury and were not influenced by progesterone, 25-Dx protein mRNA levels remained unchanged in response to injury and were upregulated by progesterone treatment in the lesioned spinal cord (Fig. 4B). The number of 25-Dx protein-positive neurons decreased after spinal cord transection and returned to control values after the administration of progesterone (Fig. 5; Labombarda et al. 2003). These results point to a new and important role for the putative progesterone membrane receptor 25-Dx in regenerative processes.

Results from a recent study provide further support for the important role of progesterone signalling mechanisms in the nervous system that do not involve the classical PR. In the mouse Schwann cell line MSC80, which does not express functional intracellular PR, a microarray analysis has indeed revealed that the progesterone analogue R5020 regulates the expression of multiple genes. Both R5020 and progesterone stimulated expression of the ChAT in MSC80 cells, which is one of the progesterone-sensitive markers of spinal motoneurons (Tomkiewicz et al. submitted for publication). This type of cell system provides an opportunity to study new signalling pathways of progesterone involved in neuroprotective and neuroregenerative processes.

## Neuroprotective effects of progesterone during spinal motoneuron degeneration

A recessive mutation on chromosome 11 results in the degeneration of motoneurons in the spinal cord and brain stem of the Wobbler mouse, making it a useful model for motoneuron diseases, including amyotrophic lateral sclerosis (ALS). The first manifestations of the disease are observed at two to three weeks of age in homozygous Wobbler mice (wr/wr) (Duchen and Strich 1968; Price et al. 1994). In two-month-old Wobbler mice, the loss of motoneurons, an increased number of vacuolated motoneurons and astrogliosis in the spinal cord are associated with severe clinical symptoms, including tremor, ambulatory difficulties and diminished muscle strength (Gonzalez Deniselle et al. 2001). At this stage, motoneurons do not die from apoptosis, but their pathology rather resembles the "type II" or "cytoplasmic form" of cell death, generally caused by oxidative stress and characterized by cytoplasmic vacuolation, damaged mitochondria, and dilatation of smooth endoplasmic reticulum cysternae, with a relative preservation of the cell nuclei (Clarke 1990).

After the treatment of two-month-old symptomatic Wobbler mice for only two weeks with subcutaneous pellets of progesterone, which produced constant high levels of the hormone, the neuropathological characteristics of spinal motoneurons were less severe, including a reduction of cell vacuolation and a better preservation of the mitochondria and endoplasmic reticulum. However, progesterone did not decrease the high number of glial fibrillary acidic protein-(GFAP) positive astrocytes in Wobbler mice. Most importantly, the progesterone treatment had a beneficial effect on muscle strength and on the survival rate of the animals. Thus, animals treated with progesterone were able to spent about three times longer on a vertical grid than control animals (Gonzalez Deniselle et al. 2002, 2003).

The effects of progesterone treatment on mRNA expression of the $\alpha3$ and $\beta1$subunits of the $Na^+/K^+$-ATPase were examined by in situ hybridization. In Wobbler motoneurons, the transcripts of both subunits were decreased, and their expression was restored by the two-week progesterone treatment

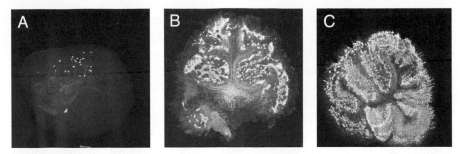

**Fig. 6.** Mifepristone prevents Purkinje cell death in organotypic slice cultures of rat cerebellum. Purkinje cells were labeled with an anti-calbindin antibody. (**A**) Only very few Purkinje cells survived in non-treated slices. Treatment of slices with 10 μM (**B**) or with 20 μM (**C**) of mifepristone allowed rescue of the neurons (adapted from Ghoumari et al. 2003a).

(Gonzalez Deniselle et al. 2002). In addition, the elevated expression of the growth-associated protein (GAP-43) mRNA, which is characteristic of Wobbler mice, was normalized by the progesterone treatment (Gonzalez Deniselle et al. 2002).

### Neuroprotective effects of mifepristone on cerebellar Purkinje cells.

A remarkable neuroprotective effect of mifepristone has been observed in cerebellar organotypic cultures, which appears to involve a novel mechanism of action. Explant cultures of cerebellar slices taken from P7 rats had previously allowed us to demonstrate a role for progesterone in CNS myelination (see above; Ghoumari et al. 2003b). As already mentioned, cerebellar Purkinje cells die by apoptosis if the explants are prepared from rat pups between P1 and P7 (Dusart et al. 1997; Ghoumari et al. 2002). Mifepristone, in a dose-dependent manner, allowed rescue of the Purkinje cells. In the absence of mifepristone, only very few Purkinje cells, immunopositively labelled for calbindin, were present in cerebellar slices taken from P3 pups (Fig. 6A). However, slices treated with 10 μM or 20 μM of mifepristone contained large numbers of Purkinje cells (Fig. 6B,C; Ghoumari et al. 2003a).

Mifepristone is a mixed antagonist/agonist for the PR and an antagonist for the glucocorticoid receptor (GR), but these receptors were obviously not involved in these neuroprotective effects. A role of the PR was excluded because progesterone and the selective PR agonist R5020 had no effect. Moreover, the protective effect of mifepristone was not influenced by the presence of progesterone in the culture medium. These observations were corroborated by the finding that mifepristone also exerted its neuroprotective effects in cerebellar slices prepared from homozygous PRKO mice (Ghoumari et al. 2003a). By using a similar experimental approach, a role for the GR could also be ruled out. The natural glucocorticoid in rodents, corticosterone, had no effect on Purkinje cell survival, and even at large concentrations, it did not inhibit the neuroprotective effects of mifepristone. Moreover, mifepristone exerted its neuroprotective effects in cerebellar explants from $GR^{Nes/Cre}$ mice, in which the GR is selectively inactivated in neurons and glial cells. These transgenic mice were prepared by using the Cre/LoxP system, with Cre expression being under the control of the nestin promoter/enhancer (Tronche et al. 1999).

The mechanism by which mifepristone promoted the survival of Purkinje cells is unknown. Previous studies have reported that mifepristone can protect against oxidative stress-induced neuronal death and against the oxidation of low-density lipoproteins (Behl et al. 1997; Parthasarathy et al. 1994). However, an antioxidant effect of mifepristone was unlikely to explain its protective effects on Purkinje cells, as several potent free-radical scavengers such as vitamin E, even at high concentrations, failed to prevent their apoptosis.

The neuroprotective effects of mifepristone are not limited to developmentally programmed cell death and could also be observed in pathological Purkinje cell death. Mifepristone also rescued Purkinje cells in organotypic cultures of cerebellar slices from pcd (Purkinje cell degeneration) mutant mice, a murine model of hereditary neurodegenerative ataxia (Ghoumari et al. 2003a). Thus, mifepristone may be a more general neuroprotective agent. A recent study has reported that pretreatment of rats with mifepristone prevented the loss of hippocampal neurons as long as 24 hours after TBI (McCullers et al. 2002). These findings, which were interpreted in terms of antiglucocorticoid effects of mifepristone, could involve alternative mechanisms of action. The novel mechanism by which mifepristone exerts its neuroprotective effects may also have implications for the use of mifepristone in the treatment of major depression and of neurodegenerative diseases such as Alzheimer's disease (Belanoff et al. 2001, 2002a,b).

## Conclusions

The classical paradigm of progesterone action involves binding of the steroid to a selective intracellular receptor and subsequent modulation of the transcription of specific target genes. This "genomic mechanism" of progesterone action remains a very intense field of research, in particular because of the recent discovery of novel PR isoforms and of nuclear coregulator proteins, which determine their transcriptional activities (Xu and O'Malley 2002). A perspective of these findings is a better understanding of the cell-specific actions of progestins and their analogs, which may be particularly relevant for the nervous system, where their pleiotropic effects differ between regions, cell types and physiopathological conditions. However, studies have so far mainly addressed the role of PR isoforms and of coregulators with respect to the reproductive functions of progesterone, and little is known concerning their functions in neurons and glial cells.

Research over the past years has also revealed the large diversity of signalling mechanisms of progestins, which not only involve intracellular PR isoforms but also neurotransmitter receptors and novel membrane receptors (mPR; Hammes 2003). Moreover, the intracellular PR is not only a ligand-dependent nuclear transcription factor; it directly interacts with cytoplasmic signalling proteins and is also targeted to the cell membrane. It can be expected that the PR exhibits distinct characteristics within different cell compartments the nucleus, the cytoplasm and the cell membrane. However, not all the rapid membrane effects of progestins can be explained by classical PRs translocated to the cell membrane. Within the nervous system, several neurotransmitter receptors mediate the rapid membrane actions of progesterone or of its metabolites, including $GABA_A$ receptors, the σ1-receptor and the nAChR. However, attempts to demonstrate direct binding of progestins to these receptors has not been successful so far, and it is possible that their effects may be mediated by accessory proteins. Several laboratories are trying to identify novel membrane receptors of progesterone (Lösel and Wehling 2003). A major breakthrough was the cloning of a novel family of mPRs, which belong to the G protein-coupled receptors (Zhu et al. 2003; Zhu and Thomas 2003).

An important issue of all these novel signalling mechanisms is the specificity and nature of progestin binding. The pharmacology of the different types of PRs may be very complex, thus providing opportunities for the development of novel ligands, which may manifest their biological activities in a specific manner depending on the cell and the physiopathological context, and which may demonstrate superior therapeutic profiles. Because of their use in contraception, in hormone replacement therapies and in the treatment of endocrine disorders, a variety of progestins are available for therapeutic applications. They differ widely in their chemical structures, structure-function relationships, metabolism, pharmacokinetics and potencies (Stanczyk 2003). SPRMs offer interesting possibilities in this regard because of their selective actions and pharmacological characteristics (Spitz 2003). These compounds could find interesting applications in protecting nerve cells, in promoting regenerative processes within the CNS and peripheral nerves and in the treatment of neurodegenerative and demyelinating diseases. These perspectives should motivate investigations of the molecular mechanisms by which progestins exert their neuroprotective and promyelinating effects in the nervous system.

## Acknowledgments

This work was partly supported by the International Agreement SEPCYT/ECOS between the Governments of France and Argentina (#A98SO1), the Commission of the European Communities (contract QLK6-CT-2000-00179), the "Myelin Project" (USA) and the "Projet Myéline" (France).

## References

Abdel-Hafiz H, Takimoto GS, Tung L, Horwitz KB (2002) The inhibitory function in human progesterone receptor N termini binds SUMO-1 protein to regulate autoinhibition and transrepression. J Biol Chem 277:33950-33956

Agarwala KL, Ganesh S, Amano K, Suzuki T, Yamakawa K (2001) DSCAM, a highly conserved gene in mammals, expressed in differentiating mouse brain. Biochem Biophys Res Commun 281:697-705

Apostolakis EM, Garai J, Fox C, Smith CL, Watson SJ, Clark JH, O'Malley BW (1996) Dopaminergic regulation of progesterone receptors: brain D5 dopamine receptors mediate induction of lordosis by D1-like agonists in rats. J Neurosci 16:4823-4834

Apostolakis EM, Ramamurphy M, Zhou D, Onate S, O'Malley BW (2002) Acute disruption of select steroid receptor coactivators prevents reproductive behavior in rats and unmasks genetic adaptation in knockout mice. Mol Endocrinol 16:1511-1523

Auger AP, Tetel MJ, McCarthy MM (2000) Steroid receptor coactivator-1 (SRC-1) mediates the development of sex-specific brain morphology and behavior. Proc Natl Acad Sci U S A 97:7551-7555

Auger AP, Perrot S, Auger CJ, Ekas LA, Tetel MJ, McCarthy MM (2002) Expression of the nuclear receptor coactivator, cAMP response element-binding protein, is sexually dimorphic and modulates sexual differentiation of neonatal rat brain. Endocrinology 143:3009-3016

Azcoitia I, Leonelli E, Magnaghi V, Veiga S, Garcia S, Melcangi RC (2003) Progesterone and its derivatives dihydroprogesterone and tetrahydroprogesterone reduce myelin fiber morphological abnormalities and myelin fiber loss in the sciatic nerve of aged rats. Neurobiol Aging 24:853-860

Bagowski CP, Myers JW, Ferrell JE (2001) The classical progesterone receptor associates with p42 MAPK and is involved in phosphatidylinositol 3-kinase signaling in Xenopus oocytes. J Biol Chem 276:37708-37714

Bai W, Rowan BG, Allgood VE, O'Malley BW, Weigel NL (1997) Differential phosphorylation of chicken progesterone receptor in hormone-dependent and ligand-independent activation. J Biol Chem 272:10457-10463

Balleine RL, Hunt SM, Clarke CL (1999) Coexpression of alternatively spliced estrogen and progesterone receptor transcripts in human breast cancer. J Clin Endocrinol Metab 84: 1370-1377

Barlow GM, Micales B, Lyons GE, Korenberg JR (2001) Down syndrome cell adhesion molecule is conserved in mouse and highly expressed in the adult mouse brain. Cytogenet Cell Genet 94:155-162

Bastianetto S, Monnet F, Junien JL, Quirion R (1999) Steroidal modulation of sigma receptor function. In: Baulieu EE, Robel P, Schumacher M (eds) Neurosteroids. A new regulatory function in the nervous system. Humana Press, Totowa, New Jersey, pp 191-205

Baulieu EE, Godeau JF, Schorderet M, Schorderet-Slatkine S (1978) Steroid induced meiotic division in Xenopus laevis oocytes: surface and calcium. Nature 275:593-598

Baulieu EE, Robel P, Schumacher M (2001) Neurosteroids: beginning of the story. Int Rev Neurobiol 46:1-32

Bayaa M, Booth RA, Sheng Y, Liu XJ (2000) The classical progesterone receptor mediates Xenopus oocyte maturation through a nongenomic mechanism. Proc Natl Acad Sci USA 97:12607-12612

Bayir H, Marion DW, Puccio AM, Wisniewski SR, Janesko KL, Clark RS, Kochanek PM (2004) Marked gender effect on lipid peroxidation after severe traumatic brain injury in adult patients. J Neurotrauma 21:1-8

Beaujean D, Do R, Galas L, Mensah N, Fredriksson R, Larhammar D, Fournier A, Luu T, Pelletier G, Vaudry H (2002) Neuropeptide Y inhibits the biosynthesis of sulfated neurosteroids in the hypothalamus through activation of Y(1) receptors. Endocrinology 143:1950-1963

Beck CA, Weigel NL, Moyer ML, Nordeen SK, Edwards DP (1993) The progesterone antagonist RU486 acquires agonist activity upon stimulation of cAMP signaling pathways. Proc Natl Acad Sci USA 90:4441-4445

Behl C, Trapp T, Skutella T, Holsboer F (1997) Protection against oxidative stress-induced neuronal cell death – a novel role for RU486. Eur J Neurosci 9:912-920

Belanoff JK, Flores BH, Kalezhan M, Sund B, Schatzberg AF (2001) Rapid reversal of psychotic depression using mifepristone. J Clin Psychopharmacol 21:516-521

Belanoff JK, Jurik J, Schatzberg LD, DeBattista C, Schatzberg AF (2002a) Slowing the progression of cognitive decline in Alzheimer's disease using mifepristone. J Mol Neurosci 19:201-206

Belanoff JK, Rothschild AJ, Cassidy F, DeBattista C, Baulieu EE, Schold C, Schatzberg AF (2002b) An open label trial of C-1073 (mifepristone) for psychotic major depression. Biol Psychiatry 52:386-392

Bergeron R, de Montigny C, Debonnel G (1996) Potentiation of neuronal NMDA response induced by dehydroepiandrosterone and its suppression by progesterone: effects mediated via sigma receptors. J Neurosci 16:1193-1202

Bergeron R, de Montigny C, Debonnel G (1999) Pregnancy reduces brain sigma receptor function. Br J Pharmacol 127:1769-1776

Betz AL, Coester HC (1990) Effects of steroid on edema and sodium uptake of the brain during focal ischemia in rats. Stroke 21:199-204

Beyer C, Damm N, Brito V, Küppers E (2002) Developmental expression of progesterone receptor isoforms in the mouse midbrain. Neuroreport 13:877-880

Blackmore PF, Beebe SJ, Danforth DR, Alexander N (1990) Progesterone and 17α-hydroxyprogesterone. Novel stimulators of calcium influx in human sperm. J Biol Chem 265:1376-1380

Boonyaratanakornkit V, Scott MP, Ribon V, Sherman L, Anderson SM, Maller JL, Miller WT, Edwards DP (2001) Progesterone receptor contains a proline-rich motif that directly interacts with SH3 domains and activates c-Src family tyrosine kinases. Mol Cell 8:269-280

Bousios S, Karandrea D, Kittas C, Kitraki E (2001) Effects of gender and stress on the regulation of steroid receptor coactivator-1 expression in the rat brain and pituitary. J Steroid Biochem Mol Biol 78:401-407

Bramley T (2003) Non-genomic progesterone receptors in the mammalian ovary: some unresolved issues. Reproduction 125:3-15

Buddhikot M, Falkenstein E, Wehling M, Meizel S (1999) Recognition of a human sperm surface protein involved in the progesterone-initiated acrosome reaction by antisera against an endomembrane progesterone binding protein from porcine liver. Mol Cell Endocrinol 158:187-193

Buisson B, Bertrand D (1999) Steroid modulation of the nicotinic acetylcholine receptor. In: Baulieu EE, Robel P, Schumacher M (eds) Neurosteroids. A new regulatory function in the nervous system. Humana Press, Totowa, pp 207-223

Camacho-Arroyo I, Perez-Palacios G, Pasapera AM, Cerbon MA (1994) Intracellular progesterone receptors are differentially regulated by sex steroid hormones in the hypothalamus and the cerebral cortex of the rabbit. J Steroid Biochem Mol Biol 50:299-303

Carlson JC, Gruber MY, Thompson JE (1983) A study of the interaction between progesterone and membrane lipids. Endocrinology 113:190

Cenedella RJ, Sexton PS, Zhu XL (1999) Lens epithelia contain a high-affinity, membrane steroid hormone-binding protein. Invest Ophthalmol Vis Sci 40:1452-1459

Cervantes M, Gonzalez-Vidal MD, Ruelas R, Escobar A, Morali G (2002) Neuroprotective effects of progesterone on damage elicited by acute global cerebral ischemia in neurons of the caudate nucleus. Arch Med Res 33:6-14

Chan JR, Phillips LJ, Glaser M (1998) Glucocorticoids and progestins signal the initiation and enhance the rate of myelin formation. Proc Natl Acad Sci USA 95:10459-10464

Chan JR, Rodriguez-Waitkus PM, Ng BK, Liang P, Glaser M (2000) Progesterone synthesized by Schwann cells during myelin formation regulates neuronal gene expression. Mol Biol Cell 11:2283-2295

Charlier TD, Balthazart J, Ball GF (2003) Sex differences in the distribution of the steroid receptor coactivator SRC-1 in the song control nuclei of male and female canaries. Brain Res 959:263-274

Chauchereau A, Amazit L, Quesne M, Guiochon M, Milgrom E (2003) Sumoylation of the progesterone receptor and of the steroid receptor coactivator SRC-1. J Biol Chem 278: 12335-12343

Choi DW (1993) Nitric oxide: foe or friend to te injured brain ? Proc Natl Acad Sci USA 90: 9741-9743

Clarke PGH (1990) Developmental cell death : morphological diversity and multiple mechanisms. Anat Embryol 181:195-213

Coirini H, Gouezou M, Liere P, Delespierre B, Pianos A, Eychenne B, Schumacher M, Guennoun R (2002) 3β-hydroxysteroid dehydrogenase expression in rat spinal cord. Neuroscience 113:883-891

Coirini H, Gouézou M, Delespierre B, Schumacher M, Guennoun R (2003a) 3β-hydroxysteroid dehydrogenase isomerase in the rat sciatic nerve: kinetic analysis and regulation by steroids. J Steroid Biochem Mol Biol 85:89-94

Coirini H, Gouezou M, Delespierre B, Liere P, Pianos A, Eychenne B, Schumacher M, Guennoun R (2003b) Characterization and regulation of the 3β-hydroxysteroid dehydrogenase isomerase enzyme in the rat sciatic nerve. J Neurochem 84:119-126

Conneely OM, Lydon JP (2000) Progesterone receptors in reproduction: functional impact of the A and B isoforms. Steroids 65:571-577

Conneely OM, Mulac J, DeMayo F, Lydon JP, O'Malley BW (2002) Reproductive functions of progesterone receptors. Recent Prog Horm Res 57:339-355

Conneely OM, Jericevic BM, Lydon JP (2003) Progesterone receptors in mammary gland development and tumorigenesis. J Mammary Gland Biol Neoplasia 8:205-214

Covey DF, Evers AS, Mennerick S, Zorumski CF, Purdy RH (2001) Recent developments in structure-activity relationships for steroid modulators of GABA(A) receptors. Brain Res Rev 37:91-97

Darbandi-Tonkabon R, Hastings WR, Zeng CM, Akk G, Manion BD, Bracamontes JR, Steinbach JH, Mennerick SJ, Covey DF, Evers AS (2003) Photoaffinity labeling with a neuroactive steroid analogue. 6-azi-pregnanolone labels voltage-dependent anion channel-1 in rat brain. J Biol Chem 278:13196-13206

Darbandi-Tonkabon R, Manion BD, Hastings WR, Craigen WJ, Akk G, Bracamontes JR, He Y, Sheiko TV, Steinbach JH, Mennerick SJ, Covey DF, Evers AS (2004) Neuroactive steroid interactions with voltage-dependent anion channels: lack of relationship to GABAA receptor modulation and anesthesia. J Pharmacol Exp Ther 308:502-511

De Nicola AF, Labombarda F, Gonzalez SL, Gonzalez Deniselle MC, Guennoun R, Schumacher M (2003) Steroid effects on glial cells: detrimental or protective for spinal cord injury? Ann N Y Acad Sci 1007:317-328.

Debonnel G, Bergeron R, de Montigny C (1996) Potentiation by dehydroepiandrosterone of the neuronal response to N-methyl-D-aspartate in the CA3 region of the rat dorsal hippocampus: an effect mediated via sigma receptors. J Endocrinol 150 Suppl:S33-S42

DeMarzo AM, Beck CA, Onate SA, Edwards DP (1991) Dimerization of mammalian progesterone receptors occurs in the absence of DNA and is related to the release of the 90-kDa heat shock protein. Proc Natl Acad Sci USA 88:72-76

DeMarzo AM, Onate SA, Nordeen SK, Edwards DP (1992) Effects of the steroid antagonist RU486 on dimerization of the human progesterone receptor. Biochemistry 31:10491-10501

Désarnaud F, Do T, Brown AM, Lemke G, Suter U, Baulieu EE, Schumacher M (1998) Progesterone stimulates the activity of the promoters of peripheral myelin protein-22 and protein zero genes in Schwann cells. J Neurochem 71:1765-1768

Dijkema R, Schoonen WG, Teuwen R, van der Struik E, de Ries RJ, van der Kar BA, Olijve W (1998) Human progesterone receptor A and B isoforms in CHO cells. I. Stable transfection of receptor and receptor-responsive reporter genes: transcription modulation by (anti)progestagens. J Steroid Biochem Mol Biol 64:147-156

Djebaili M, Hoffman SW, Stein DG (2004) Allopregnanolone and progesterone decrease cell death and cognitive deficits after contusion of the rat pre-frontal cortex. Neuroscience 123:349-359

Duchen LW, Strich SJ (1968) An hereditary motor neurone disease with progressive denervation of muscle in the mouse: the mutant 'wobbler'. J Neurol Neurosurg Psychiat 31:535-542

Dusart I, Airaksinen MS, Sotelo C (1997) Purkinje cell survival and axonal regeneration are age dependent: an in vitro study. J Neurosci 17:3710-3726

Edwards DP, Leonhardt SA, Gass H (2000) Novel mechanisms of progesterone antagonists and progesterone receptor. J Soc Gynecol Investig 7:S22-S24

Edwards DP, Wardell SE, Boonyaratanakornkit V (2003) Progesterone receptor interacting coregulatory proteins and cross talk with cell signaling pathways. J Steroid Biochem Mol Biol 83:173-186

Ekins S, Schuetz E (2002) The PXR crystal structure: the end of the beginning. Trends Pharmacol Sci 23:49-50

Falkenstein E, Meyer C, Eisen C, Scriba PC, Wehling M (1996) Full-length cDNA sequence of a progesterone membrane-binding protein from porcine vascular smooth muscle cells. Biochem Biophys Res Commun 229:86-89

Falkenstein E, Heck M, Gerdes D, Grube D, Christ M, Weigel M, Buddhikot M, Meizel S, Wehling M (1999) Specific progesterone binding to a membrane protein and related nongenomic effects on Ca2+-fluxes in sperm. Endocrinology 140:5999-6002

Fang X, Wong S, Mitchell BF (2002) Messenger RNA for progesterone receptor isoforms in the late-gestation rat uterus. Am J Physiol Endocrinol Metab 283:E1167-E1172

Ferrell JEJ (1999) Xenopus oocyte maturation: new lessons from a good egg. BioEssays 21:833-842

Finidori-Lepicard J, Schorderet-Slatkine S, Hanoune J, Baulieu EE (1981) Progesterone inhibits membrane-bound adenylate cyclase in Xenopus laevis oocytes. Nature 292:255

Frye CA (1995) The neurosteroid 3α,5α-THP has antiseizure and possible neuroprotective effects in an animal model of epilepsy. Brain Res 696:113-120

Garcia-Estrada J, Del Rio JA, Luquin S, Soriano E, Garcia-Segura LM (1993) Gonadal hormones down-regulate reactive gliosis and astrocyte proliferation after a penetrating brain injury. Brain Res 628:271-278

Gehin M, Mark M, Dennefeld C, Dierich A, Gronemeyer H, Chambon P (2002) The function of TIF2/GRIP1 in mouse reproduction is distinct from those of SRC-1 and p/CIP. Mol Cell Biol 22:5923-5937

Gerdes D, Wehling M, Leube B, Falkenstein E (1998) Cloning and tissue expression of two putative steroid membrane receptors. Biol Chem 379:907-911

Ghoumari AM, Dusart I, el-Etr M, Tronche F, Sotelo C, Schumacher M, Baulieu EE (2003a) Mifepristone (RU486) protects Purkinje cells from cell death in organotypic slice cultures of postnatal rat and mouse cerebellum. Proc Natl Acad Sci U S A 100:7953-7958

Ghoumari AM, Ibanez C, El E, Leclerc P, Eychenne B, O'Malley BW, Baulieu EE, Schumacher M (2003b) Progesterone and its metabolites increase myelin basic protein expression in organotypic slice cultures of rat cerebellum. J Neurochem 86:848-859

Ghoumari AM, Wehrle R, De Zeeuw CI, Sotelo C, Dusart I (2002) Inhibition of protein kinase C prevents Purkinje cell death but does not affect axonal regeneration. J Neurosci 22: 3531-3542

Giangrande PH, Pollio G, Mcdonnell DP (1997) Mapping and characterization of the functional domains responsible for the differential activity of the A and B isoforms of the human progesterone receptor. J Biol Chem 272:32889-32900

Giangrande PH, Mcdonnell DP (1999) The A and B isoforms of the human progesterone receptor: two functionally different transcription factors encoded by a single gene. Recent Prog Horm Res 54:291-314

Giangrande PH, Kimbrel EA, Edwards DP, Mcdonnell DP (2000) The opposing transcriptional activities of the two isoforms of the human progesterone receptor are due to differential cofactor binding. Mol Cell Biol 20:3102-3115

Giannoukos G, Szapary D, Smith CL, Meeker JE, Simons SS (2001) New antiprogestins with partial agonist activity: potential selective progesterone receptor modulators (SPRMs) and probes for receptor- and coregulator-induced changes in progesterone receptor induction properties. Mol Endocrinol 15:255-270

Glass CK, Rosenfeld MG (2000) The coregulator exchange in transcriptional functions of nuclear receptors. Genes Dev 14:121-141

Godeau JF, Schorderet-Slatkine S, Hubert P, Baulieu EE (1978) Induction of maturation in Xenopus laevis oocytes by a steroid linked to a polymer. Proc Natl Acad Sci USA 75:2353-2357

Gonzalez SL, Labombarda F, Gonzalez Deniselle MC, Guennoun R, Schumacher M, De Nicola AF (2004) Progesterone up-regulates neuronal brain-derived neurotrophic factor in the injured spinal cord. Neuroscience 125:605-614.

Gonzalez Deniselle MC, Gonzalez S, De Nicola AF (2001) Cellular basis of steroid neuroprotection in the Wobbler mouse, a model of motoneuron disease. Cell Mol Neurobiol 21:237-254

Gonzalez Deniselle MC, Lopez-Costa JJ, Saavedra JP, Pietranera L, Gonzalez SL, Garay L, Guennoun R, Schumacher M, De Nicola AF (2002) Progesterone neuroprotection in the wobbler mouse, a genetic model of spinal cord motor neuron disease. Neurobiol Dis 11: 457-468

Gonzalez Deniselle MC, Lopez Costa JJ, Gonzalez SL, Labombarda F, Garay L, Guennoun R, Schumacher M, De Nicola AF (2003) Basis of progesterone protection in spinal cord neurodegeneration. J Steroid Biochem Mol Biol 83:199-209

Gonzalez-Vidal MD, Cervera-Gaviria M, Ruelas R, Escobar A, Morali G, Cervantes M (1998) Progesterone : protective effects on the cat hippocampal neuronal damage due to acute global cerebral ischemia. Arch Med Res 29:117-124

Guennoun R, Fiddes RJ, Gouézou M, Lombès M, Baulieu EE (1995) A key enzyme in the biosynthesis of neurosteroids, $3\beta$-hydroxysteroid dehydrogenase/$\Delta 5$-$\Delta 4$-isomerase ($3\beta$-HSD), is expressed in rat brain. Brain Res Mol Brain Res 30:287-300

Guennoun R, Schumacher M, Robert F, Delespierre B, Gouézou M, Eychenne B, Akwa Y, Robel P, Baulieu EE (1997) Neurosteroids: expression of functional $3\beta$-hydroxysteroid dehydrogenase by rat sensory neurons and Schwann cells. Eur J Neurosci 9:2236-2247

Guerra-Araiza C, Coyoy-Salgado A, Camacho-Arroyo I (2002) Sex differences in the regulation of progesterone receptor isoforms expression in the rat brain. Brain Res Bull 59:105-109

Guerra-Araiza C, Villamar-Cruz O, Gonzalez-Arenas A, Chavira R, Camacho-Arroyo I (2003) Changes in progesterone receptor isoforms content in the rat brain during the oestrous cycle and after oestradiol and progesterone treatments. J Neuroendocrinol 15:984-990

Guiochon-Mantel A, Loosfelt H, Lescop P, Sar S, Atger M, Perrot-Applanat M, Milgrom E (1989) Mechanisms of nuclear localization of the progesterone receptor: evidence for interaction between monomers. Cell 57:1147-1154

Guiochon-Mantel A, Milgrom E (1993) Cytoplasmic-nuclear trafficking of steroid hormone receptors. Trends Endocrinol Metab 4:322-328

Guiochon-Mantel A (2000) Structure of the progesterone receptor and mode of action of progesterone. In: Sitruk-Ware R, Mishell DR (eds) Progestins and antiprogestins in clinical practice. Marcel Dekker, Basel, pp 1-13

Gutai JP, Meyer WJ, Kowarski AA, Migeon CJ (1977) Twenty-four hour integrated concentrations of progesterone, 17-hydroxyprogesterone and cortisol in normal male subjects. J Clin Endocrinol Metab 44:116-120

Hagihara K, Hirata S, Osada T, Hirai M, Kato J (1992) Distribution of cells containing progesterone receptor mRNA in the female rat di- and telencephalon: an in situ hybridization study. Brain Res Mol Brain Res 14:239-249

Hamano K, Iwasaki N, Takeya T, Takita H (1996) A quantitative analysis of rat central nervous system myelination using the immunohistochemical method for MBP. Brain Res Dev Brain Res 93:18-22

Hammes SR (2003) The further redefining of steroid-mediated signalling. Proc Natl Acad Sci USA 100:2168-2170

Hammond GL, Hirvonen J, Vihko R (1983) Progesterone, androstenedione, testosterone, 5α-dihydrotestosterone and androsterone concentrations in specific regions of the human brain. J Steroid Biochem 18:185-189

Hanner M, Moebius FF, Flandorfer A, Knaus HG, Striessnig J, Kempner E, Glossmann H (1996) Purification, molecular cloning, and expression of the mammalian sigma1-binding site. Proc Natl Acad Sci USA 93:8072-8077

Hernandez MC, Andres B, Holt I, Israel MA (1998) Cloning of human ENC-1 and evaluation of its expression and regulation in nervous system tumors. Exp Cell Res 242:470-477

Hirata S, Shoda T, Kato J, Hoshi K (2000) The novel isoform of the progesterone receptor cDNA in the human testis and detection of its mRNA in the human uterine endometrium. Oncology 59:39-44

Hirata S, Shoda T, Kato J, Hoshi K (2003a) Isoform/variant mRNAs for sex steroid hormone receptors in humans. Trends Endocrinol Metab 14:124-129

Hirata S, Shoda T, Kato J, Hoshi K (2003b) Novel isoforms of the mRNA for human female sex steroid hormone receptors. J Steroid Biochem Mol Biol 83:25-30

Hodges YK, Richer JK, Horwitz KB, Horwitz LD (1999) Variant estrogen and progesterone receptor messages in human vascular smooth muscle. Circulation 99:2688-2693

Horwitz KB, Sartorius CA, Hovland AR, Jackson TA, Groshong SD, Tung L, Takimoto GS (1995) Surprises with antiprogestins: novel mechanisms of progesterone receptor action. In: Bock GR, Goode JA (eds) Non reproductive actions of sex steroids (CIBA Foundation Symposium 191). John Wiley, Chichester, pp 235-253

Hovland AR, Powell RL, Takimoto GS, Tung L, Horwitz KB (1998) An N-terminal inhibitory function, IF, suppresses transcription by the A-isoform but not the B-isoform of human progesterone receptors. J Biol Chem 273:5455-5460

Ibanez C, Shields SA, Liere P, el-Etr M, Baulieu EE, Schumacher M, Franklin RJM (2004) Systemic progesterone administration results in a partial reversal of the age-associated decline in CNS remyelination following toxin-induced demyelination in male rats. Neuropathol Appl Neurobiol 30:80-89

Ikeda K, Klinkosz B, Greene T, Cedarbaum JM, Wong V, Lindsay RM, Mitsumoto H (1995) Effects of brain-derived neurotrophic factor on motor dysfunction in wobbler mouse motor neuron disease. Ann Neurol 37:505-511

Inoue T, Akahira JI, Takeyama J, Suzuki T, Darnel AD, Kaneko C, Kurokawa Y, Satomi S, Sasano H (2001) Spatial and topological distribution of progesterone receptor A and B isoforms during human development. Mol Cell Endocrinol 182:83-89

Inoue T, Akahira J, Suzuki T, Darnel AD, Kaneko C, Takahashi K, Hatori M, Shirane R, Kumabe T, Kurokawa Y, Satomi S, Sasano H (2002) Progesterone production and actions in the human central nervous system and neurogenic tumors. J Clin Endocrinol Metab 87:5325-5331

Jackson TA, Richer JK, Bain DL, Takimoto GS, Tung L, Horwitz KB (1997) The partial agonist activity of antagonist-occupied steroid receptors is controlled by a novel hinge domain-binding coactivator L7/SPA and the corepressors N-CoR or SMRT. Mol Endocrinol 11: 693-705

Jacobsen BM, Richer JK, Schittone SA, Horwitz KB (2002) New human breast cancer cells to study progesterone receptor isoform ratio effects and ligand-independent gene regulation. J Biol Chem 277:27793-27800

Jezierski MK, Sohrabji F (2001) Neurotrophin expression in the reproductively senescent forebrain is refractory to estrogen stimulation. Neurobiol Aging 22:311-321

Jiang N, Chopp M, Stein DG, Feldblum S (1996) Progesterone is neuroprotective after transient middle cerebral artery occlusion in male rats. Brain Res 735:101-107

Jung-Testas I, Schumacher M, Robel P, Baulieu EE (1996) Demonstration of progesterone receptors in rat Schwann cells. J Steroid Biochem Mol Biol 58:77-82

Jung-Testas I, Do-Thi A, Koenig H, Desarnaud F, Shazand K, Schumacher M, Baulieu EE (1999) Progesterone as a neurosteroid: synthesis and actions in rat glial cells. J Steroid Biochem Mol Biol 69:97-107

Kalkhoven E, Wissink S, van der Saag PT, Van der Burg B (1996) Negative interaction between the RelA(p65)subunit of NF-kB and the progesterone receptor. J Biol Chem 271:6217-6224

Kalra PS, Kalra SP (1977) Circadian periodicities of serum androgens, progesterone, gonadotropins and luteinizing hormone-releasing hormone in male rats: the effects of hypothalamic deafferentation, castration and adrenalectomy. Endocrinology 101:1821-1827

Kastner P, Krust A, Turcotte B, Stropp U, Tora L, Gronemeyer H, Chambon P (1990) Two distinct estrogen-regulated promoters generate transcripts encoding the two functionally different human progesterone receptor forms A and B. EMBO J 9:1603-1614

Kato J, Hirata S, Nozawa A, Mouri N (1993) The ontogeny of gene expression of progestin receptors in the female rat brain. J Steroid Biochem Mol Biol 47:173-182

Katzenellenbogen BS, Katzenellenbogen JA (2002) Defining the "S" in SERMs. Science 295: 2380-2381

Ke FC, Ramirez VD (1990) Binding of progesterone to nerve cell membranes of rat brain using progesterone conjugated to 125I-bovine serum albumin as a ligand. J Neurochem 54: 467-472

Kekuda R, Prasad PD, Fei YJ, Leibach FH, Ganapathy V (1996) Cloning and functional expression of the human type 1 sigma receptor (hSigmaR1). Biochem Biophys Res Commun 229:553-558

Kirkman-Brown JC, Barratt CLR, Publicover SJ (2003) Nifedipine reveals the existence of two discrete components of the progesterone-induced [Ca2+]i transient in human spermatozoa. Dev Biol 259:71-82

Kliewer SA, Moore JT, Wade L, Staudinger JL, Watson MA, Jones SA, McKee DD, Oliver BB, Willson TM, Zetterström RH, Perlmann T, Lehmann JM (1998) An orphan nuclear receptor activated by pregnanes defines a novel steroid signaling pathway. Cell 92:73-82

Kliewer SA, Goodwin B, Willson TM (2002) The nuclear pregnane X receptor: a key regulator of xenobiotic metabolism. Endocrinol Rev 23:687-702

Knotts TA, Orkiszewski RS, Cook RG, Edwards DP, Weigel NL (2001) Identification of a phosphorylation site in the hinge region of the human progesterone receptor and additional amino-terminal phosphorylation sites. J Biol Chem 276:8475-8483

Koenig HL, Schumacher M, Ferzaz B, Do Thi AN, Ressouches A, Guennoun R, Jung-Testas I, Robel P, Akwa Y, Baulieu EE (1995) Progesterone synthesis and myelin formation by Schwann cells. Science 268:1500-1503

Koliatsos VE, Clatterbuck RE, Winslow JW, Cayouette MH, Price DL (1993) Evidence that brain-derived neurotrophic factor is a trophic factor for motor neurons in vivo. Neuron 10:359-367

Kraus WL, Weis KE, Katzenellenbogen BS (1995) Inhibitory cross-talk between steroid hormone receptors: differential targeting of estrogen receptor in the repression of its transcriptional activity by agonist- and antagonist-occupied progestin receptors. Mol Cell Biol 15:1847-1857

Krebs CJ, Jarvis ED, Chan J, Lydon JP, Ogawa S, Pfaff DW (2000) A membrane-associated progesterone-binding protein, 25-Dx, is regulated by progesterone in brain regions involved in female reproductive behavior. Proc Natl Acad Sci USA 97:12816-12821

Labombarda F, Gonzalez S, Roig P, Lima A, Guennoun R, Schumacher M, De Nicola AF (2000a) Modulation of NADPH-diaphorase and glial fibrillary acidic protein by progesterone in astrocytes from normal and injured rat spinal cord. J Steroid Biochem Mol Biol 73:159-169

Labombarda F, Guennoun R, Gonzalez S, Roig P, Lima A, Schumacher M, De Nicola AF (2000b) Immunocytochemical evidence for a progesterone receptor in neurons and glial cells of the rat spinal cord. Neurosci Lett 288:29-32

Labombarda F, Gonzalez SL, Gonzalez DM, Guennoun R, Schumacher M, De Nicola AF (2002) Cellular basis for progesterone neuroprotection in the injured spinal cord. J Neurotrauma 19:343-355

Labombarda F, Gonzalez SL, Deniselle MC, Vinson GP, Schumacher M, De Nicola AF, Guennoun R (2003) Effects of injury and progesterone treatment on progesterone receptor and progesterone binding protein 25-Dx expression in the rat spinal cord. J Neurochem 87:902-913

Lambert JJ, Belelli D, Peden DR, Vardy AW, Peters JA (2003) Neurosteroid modulation of GABAA receptors. Prog Neurobiol 71:67-80

Landgren S, Wang MD, Bäckström T, Johansson S (1998) Interaction between 3α-hydroxy-5α-pregnan-20-one and carbachol in the control of neuronal excitability in hippocampal slices of female rats in defined phases of the oestrus. Acta Physiol Scand 162:77-88

Lauber AH, Romano GJ, Pfaff DW (1991) Gene expression for estrogen and progesterone receptor mRNAs in rat brain and possible relations to sexually dimorphic functions. J Steroid Biochem Mol Biol 40:53-62

Léna C, Changeux JP (1993) Allosteric modulations of the nicotinic acetylcholine receptor. Trends Neurosci 16:181-186

Leo C, Chen JD (2000) The SRC family of nuclear receptor coactivators. Gene 245:1-11

Leonhardt SA, Boonyaratanakornkit V, Edwards DP (2003) Progesterone receptor transcription and non-transcription signaling mechanisms. Steroids 68:761-770

Li X, O'Malley BW (2003) Unfolding the action of progesterone receptors. J Biol Chem 278: 39261-39264

Liu Z, Auboeuf D, Wong J, Chen JD, Tsai SY, Tsai MJ, O'Malley BW (2002) Coactivator/corepressor ratios modulate PR-mediated transcription by the selective receptor modulator RU486. Proc Natl Acad Sci U S A 99:7940-7944

Lösel R, Falkenstein E, Feuring M, Schultz A, Tillmann HC, Rossol H, Wehling M (2003) Nongenomic steroid action: controversies, questions, and answers. Physiol Rev 83:965-1016

Lösel R, Wehling M (2003) Nongenomic actions of steroid hormones. Nat Rev Mol Cell Biol 4:46-56

Luconi M, Bonaccorsi L, Bini L, Liberatori S, Pallini V, Forti G, Baldi E (2002) Characterization of membrane nongenomic receptors for progesterone in human spermatozoa. Steroids 67: 505-509

MacLusky NJ, McEwen BS (1980) Progestin receptors in rat brain: distribution and properties of cytoplasmic progestin-binding sites. Endocrinology 106:192-202

Magnaghi V, Cavarretta I, Zucchi I, Susani L, Rupprecht R, Hermann B, Martini L, Melcangi RC (1999) Po gene expression is modulated by androgens in the sciatic nerve of adult male rats. Mol Brain Res 70:36-44

Magnaghi V, Cavarretta I, Galbiati M, Martini L, Melcangi RC (2001) Neuroactive steroids and peripheral myelin proteins. Brain Res Rev 37:360-371

Maller JL (2001) The elusive progesterone receptor in Xenopus oocytes. Proc Natl Acad Sci USA 98:8-10

Mani SK, Allen JM, Clark JH, Blaustein JD, O'Malley BW (1994) Convergent pathways for steroid hormone- and neurotransmitter- induced rat sexual behavior. Science 265:1246-1249

Mani SK, Allen JM, Lydon JP, Mulac-Jericevic B, Blaustein JD, DeMayo FJ, Conneely O, O'Malley BW (1996) Dopamine requires the unoccupied progesterone receptor to induce sexual behavior in mice. Mol Endocrinol 10:1728-1737

Masuyama H, Hiramatsu Y, Mizutani Y, Inoshita H, Kudo T (2001) The expression of pregnane X receptor and its target gene, cytochrome P450 3A1, in perinatal mouse. Mol Cell Endocrinol 172:47-56

Matsumoto A (2002) Age-related changes in nuclear receptor coactivator immunoreactivity in motoneurons of the spinal nucleus of the bulbocavernosus of male rats. Brain Res 943: 202-205

McCann DJ, Weissman AD, Su TP (1994) Sigma-1 and sigma-2 sites in rat brain: comparison of regional, ontogenetic, and subcellular patterns. Synapse 17:182-189

McCullers DL, Sullivan PG, Scheff SW, Herman JP (2002) Mifepristone protects CA1 hippocampal neurons following traumatic brain injury in rat. Neuroscience 109:219-230

Mcdonnell DP, Goldman ME (1994) RU486 exerts antiestrogenic activities through a novel progesterone receptor A form-mediated mechanism. J Biol Chem 269:11945-11949

Mcdonnell DP, Shahbaz MM, Vegeto E, Goldman ME (1994) The human progesterone receptor A-form functions as a transcriptional modulator of mineralocorticoid receptor transcriptional activity. J Steroid Biochem Mol Biol 48:425-432

McKenna NJ, Lanz RB, O'Malley BW (1999) Nuclear receptor coregulators: cellular and molecular biology. Endocrinol Rev 20:321-344

Meijer OC, Steenbergen PJ, De K (2000) Differential expression and regional distribution of steroid receptor coactivators SRC-1 and SRC-2 in brain and pituitary. Endocrinology 141: 2192-2199

Melcangi RC, Magnaghi V, Cavarretta I, Martini L, Piva F (1998) Age-induced decrease of glycoprotein Po and myelin basic protein gene expression in the rat sciatic nerve. Repair by steroid derivatives. Neuroscience 85:569-578

Melcangi RC, Azcoitia I, Ballabio M, Cavarretta I, Gonzalez LC, Leonelli E, Magnaghi V, Veiga S, Garcia-Segura LM (2003) Neuroactive steroids influence peripheral myelination: a promising opportunity for preventing or treating age-dependent dysfunctions of peripheral nerves. Prog Neurobiol 71:57-66

Mellon SH, Vaudry H (2001) Biosynthesis of neurosteroids and regulation of their synthesis. Int Rev Neurobiol 46:33-78

Meyer C, Schmid R, Schmieding K, Falkenstein E, Wehling M (1998) Characterization of high affinity progesterone-binding membrane proteins by anti-peptide antiserum. Steroids 63:111-116

Meyer C, Schmid R, Scriba PC, Wehling M (1996) Purification and partial sequencing of high-affinity progesterone-binding site(s) from porcine liver membranes. Eur J Biochem 239: 726-731

Meyer ME, Pornon A, Ji J, Bocquel MT, Chambon P, Gronemeyer H (1990) Agonistic and antagonistic activities of RU486 on the function of the human progesterone receptor. EMBO J 9:3923-3932

Migliaccio A, Piccolo D, Castoria G, Di Domenico M, Bilancio A, Lombardi M, Gong W, Beato M, Auricchio F (1998) Activation of the Src/p21ras/Erk pathway by progesterone receptor via cross talk with estrogen receptor. EMBO J 17:2008-2018

Misao R, Sun WS, Iwagaki S, Fujimoto J, Tamaya T (1998) Identification of various exon-deleted progesterone receptor mRNAs in human endometrium and ovarian endometriosis. Biochem Biophys Res Commun 252:302-306

Misao R, Nakanishi Y, Sun WS, Iwagaki S, Fujimoto J, Tamaya T (2000) Identification of exon-deleted progesterone receptor mRNAs in human uterine endometrial cancers. Oncology 58:60-65

Misiti S, Schomburg L, Yen PM, Chin WW (1998) Expression and hormonal regulation of coactivator and corepressor genes. Endocrinology 139:2493-2500

Misrahi M, Venencie PY, Saugier-Veber P, Sar S, Dessen P, Milgrom E (1993) Structure of the human progesterone receptor gene. Biochem Biophys Acta 1216, 289-292

Mitev YA, Wolf SS, Almeida OF, Patchev VK (2003) Developmental expression profiles and distinct regional estrogen responsiveness suggest a novel role for the steroid receptor coactivator SRC-1 as a discriminative amplifier of estrogen signalling in the rat brain. FASEB J, express article 10.1096/fj.02-0513fge published online

Molenda HA, Griffin AL, Auger AP, McCarthy MM, Tetel MJ (2002) Nuclear receptor coactivators modulate hormone-dependent gene expression in brain and female reproductive behavior in rats. Endocrinology 143:436-444

Monnet FP, Mahe V, Robel P, Baulieu EE (1995) Neurosteroids, via sigma receptors, modulate the [3H]norepinephrine release evoked by N-methyl-D-aspartate in the rat hippocampus. Proc Natl Acad Sci USA 92:3774-3778

Moore LB, Maglich JM, McKee DD, Wisely B, Willson TM, Kliewer SA, Lambert MH, Moore JT (2002) Pregnane X receptor (PXR), constitutive androstane receptor (CAR), and benzoate X receptor (BXR) define three pharmacologically distinct classes of nuclear receptors. Mol Endocrinol 16:977-986

Morrow AL, VanDoren MJ, Fleming R, Penland S (2001) Ethanol and neurosteroid interactions in the brain. Int Rev Neurobiol 46:349-377

Mote PA, Balleine RL, McGowan EM, Clarke CL (1999) Colocalization of progesterone receptors A and B by dual immunofluorescent histochemistry in human endometrium during the menstrual cycle. J Clin Endocrinol Metab 84:2963-2971

Mote PA, Bartow S, Tran N, Clarke CL (2002) Loss of co-ordinate expression of progesterone receptors A and B is an early event in breast carcinogenesis. Breast Cancer Res Treat 72: 163-172

Mulac-Jericevic B, Mullinax RA, DeMayo FJ, Lydon JP, Conneely OM (2000) Subgroup of reproductive functions of progesterone mediated by progesterone receptor-B isoform. Science 289:1751-1754

Muller S, Hoege C, Pyrowolakis G, Jentsch S (2001) SUMO, ubiquitin's mysterious cousin. Nat Rev Mol Cell Biol 2:202-210

Muse ED, Jurevics H, Toews AD, Matsushima GK, Morell P (2001) Parameters related to lipid metabolism as markers of myelination in mouse brain. J Neurochem 76:77-86

Nishihara E, Yoshida-Komiya H, Chan CS, Liao L, Davis RL, O'Malley BW, Xu J (2003) SRC-1 null mice exhibit moderate motor dysfunctions and delayed development of cerebellar Purkinje cells. J Neurosci 23:213-222

Nordeen SK, Bona BJ, Moyer ML (1993) Latent agonist activity of the steroid antagonist, RU486, is unmasked in cells treated with activators of protein kinase A. Mol Endocrinol 7:731-742

Notterpek LM, Bullock PN, Malek H, Fisher R, Rome LH (1993) Myelination in cerebellar slice cultures: development of a system amenable to biochemical analysis. J Neurosci Res 36: 621-634

Ogata T, Nakamura Y, Tsuji K, Shibata T, Kataoka K (1993) Steroid hormones protect spinal cord neurons from glutamate toxicity. Neuroscience 55:445-449

Ogawa H, Nishi M, Kawata M (2001) Localization of nuclear coactivators p300 and steroid receptor coactivator 1 in the rat hippocampus. Brain Res 890:197-202

Ogle TF (2002) Progesterone-action in the decidual mesometrium of pregnancy. Steroids 67: 1-14

Ogle TF, Dai D, George P, Mahesh VB (1998) Regulation of the progesterone receptor and estrogen receptor in decidua basalis by progesterone and estradiol during pregnancy. Biol Reprod 58:1188-1198

Onate SA, Tsai SY, Tsai MJ, O'Malley BW (1995) Sequence and characterization of a coactivator for the steroid hormone receptor superfamily. Science 270:1354-1357

Onate SA, Boonyaratanakornkit V, Spencer TE, Tsai SY, Tsai MJ, Edwards DP, O'Malley BW (1998) The steroid receptor coactivator-1 contains multiple receptor interacting and activation domains that cooperatively enhance the activation function 1 (AF1) and AF2 domains of steroid receptors. J Biol Chem 273:12101-12108

Osman RA, Andria ML, Jones AD, Meizel S (1989) Steroid induced exocytosis: the human sperm acrosome reaction. Biochem Biophys Res Commun 160:828-833

Parthasarathy S, Morales AJ, Murphy AA (1994) Antioxidant: a new role for RU-486 and related compounds. J Clin Invest 94:1990-1995

Phan VL, Urani A, Romieu P, Maurice T (2002) Strain differences in sigma(1) receptor-mediated behaviours are related to neurosteroid levels. Eur J Neurosci 15:1523-1534

Poukka H, Karvonen U, Janne OA, Palvimo JJ (2000) Covalent modification of the androgen receptor by small ubiquitin-like modifier 1 (SUMO-1). Proc Natl Acad Sci U S A 97:14145-14150

Power RF, Conneely OM, O'Malley BW (1992) New Insights into Activation of the Steroid Hormone Receptor Superfamily. Trends Pharmacol Sci 13:318-323

Prasad PD, Li HW, Fei YJ, Ganapathy ME, Fujita T, Plumley LH, Yang-Feng TL, Leibach FH, Ganapathy V (1998) Exon-intron structure, analysis of promoter region, and chromosomal localization of the human type 1 sigma receptor gene. J Neurochem 70:443-451

Price DL, Cleveland DW, Koliatsos VE (1994) Motor neurone disease and animal models. Neurobiol Dis 1:3-11

Qiu M, Lange CA (2003) MAP kinases couple multiple functions of human progesterone receptors: degradation, transcriptional synergy, and nuclear association. J Steroid Biochem Mol Biol 85:147-157

Quirion R, Bowen WD, Itzhak Y, Junien JL, Musacchio JM, Rothman RB, Su TP, Tam SW, Taylor DP (1992) A proposal for the classification of sigma binding sites. Trends Pharmacol Sci 13:85-86

Raza FS, Takemori H, Tojo H, Okamoto M, Vinson GP (2001) Identification of the rat adrenal zona fasciculata/reticularis specific protein, inner zone antigen (IZAg), as the putative membrane progesterone receptor. Eur J Biochem 268:2141-2147

Reyna-Neyra A, Camacho-Arroyo I, Ferrera P, Arias C (2002) Estradiol and progesterone modify microtubule associated protein 2 content in the rat hippocampus. Brain Res Bull 58:607-612

Richer JK, Lange CA, Wierman AM, Brooks KM, Tung L, Takimoto GS, Horwitz KB (1998) Progesterone receptor variants found in breast cells repress transcription by wild-type receptors. Breast Cancer Res Treat 48:231-241

Richer JK, Jacobsen BM, Manning NG, Abel MG, Wolf DM, Horwitz KB (2002) Differential gene regulation by the two progesterone receptor isoforms in human breast cancer cells. J Biol Chem 277:5209-5218

Robel P, Schumacher M, Baulieu EE (1999) Neurosteroids : from definition and biochemistry to physiological function. In: Baulieu EE, Robel P, Schumacher M (eds) Neurosteroids. A new regulatory function in the nervous system. Humana Press, Totowa, pp 1-25

Robert F, Guennoun R, Desarnaud F, Do-Thi A, Benmessahel Y, Baulieu EE, Schumacher M (2001) Synthesis of progesterone in Schwann cells: regulation by sensory neurons. Eur J Neurosci 13:916-924

Robyr D, Wolffe AP, Wahli W (2000) Nuclear hormone receptor coregulators in action: diversity for shared tasks. Mol Endocrinol 14:329-347

Roof RL, Duvdevani R, Stein DG (1993) Gender influences outcome of brain injury: progesterone plays a protective role. Brain Res 607:333-336

Roof RL, Duvdevani R, Braswell L, Stein DG (1994) Progesterone facilitates cognitive recovery and reduces secondary neuronal loss caused by cortical contusion injury in male rats. Exp Neurol 129:64-69

Roof RL, Duvdevani R, Heyburn JW, Stein DG (1996) Progesterone rapidly decreases brain edema: treatment delayed up to 24 hours is still effective. Exp Neurol 138:246-251

Roof RL, Hoffman SW, Stein DG (1997) Progesterone protects against lipid peroxidation following traumatic brain injury in rats. Mol Chem Neuropathol 31:1-11

Rousseau-Merck MF, Misrahi M, Loosfelt H, Milgrom E, Berger R (1987) Localization of the human progesterone receptor gene to chromosome 11q22-q23. Hum Genet 77:280-282

Rowan BG, O'Malley BW (2000) Progesterone receptor coactivators. Steroids 65:545-549

Rowan BG, Garrison N, Weigel NL, O'Malley BW (2000) 8-Bromo-cyclic AMP induces phosphorylation of two sites in SRC-1 that facilitate ligand-independent activation of the chicken progesterone receptor and are critical for functional cooperation between SRC-1 and CREB binding protein. Mol Cell Biol 20:8720-8730

Saner KJ, Welter BH, Zhang F, Hansen E, Dupont B, Wei Y, Price TM (2003) Cloning and expression of a novel, truncated, progesterone receptor. Mol Cell Endocrinol 200:155-163

Sartorius CA, Tung L, Takimoto GS, Horwitz KB (1993) Antagonist-Occupied Human Progesterone Receptors Bound to DNA Are Functionally Switched to Transcriptional Agonists by cAMP. J Biol Chem 268:9262-9266

Sartorius CA, Melville MY, Hovland AR, Tung L, Takimoto GS, Horwitz KB (1994) A third transactivation function (AF3) of human progesterone receptors located in the unique N-terminal segment of the B- isoform. Mol Endocrinol 8:1347-1360

Schmidt BM, Gerdes D, Feuring M, Falkenstein E, Christ M, Wehling M (2000) Rapid, nongenomic steroid actions: A new age? Front Neuroendocrinol 21:57-94

Schumacher M, Coirini H, Robert F, Guennoun R, el-Etr M (1999) Genomic and membrane actions of progesterone: implications for reproductive physiology and behavior. Behav Brain Res 105:37-52

Schumacher M, Guennoun R, Mercier G, Desarnaud F, Lacor P, Benavides J, Ferzaz B, Robert F, Baulieu EE (2001) Progesterone synthesis and myelin formation in peripheral nerves. Brain Res Rev 37:343-359

Schumacher M, Robert F (2002) Progesterone : synthesis, metabolism, mechanisms of action and effects in the nervous system. In: Pfaff D, Arnold A, Etgen A, Fahrbach S, Rubin R (eds) Hormones, Brain and Behavior (vol. 3). Academic Press, San Diego, pp 683-745

Selmin O, Lucier GW, Clark GC, Tritscher AM, Vanden Heuvel JP, Gastel JA, Walker NJ, Sutter TR, Bell DA (1996) Isolation and characterization of a novel gene induced by 2,3,7,8-tetrachlorodibenzo-p-dioxin in rat liver. Carcinogenesis 17:2609-2615

Sendtner M, Holtmann B, Kolbeck R, Thoenen H, Barde YA (1992) Brain-derived neurotrophic factor prevents the death of motoneurons in newborn rats after nerve section. Nature 360: 757-759

Sereda MW, Meyer Z, Suter U, Uzma N, Nave KA (2003) Therapeutic administration of progesterone antagonist in a model of Charcot-Marie-Tooth disease (CMT-1A). Nat Med 9:1533-1537

Seth P, Fei YJ, Li HW, Huang W, Leibach FH, Ganapathy V (1998) Cloning and functional characterization of a sigma receptor from rat brain. J Neurochem 70:922-931

Seyle H (1942) The anatgonism between anesthetic steroid hormones and pentamethylenetetrazol (metrazol). J Lab Clin Med 27:1051-1053

Shi QX, Yuan YY, Roldan ER (1997) gamma-Aminobutyric acid (GABA) induces the acrosome reaction in human spermatozoa. Mol Hum Reprod 3:677-683

Shiozawa T, Shih HC, Miyamoto T, Feng YZ, Uchikawa J, Itoh K, Konishi I (2003) Cyclic changes in the expression of steroid receptor coactivators and corepressors in the normal human endometrium. J Clin Endocrinol Metab 88:871-878

Shyamala G, Yang X, Silberstein G, Barcellos H, Dale E (1998) Transgenic mice carrying an imbalance in the native ratio of A to B forms of progesterone receptor exhibit developmental abnormalities in mammary glands. Proc Natl Acad Sci USA 95:696-701

Shyamala G, Yang X, Cardiff RD, Dale E (2000) Impact of progesterone receptor on cell-fate decisions during mammary gland development. Proc Natl Acad Sci USA 97:3044-3049

Simons SS (2003) The importance of being varied in steroid receptor transactivation. Trends Pharmacol Sci 24:253-259

Smith SS (1991) Progesterone administration attenuates excitatory amino acid responses of cerebellar Purkinje cells. Neuroscience 42:309-320

Spencer TE, Jenster G, Burcin MM, Allis CD, Zhou J, Mizzen CA, McKenna NJ, Onate SA, Tsai SY, Tsai MJ, O'Malley BW (1997) Steroid receptor coactivator-1 is a histone acetyltransferase. Nature 389:194-198

Spitz IM (2003) Progesterone antagonists and progesterone receptor modulators : an overview. Steroids 68:981-993

Stanczyk FZ (2003) All progestins are not created equal. Steroids 68:879-890

Stein DG (2001) Brain damage, sex hormones and recovery : a new role for progesterone and estrogen? Trends Neurosci 24:386-391

Su TP, London ED, Jaffe JH (1988) Steroid binding at s receptors suggests a link between endocrine, nervous, and immune systems. Science 240:219-221

Suzuki Y, Shimozawa N, Imamura A, Kondo N, Orii T (1996) Peroxisomal disorders: clinical aspects. Ann NY Acad Sci 804:442-449

Szabo M, Kilen SM, Nho SJ, Schwartz NB (2000) Progesterone receptor A and B messenger ribonucleic acid levels in the anterior pituitary of rats are regulated by estrogen. Biol Reprod 62:95-102

Takimoto GS, Tung L, Abdel H, Abel MG, Sartorius CA, Richer JK, Jacobsen BM, Bain DL, Horwitz KB (2003) Functional properties of the N-terminal region of progesterone receptors and their mechanistic relationship to structure. J Steroid Biochem Mol Biol 85: 209-219

Thomas AJ, Nockels RP, Pan HQ, Shaffrey CI, Chopp M (1999) Progesterone is neuroprotective after acute experimental spinal cord trauma in rats. Spine 24:2134-2138

Tischkau SA, Ramirez VD (1993) A specific membrane binding protein for progesterone in rat brain: sex differences and induction by estrogen. Proc Natl Acad Sci U S A 90:1285-1289

Tronche F, Kellendonk C, Kretz O, Gass P, Anlag K, Orban PC, Bock R, Klein R, Schütz G (1999) Disruption of the glucocorticoid receptor gene in the nervous system results in reduced anxiety. Nat Genet 23:99-103

Tsai MJ, O'Malley BW (1994) Molecular mechanisms of action of steroid/thyroid receptor superfamily members. Annu Rev Biochem 63:451-486

Tsuzaka K, Ishiyama T, Pioro EP, Mitsumoto H (2001) Role of brain-derived neurotrophic factor in wobbler mouse motor neuron disease. Muscle Nerve 24:474-480

Tyagi RK, Amazit L, Lescop P, Milgrom E, Guiochon-Mantel A (1998) Mechanisms of progesterone receptor export from nuclei: role of nuclear localization signal, nuclear export signal, and ran guanosine triphosphate. Mol Endocrinol 12:1684-1695

Ukena K, Kohchi C, Tsutsui K (1999) Expression and activity of 3β-hydroxysteroid dehydrogenase/Δ5-Δ4-isomerase in the rat Purkinje neuron during neonatal life. Endocrinology 140:805-813

Valera S, Ballivet M, Bertrand D (1992) Progesterone modulates a neuronal nicotinic acetylcholine receptor. Proc Natl Acad Sci USA 89:9949-9953

Vegeto E, Shahbaz MM, Wen DX, Goldman ME, O'Malley BW, Mcdonnell DP (1993) Human progesterone receptor A form is a cell- and promoter-specific repressor of human progesterone receptor B function. Mol Endocrinol 7:1244-1255

Wagner AK, Bayir H, Ren D, Puccio AM, Zafonte RD, Kochanek PM (2004) Relationship between cerebrospinal fluid markers of excitotoxicity, ischemia, and oxidative damage after severe TBI: the impact of gender, age and hypothermia. J Neurotrauma 21:125-136

Wagner BL, Norris JD, Knotts TA, Weigel NL, Mcdonnell DP (1998) The nuclear corepressors NCoR and SMRT are key regulators of both ligand- and 8-bromo-cyclic AMP-dependent transcriptional activity of the human progesterone receptor. Mol Cell Biol 18:1369-1378

Wardell SE, Boonyaratanakornkit V, Adelman JS, Aronheim A, Edwards DP (2002) Jun dimerization protein 2 functions as a progesterone receptor N-terminal domain coactivator. Mol Cell Biol 22:5451-5466

Watkins RE, Wisely GB, Moore LB, Collins JL, Lambert MH, Williams SP, Willson TM, Kliewer SA, Redinbo MR (2001) The human nuclear xenobiotic receptor PXR: structural determinants of directed promiscuity. Science 292:2329-2333

Watkins RE, Davis S, Lambert MH, Redinbo MR (2003) Coactivator binding promotes the specific interaction between ligand and the pregnane X receptor. J Mol Biol 331:815-828

Wei LL, Hawkins P, Baker C, Norris B, Sheridan PL, Quinn PG (1996) An amino-terminal truncated progesterone receptor isoform, PRc, enhances progestin-induced transcriptional activity. Mol Endocrinol 10:1379-1387

Weigel NL (1996) Steroid hormone receptors and their regulation by phosphorylation. Biochem J 319:657-667

Weill-Engerer S, David JP, Sazdovitch V, Liere P, Eychenne B, Pianos A, Schumacher M, Delacourte A, Baulieu EE, Akwa Y (2002) Neurosteroid quantification in human brain regions : comparison between Alzheimer's and non-demented patients. J Clin Endocrinol Metab 87:5138-5143

Wen DX, Xu YF, Mais DE, Goldman ME, Mcdonnell DP (1994) The A and B isoforms of the human progesterone receptor operate through distinct signaling pathways within target cells. Mol Cell Biol 14:8356-8364

Xu J, Qiu Y, DeMayo FJ, Tsai SY, Tsai MJ, O'Malley BW (1998) Partial hormone resistance in mice with disruption of the steroid receptor coactivator-1 (SRC-1) gene. Science 279: 1922-1925

Xu J, O'Malley BW (2002) Molecular mechanisms and cellular biology of the steroid receptor coactivator (SRC) family in steroid receptor function. Rev Endocr Metab Disord 3:185-192

Yan Q, Elliott J, Snider WD (1992) Brain-derived neurotrophic factor rescues spinal motor neurons from axotomy-induced cell death. Nature 360:753-755

Yang J, Serres C, Philibert D, Robel P, Baulieu EE (1994) Progesterone and RU486: opposing effects on human sperm. Proc Natl Acad Sci USA 91:529-533

Yeates C, Hunt SM, Balleine RL, Clarke CL (1998) Characterization of a truncated progesterone receptor protein in breast tumors. J Clin Endocrinol Metab 83:460-467

Yu WH (1989) Survival of motoneurons following axotomy is enhanced by lactation or by progesterone treatment. Brain Res 491:379-382

Zhang X, Jeyakumar M, Petukhov S, Bagchi MK (1998) A nuclear receptor corepressor modulates transcriptional activity of antagonist-occupied steroid hormone receptor. Mol Endocrinol 12:513-524

Zhu Y, Thomas P (2003) Identification, classification, and partial characterization of genes in humans and other vertebrates homologous to a fish membrane progestin receptor. Proc Natl Acad Sci USA 100:2237-2242

Zhu Y, Rice CD, Pang Y, Pace M, Thomas P (2003) Cloning, expression, and characterization of a membrane progestin receptor and evidence it is an intermediary in meiotic maturation of fish oocytes. Proc Natl Acad Sci USA 100:2231-2236

# Rapid Effects of Estradiol on Motivated Behaviors

*Jill B. Becker\**

## Summary

Estradiol can act extracellularly to rapidly enhance dopamine (DA) activity in striatum and nucleus accumbens (NAcc) as well as the behavioral response to psychomotor stimulants. Considerable research has demonstrated that the effects of estradiol on behavioral and neurochemical indices of DA activity in the striatum are found in female but not male rats. Furthermore, natural variation in circulating hormones modulates this neural system. During naturally occurring behavioral estrus, amphetamine (AMPH)-induced striatal DA release and AMPH-induced behaviors are potentiated relative to other days of the estrous cycle. Ovariectomy (OVX) attenuates, whereas estradiol treatment in OVX rats rapidly enhances, striatal DA release and behaviors that are thought to be mediated by striatal DA activity. Estradiol has similar effects on dopamine activity in the NAcc.

Sex differences in, and hormonal influences on, the ascending DA system have implications for drug abuse. In adult rats, there are sex differences in the rate of behavioral sensitization to cocaine and in the acquisition of cocaine self-administration behavior. These sex differences occur independent of circulating gonadal hormones: OVX females exhibit greater sensitization and more rapid onset of cocaine self-administration than do castrated males. Furthermore, estradiol treatment to OVX females, but not to castrated male rats, enhances both sensitization and acquisition of cocaine self-administration. We postulate that hormonal modulation of this pathway evolved because of its role in the motivation to engage in sexual behavior, since extracellular dopamine increases during sexual behavior in the female rat. A model is proposed to describe the mechanism through which estradiol enhances stimulated DA release.

\* Psychology Department Neuroscience Program and Reproductive Sciences Program, University of Michigan, Ann Arbor, MI 48109

Kordon et al.
Hormones and the Brain
© Springer-Verlag Berlin Heidelberg 2005

## Introduction

The pattern of cocaine use and onset of addiction to cocaine is more rapid in women than in men (Lynch and Carroll 1999). Women begin using cocaine and enter treatment at earlier ages than men (Griffin et al. 1989; Mendelson et al. 1991) and have more severe cocaine use at intake than men (Kosten et al. 1993). Furthermore, cocaine cues induce more drug craving in female than male addicts (Robbins et al. 1999). Among women who have used cocaine (approximately 9% of the population of the USA), the prevalence of lifetime dependence for cocaine is 14.9±2.0% (mean ±S.D.). This finding is in contrast to alcohol, where 79% have used alcohol but only 9.2±0.8% have developed lifetime dependence (Kandel et al. 1995). The use of all illicit drugs has been increasing among women in the past decade, and cocaine dependence among women, in particular, is a growing public health concern in the USA (Wetherington and Roman 1995; Lynch et al. 2002). Recent trends in drug-taking behavior, therefore, suggest that women may be more sensitive to the addictive properties of cocaine than men. To begin to understand the neurobiological bases of sex differences in drug abuse, this review will discuss research on the role of sex-related differences and the influence of ovarian hormones on the neurochemical and behavioral responses to acute and repeated exposure to the psychomotor stimulants, cocaine and amphetamine (AMPH). Data from this laboratory indicate that these sex-related differences may be due, at least in part, to the effect of the ovarian hormone, estradiol, on the neural systems that mediate motivated behaviors. The possible mechanisms through which ovarian hormones induce these effects will be discussed.

The issues involved are complex. First, adult males and females do not differ solely in their genetic composition but also in the hormones secreted by their gonads and the patterns of hormone secretion (i.e., females exhibit a cyclic release of estradiol and progesterone, whereas males exhibit a tonic release of testosterone). These patterns of hormone release are a consequence of hormone exposure during sexual differentiation of the brain. Thus there are three different ways that males and females can be different: 1) sex differences independent of circulating gonadal hormones in the adult, due to sex differences in the organization of the brain caused by hormonal and/or genetic signals; 2) sex differences in the functional effects of gonadal hormones acting on a sexually dimorphic brain; and 3) actions of gonadal hormones on brain and behavior that are different because males and females produce different hormones.

In addition to the complexity of investigating when gonadal hormones act on the brain to impact behavior (i.e., during development or in the adult), the mechanisms through which, in the adult, they exert their effects on the behavioral and neurochemical responses to the psychomotor stimulants are novel. Estradiol appears to be acting on a membrane-associated receptor in the nucleus accumbens (NAcc) and the striatum to influence dopaminergic neurotransmission. Not only is the mechanism novel but also these areas of the brain are not typically thought of as targets for gonadal steroid hormones.

Dopamine (DA) neurons in the midbrain ventral tegmental area and substantia nigra project to the NAcc and the striatum in the forebrain, respectively. These brain regions are involved in the initiation and control of sensorimotor behavior, learning and memory, and in motivated behaviors. The acute stimulation of the ascending DA systems by DA agonists produces behavioral activation. For example, treatment with a low dose of the indirect agonist AMPH or the direct agonist apomorphine induces locomotion and exploratory behavior. With higher doses of these drugs, the locomotor phase is followed by a phase in which the animal or individual exhibits "stereotyped behaviors." These stereotyped behaviors in rodents include repetitive movements of the head and forelimbs and are thought to be due to activation of the striatal DA system along with increased DA activity in the NAcc and olfactory tubercle. The systemic administration of AMPH results in a behavioral syndrome that is predominantly mediated by the activity of DA in the striatum and NAcc. This effect has been demonstrated in experiments in which these DA systems are either lesioned or blocked pharmacologically (e.g., Arbuthnott and Crow 1971; Ungerstedt 1971; Costall and Naylor 1977; Fink and Smith 1980). By contrast, treatment with DA antagonists such as chlorpromazine or haloperidol results in reduced locomotor activity and, at high doses, catalepsy (Fog 1972). It is the role of these DA projections in motivation, however, that has contributed to our understanding of the neural basis of sexual motivation, motivation to take drugs and other motivated behaviors (Meisel et al. 1993; Fiorino and Phillips 1999; Becker et al. 2001b; Robinson and Berridge 2001; Hu et al. 2003). As you will see, behaviors mediated by the ascending DA systems in the brain are sexually dimorphic. Furthermore, in females, behaviors that are mediated by the ascending DA systems are modulated by ovarian hormones.

## Sex-related differences in striatum and NAcc

The acute behavioral response to psychomotor stimulants in rats reflects sex-related differences and is modulated differentially by gonadal hormones in males and females (for review, see Becker 1999). Intact female rats show more intense and prolonged stereotyped behavior after AMPH or apomorphine administration than do males (Beatty et al. 1982; Hruska and Pitman 1982). They also exhibit a greater decrease in activity in response to chlorpromazine or haloperidol (Mislow and Freidhoff 1973; Beatty and Holzer 1978) and greater AMPH-stimulated rotational behavior than do males (Robinson et al. 1980). While male rats metabolize some drugs more rapidly than do females, the sex difference in rotational behavior persists even when brain levels of AMPH are equivalent (Becker et al. 1982). This finding suggests that, while most reported sex differences in response to AMPH may be greater in magnitude than would be found if concentrations were equalized, there are sex-related differences in the organization of the striatal DA system. This idea is supported by research on sex differences in the behavioral response to cocaine, where males and females experience equivalent brain concentrations of cocaine after systemic administration (Bowman et al., 1999), but female rats exhibit greater locomotor activation in response to cocaine than do male rats under certain testing conditions (e.g., van Haaren and Meyer 1991; Walker et al., 2001).

In addition to sex differences in the behavioral response to psychomotor stimulants, there are more D1 DA receptors in the striatum of male rats than in intact female or ovariectomized (OVX) female rats, but no sex difference in striatal D2 DA receptors (Hruska et al. 1982; Levesque and Di Paolo 1988). There are, however, sex-related differences in the effect of estradiol on D2 DA receptors, where estradiol rapidly down-regulates D2 DA receptor binding in striatum of females but not males (Bazzett and Becker 1994). When DA release from striatal tissue is studied in vitro, the AMPH-stimulated increase in DA efflux is comparable for tissue from intact male rats and intact female rats in estrus (Becker and Ramirez 1981b). Nevertheless, in the absence of gonadal hormones, the AMPH-induced increase in striatal DA release from striatal tissue from OVX females in vitro is significantly less than the response of tissue from castrated (CAST) males (Becker and Ramirez 1981b). Furthermore, results from in vivo microdialysis studies in freely moving rats have found that the basal extracellular concentrations of DA are twice as high in striatum of CAST males as in OVX females (Xiao and Becker 1994). These sex-related differences in striatal DA release and DA receptor binding reflect an underlying sexual dimorphism in the organization of the striatum.

**Females.** It is well known that estradiol and progesterone influence neural activity in the female rat, so that when confronted by a sexually active male rat, lordosis behavior is exhibited. The female rat will not exhibit lordosis in the absence of appropriate activating stimuli (McCarthy and Becker 2002). Similarly, estradiol treatment does not directly activate locomotor activity or DA release, but given the proper environment (e.g., a running wheel) or drug treatment, estradiol enhances the behavioral response that is induced.

During the four-day estrous cycle of the female rat, circulating estradiol is low during diestrus 1 and increases gradually during diestrus 2. The endogenous surges of estradiol and progesterone occur on the afternoon of the next day (proestrus) and are followed 6-12 hours later by the onset of behavioral estrus (estrus). Female rats show a greater behavioral response to striatal DA activation on the evening of behavioral estrus (6-12 hours after the surges of estradiol and progesterone) than 24 hours later on diestrus; neurochemical markers of DA activity are also elevated at this time (for summary, see Becker 1999). In addition, during naturally occurring behavioral estrus, AMPH-induced

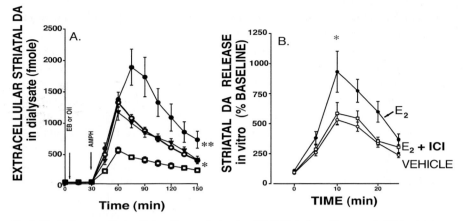

**Fig. 1.** The influence of estradiol on the amphetamine (AMPH)-induced increase in DA in striatum. **A.** The effect of estradiol benzoate (EB) with or without EB priming on the AMPH-induced (2.5 mg/kg) increase in DA in dialysate from dorsolateral striatum. DA concentrations are expressed in fmole/15 min sample (mean ± SEM). OVX female rats were treated with oil (open squares), 5 μg EB 30 min before AMPH (closed triangles), three treatments with 5 μg EB 72, 48, and 24 hr prior to dialysis + oil 30 min before AMPH (open circles), or three treatments with 5 μg EB 72, 48, and 24 hr prior to dialysis + 5 μg EB 30 min before AMPH (closed circles). **Rats that received EB PRIMED + EB showed significantly greater AMPH-induced DA in dialysate than all EB-treated groups for the entire two-hour period of sample collection (Overall ANOVA; p < 0.05). * EB PRIMED + OIL and OIL PRIMED + EB groups showed a greater increase (p < 0.05) in AMPH-induced DA in dialysate than did the OIL PRIMED + OIL. (Adapted from Becker and Rudick 1999). **B.** Effects of 370 pM ICI + 370 pM estradiol, 370 pM estradiol or vehicle on AMPH-induced striatal DA release. *$E_2$ enhanced AMPH-induced DA release and this was significantly greater than the response from the ICI+ $E_2$ (p<0.03) or the vehicle-treated groups (p<0.01). Bars indicate the SEM. (Methods: Striatal tissue obtained from OVX animals placed into superfusion chambers containing Ringer's solution. Following a 60-min stabilization period with Ringer's, three baseline samples were collected. The chambers were then assigned to one of three treatment groups: 1) 15-min infusion with ICI followed by 60-min infusion with a solution containing both ICI and E2; 2) 15-min infusion with Ringer's followed by 60-min infusion with $E_2$, and 3) 75-min infusion with vehicle (0.001% ethanol in Ringer's). Effluent samples were collected throughout the experiment at five-min intervals. A 2.5-min infusion of 10 μM $d$-AMPH was then delivered to all the chambers 45 min after collection of the baseline samples was initiated, in the presence of test or control compounds. All media were continually infused into the chambers at a flow rate of 100 μl/min and warmed to 37° C in a water bath prior to reaching the chambers. (Adapted from Xiao et al. 2003)

behaviors are potentiated relative to other days of the estrous cycle (Becker et al. 1982; Becker and Cha 1989).

To determine which hormones are influencing striatal DA activity during the estrous cycle, it is necessary to remove the endogenous sources of hormones (the ovaries) and then selectively replace estradiol and/or progesterone. Following OVX, rotational behavior is attenuated two to three weeks later (Robinson et al. 1981; Becker and Beer 1986; Camp et al. 1986). OVX also severely attenuates basal extracellular striatal DA concentrations (Xiao and Becker 1994) and AMPH-stimulated striatal DA release (Becker and Ramirez 1981a, b). Replacement with estradiol induces both rapid and long-term effects of estradiol on the striatum. The acute administration of estradiol to OVX rats induces a rapid increase in AMPH-induced striatal DA release, as detected by in vivo microdialysis (Fig. 1A; Becker 1990b; Castner and Becker 1990; Becker and Rudick 1999). In addition, prior treatment with estradiol enhances the effect of administering estradiol 30 min before giving AMPH (Becker and Rudick 1999). These effects on pre-synaptic DA activity are due to a direct effect of estradiol on the striatum, as physiological concentrations of estradiol in vitro enhance the AMPH-induced release of DA from striatal tissue in superfusion, whereas the estradiol-antagonist ICI 182,780 blocks this effect (Fig. 1B; Becker 1990a; Xiao et al. 2003). In cultured striatal neurons from embryonic mouse, estradiol induces changes in adenylate cyclase activity stimulated by D1 and D2 DA receptor agonists by apparently modifying the G-protein coupling process (Maus et al. 1989a, b). Furthermore, the pulsatile administration of physiological concentrations of estradiol to striatal slices directly stimulates DA release in vitro (Becker 1990a). Thus, estradiol acts directly on the striatum to induce changes in DA release and DA receptor activity.

Estradiol also acts directly on the NAcc to rapidly enhance $K^+$-stimulated DA release (Thompson and Moss 1994; Thompson et al. 2001). Local injection of 20-50 pg 17β-estradiol, but not 17α-estradiol, produces a rapid (within two minutes) and dramatic increase in stimulated DA overflow detected by in vivo voltammetry. Although there has been less research on estradiol DA interaction in the NAcc, the work of Thompson (Thompson and Moss 1995, 1997; Wong et al. 1996; Thompson, 1999; Thompson et al., 2000, 2001) suggests that the mechanism(s) mediating the effects of estradiol in the NAcc and striatum are similar.

Progesterone has also been shown to affect striatal DA release in tissue from estradiol-primed OVX rats (Dluzen and Ramirez 1984, 1987, 1989, 1990, 1991). Furthermore, after estradiol priming, a membrane-associated protein with high affinity for progesterone has been isolated from the striatum (Ke and Ramirez 1990). The effect of progesterone on striatal DA release is not seen without estradiol priming; neither are the progesterone receptors present in striatum in the absence of estradiol priming. Thus, there are acute effects of estradiol on the striatum as well as a long-term effect of estradiol that enhances the effects of subsequent estradiol or progesterone treatments on AMPH-stimulated DA in dialysate from dorsolateral striatum (Becker 1999).

**Males.** There are no differences between intact and CAST males in the efficacy of AMPH or apomorphine to induce stereotyped behaviors (Savageau and Beatty 1981; Verimer et al. 1981). While some studies have reported that CAST increases AMPH-induced stereotypy (Beatty et al. 1982) or prolongs chlorpromazine-induced catalepsy (Mislow and Freidhoff 1973), it is difficult to dissociate these increases in drug-induced behaviors from the decreased rate of liver microsomal enzyme activity that accompanies CAST (Conney1967). When different systemic doses are used to produce equivalent brain concentrations in CAST and intact males, the two groups do not differ in AMPH-induced rotational behavior or stereotypy (Camp et al., 1986) or cocaine-induced rotational behavior or stereotyped behavior (Becker et al. 2001a; Hu and Becker, 2003). CAST also does not alter rotational behavior induced by unilateral electrical stimulation of the ascending nigrostriatal bundle (Robinson et al. 1982), indicating that the acute activation of this neural system is not modulated by testicular hormones.

To summarize the above discussion, the neural systems mediating the behavioral response to psychomotor stimulants are sexually dimorphic and, in the female rat, are modulated by the gonadal steroid hormones. Estradiol enhances the acute behavioral and neurochemical responses to AMPH or cocaine in female rats, and female rats exhibit a greater increase in psychomotor behavior in response to these drugs than do males.

## Motivated Behaviors

### Pacing of sexual behavior

Demonstrating that estradiol modulates sensorimotor function and DA-induced behaviors through its effects on the striatum has been important for understanding how estradiol affects this neural system. Research on the role of the ascending DA systems in sexual behavior of the male rat suggests that DA in the NAcc is important for anticipatory or motivational components of sexual behavior, whereas the striatum is important for consummatory aspects of sexual behavior. In male rats, extracellular DA concentrations detected by microdialysis or voltammetry increase in the NAcc when a sexually receptive female rat is presented. DA increases in both NAcc and striatum during copulation (Pfaus et al. 1990; Pleim et al. 1990; Phillips et al. 1991; Damsma et al. 1992).

To study the possible role of the ascending DA system in sexual motivation of the female rat, however, testing conditions need to be optimized for the expression of female-initiated behaviors. Sexual behavior in the female rat has typically been studied in the laboratory under conditions where the male rat is able to copulate with the female rat at will, resulting in low levels of female proceptive behaviors. In semi-natural conditions, however, the female rat will actively control the pace of copulatory behavior (i.e., show pacing behavior) by exhibiting proceptive behaviors and actively withdrawing from the male (McClintock 1984). This is important, as the optimal rate of intromissions for males and females are different. For the male rat, a rapidly paced series of intromissions (about 0.5–1 minutes between intromissions) is optimal to induce ejaculation in the fewest number of intromissions (Adler 1978). The

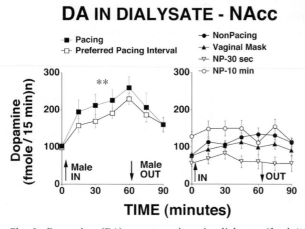

**DA IN DIALYSATE - NAcc**

**Fig. 2.** Dopamine (DA) concentrations in dialysate (fmole/15 min) obtained from nucleus accumbens (NAcc) of sexually receptive female rats. The value obtained for time zero is the mean of two 15-min baseline samples obtained immediately prior to the introduction of the male rat into the chamber. Values indicate the mean ± SEM. OVX female rats were randomly assigned to one of the following groups: Pacing (N = 8), Preferred Pacing Interval (PPI; N = 9), Vaginal Mask (N = 8), NonPacing (N = 9), NonPacing – 30 sec Interval (NP-30sec; N = 8), or NonPacing 10 min Interval (NP-10 min; N = 8). Prior to dialysis, all OVX rats were treated with EB and progesterone as described above. The Pacing group was tested during dialysis in a chamber where the female could pace the rate of intromission. The PPI group was tested in the same chamber with the barrier removed, and the male rat was removed from the chamber after an intromission or ejaculation and returned at the female's preferred interval (87–120 sec; mean = 100.1 sec), as determined in previous pacing situations. The Vaginal Mask group was tested under pacing conditions, but with a small piece of masking tape occluding the vagina. The tape was put in place prior to the initial collection of baseline samples and remained in place throughout dialysis. The NonPacing group was placed in the testing chamber without the opaque barrier, so the male had free access to the female during the time he was in the chamber. The NonPacing-interval groups were also tested without the barrier in place, but the male was removed after an intromission or ejaculation and returned either 30 sec later or 10 min later. ** The increase in DA in dialysate during the time the male was present was significantly greater for the Pacing and the preferred pacing interval (PPI) Group than for all other groups (P<0.003). There were no other differences among the groups. (Adapted from Becker et al. 2001b)

female rat, on the other hand, requires behavioral activation of a progestational response in order to facilitate pregnancy. When intromissions are spaced two to four minutes apart, the chance that insemination will result in pregnancy is significantly enhanced (Adler 1978). In addition, when a female rat is allowed to pace sexual behavior, she will develop a conditioned place preference for places where she has had paced sexual behavior over places where sexual behavior was not paced (Paredes and Vazquez 1999; Jenkins and Becker 2003b).

***The role of DA in pacing behavior.*** The possible role of the ascending DA systems in female rat sexual behavior has been a topic of investigation in this laboratory. We find that there is enhanced DA in dialysate from striatum and NAcc during sexual behavior in female rats that are pacing sexual behavior, as compared to females that are having sex but not pacing, or other control groups (Mermelstein and Becker 1995). DA in the NAcc also increases if the male rat is removed by the experimenter and then returned to the female at her preferred pacing interval, so she receives coital stimulation at her preferred interval (but not if the male is returned at intervals substantially longer or shorter; Fig. 2; Becker et al. 2001b). These results support the idea that DA in the striatum and NAcc are important for coding specific aspects of the sexual experience, rather than being related to specific motor behaviors (Becker et al. 2001b; Jenkins and Becker 2003a). Furthermore, female rats develop a conditioned place preference for places where sex occurred at their preferred pacing interval over non-paced sexual behavior, whether or not the female is actively pacing sexual behavior (Jenkins and Becker 2003b).

*The roles of the striatum and NAcc in pacing behavior.* Support for the functional dissociation of the roles of the striatum and NAcc in pacing behavior comes from studies in which female rats were induced into behavioral estrus via bilateral VMH hormonal treatments and then received estradiol bilaterally into the striatum or NAcc (Xiao and Becker 1997). Intrastriatal estradiol was found to facilitate percent exits after a copulatory contact (percentage of times the female exits the male side after contact), whereas intra-NAcc implants affected return latency (time from contact until the female returns to the male's side). Conversely, the antiestrogen ICI 182,780, but not tamoxifen, applied to the striatum decreased percent exits, and in the Nacc, it affected return latency (Xiao et al. 2003). Finally, after lesions of the medial shell of the NAcc, female rats did not approach a male to engage in copulatory behavior, even though they were behaviorally receptive (Jenkins and Becker 2001). Together these results suggest that estradiol acts in the striatum and NAcc to differentially modulate specific components of sexual behavior in the female rat. Estradiol is postulated to act in the striatum to enhance integration of sensorimotor activity (i.e., interpreting the intensity of the coital stimulation) and in the NAcc to enhance motivational aspects of sexual behavior (i.e., initiating the female's return to the male).

## Sex differences and effects of estradiol in drug abuse

We hypothesize that the hormonal modulation of the striatum and Nacc, which is important for the female's participation in sexual behavior, influences the behavioral and motivation-related consequences of exposure to drugs of abuse and, in particular, to drugs that act directly on the DA system. As discussed above, male-female differences in the pattern of cocaine abuse and behavioral responses to cocaine indicate that the pattern of cocaine use and onset of addiction to cocaine are more rapid in women than men (Lynch et al. 2002). Women begin using cocaine and enter treatment at earlier ages than men do and have more severe cocaine use at intake than men. Furthermore, as discussed above, cocaine cues induce more drug craving in female than male addicts. Collectively, these results suggest that women may be more sensitive to the addictive properties of cocaine than men.

The effects of drugs of abuse can change with repeated administration. These changes take two general forms: tolerance or sensitization. Historically, tolerance, and its role in the development of physical dependence, has been a central focus of research on addiction. Until recently, much less attention has been paid to the possible role of sensitization in addiction. Behavioral sensitization refers to an increase in a drug effect with repeated drug administration and is typically quantified as a progressive increase in drug effect with successive injections of a constant dose of a drug. Given the effects of estradiol on the ascending DA systems and the influence of this neural system on motivated behaviors, we have begun to investigate the influence of estradiol as well as sex-related differences in behavioral indices of drug abuse: behavioral sensitization and self-administration of cocaine.

In a recent experiment, animals with unilateral DA denervation underwent behavioral testing for rotational behavior with 0, 5, 10 or 20 mg/kg cocaine (Hu and Becker 2003); Fig. 3). In the unilateral DA-denervated rat, the amount of rotational behavior (turning in circles, like a dog chasing its tail) is linearly related to the dose of cocaine (Crombag et al. 1999). We compared intact male rats (SHAM), CAST male rats, OVX females, and OVX females treated with 5 µg estradiol benzoate 30 min before testing (OVX+E; all other groups received vehicle 30 min before testing). As shown in Figure 3A, there were both sex differences and effects of estradiol on sensitization of rotational behavior induced by repeated treatment with 20 mg/kg cocaine. First, all of the groups showed sensitization of rotational behavior, but the OVX+E group exhibited a greater increase in rotational behavior over the 12 testing days than did the other groups ($p < 0.001$), and the OVX rats exhibited a greater increase in rotational behavior than the CAST or SHAM males ($p < 0.001$). As illustrated in Figure 3B, on post-hoc comparisons the rate of sensitization of the OVX+E group was greater than for the OVX group ($p < 0.0378$), the CAST group ($p < 0.0021$) and the SHAM group ($p < 0.001$). There was no significant difference between OVX and CAST groups and no significant difference between the two male groups in the rate of sensitization.

The results of this study demonstrate that there are sex differences in behavioral sensitization in the absence of the milieu of gonadal hormones (OVX females exhibit a greater rate of rotational behavior after repeated cocaine treatment at 20 mg/kg than CAST males) and that estradiol treatment prior to cocaine enhances sensitization of cocaine-induced rotational behavior in OVX female rats at all doses of cocaine tested. On the challenge day (10 days after the last day of the original test schedule), all rats received 10 mg/kg cocaine but no groups were treated with estradiol. The OVX+E groups showed significantly

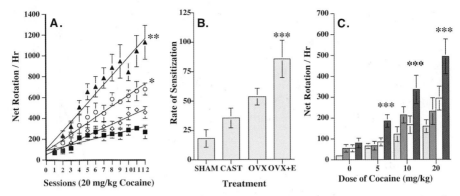

**Fig 3.** Sex differences and effect of estradiol (E) on sensitization to cocaine. **A.** Net rotations/hr exhibited by OVX that received E (OVX+E closed triangles, N = 8) followed 30 min later by 20 mg/ kg cocaine vs OVX (open circles, N = 8), intact males (SHAM; closed squares, N = 7) and castrated males (CAST; open diamonds, N = 8) who received oil followed by cocaine as described above. **OVX+E made more net rotations than did all other groups (p<0.001); *OVX group exhibited more net rotations than CAST males or SHAM males (p<0.01). **B.** Group differences for the rate of sensitization at 20 mg/kg cocaine. ***OVX+E females exhibited a faster rate of sensitization than all other groups (p<00.05). **C.** Results of a challenge dose of 10 mg/kg administered after 10 days withdrawal from E and cocaine. Animals were sensitized for 12 sessions with 0, 5, 10, or 20 mg/kg cocaine. All animals were tested without hormone treatment. ***OVX+E exhibited a greater magnitude of sensitization (Hu and Becker 2003).

more net rotations on the challenge day than the other three groups, regardless of previous cocaine history (Fig. 3C). When net rotations were compared there was a significant effect of group, p<0.0001) and no interaction between previous dose and group). When the response on the challenge day for each cocaine-treated group is compared with the response of the comparable saline-treated groups, all groups showed sensitization after pretreatment with 10 or 20 mg/kg, but after pretreatment with 5 mg/kg, the mean responses to 10 mg/kg were not different from the response of the saline- pretreated animals, except for the OVX+E treated animals (Fig. 3C).

The finding that there were both sex differences independent of concurrent gonadal hormones and an effect of estradiol on behavioral sensitization to cocaine lead us to examine whether there would also be effects of these factors on the self-administration of cocaine. The same four groups that were tested in the sensitization experiment were tested in a paradigm looking at the acquisition of cocaine self-administration (i.e., OVX+E, OVX, CAST and SHAM). During the first five self-administration sessions, rats received 0.3 mg/kg/infusion and then had two days off. During the second five sessions, animals received 0.4 mg/kg/infusion followed by two days off, and during the last five sessions, 0.5 mg/kg/infusion.

At the lowest dose tested, the OVX group self-administered more cocaine than the CAST group (p<0.05) and OVX+E group self-administered more cocaine

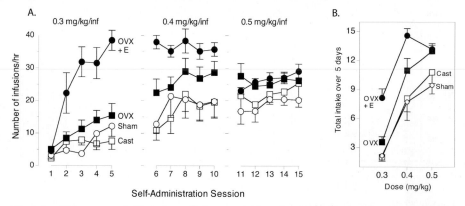

**Fig. 4.** Sex differences and effect of estradiol on acquisition of cocaine self-administration. Rats were tested on a FR1 schedule for five days followed by two days off each week. Rats received 0.3 mg/kg/inj cocaine for the first week, 0.4 mg/kg/inj cocaine for the second week and 0.5 mg/kg/inj cocaine for the third week. **A.** The mean (± SE) number of cocaine infusions per day for 15 testing sessions. The OVX+E group was treated with 5 µg EB 30 min prior to testing. OVX, CAST and SHAM male groups received 0.1 ml peanut oil 30 min prior to testing. Estradiol enhanced the number of cocaine infusions during the first week (p <0.001), with OVX+E greater than OVX, CAST and SHAM rats (p < 0.001). and OVX greater than CAST and SHAM rats (p < 0.0489). During week 3, the two female groups were greater than the two male groups (p < 0.028)). **B.** The mean (±SEM) amount of cocaine received (mg/kg/session) averaged over the three five-day blocks of testing. ANOVA with repeated measures were conducted for data at each dose(Adapted from Hu et al. 2003).

than all other groups (p<0.001; Fig. 4A; Hu et al. 2003). At 0.4 mg/kg/infusion, the OVX group self-administered more cocaine than the CAST (p<0.001) or the SHAM group (p<0.004), and the OVX+E group again self-administered more cocaine than all other groups (p<0.001). At 0.5 mg/kg/infusion, both the OVX and OVX+E groups self-administered more cocaine than the CAST (p<0.02) or SHAM groups (p<0.001). CAST and SHAM did not differ at any of the doses tested. Figuew 4B shows the mean (±SEM) amount of cocaine received (mg/kg/ session) during each three five-day blocks of testing.

The results from both the behavioral sensitization study and the study looking at self-administration of cocaine indicate that there are sex differences in cocaine-induced behaviors that are present in adult rats, independent of circulating gonadal hormones. This finding indicates that the neural systems mediating the behavioral response to cocaine are sexually dimorphic even without gonadal hormone activation. In other words, independent of concurrent circulating gonadal hormones in adulthood, OVX rats acquire cocaine self-administration more rapidly than males and exhibit a greater increase in cocaine-induced turning with repeated cocaine treatments than do males. Second, in female rats, but not males, circulating gonadal hormones modulate the behavioral response to cocaine and cocaine-taking behavior. In fact, estradiol promotes avid drug self-administration. These results are consistent

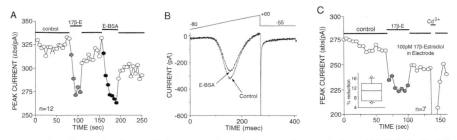

**Fig. 5.** The effects of 17β-estradiol occur at the cellular membrane. **A.** Estradiol (17β-E; 52 pM) or estradiol conjugated to the large protein bovine serum albumin (E-BSA; 52 pM) inhibits $Ca^{+2}$ current (as indicated by reduced $Ba^{+2}$ current ) in whole-cell clamp experiments with acutely dissociated striatal neurons, indicating that the actions of estradiol occur at the membrane surface. **B.** Individual traces taken from the data used to generate A. **C.** Dialyzing the inside of the cell with 100 pM 17β-E did not influence the response to 17β-E (1 pM) administered to the external membrane surface. Inset. Statistical summary of the percentage reduction of the whole-cell $Ca^{+2}$ current inhibited by 1 pM 17β-E after intracellular dialysis with 100 pM 17β-E. (Adapted from Mermelstein et al. 1996).

with results from other laboratories that have investigated sex differences and the influence of estradiol on sensitization and self-administration behavior (for a review, see Lynch et al. 2002).

## Mechanisms mediating the effects of estradiol on the striatum

Electrophysiological studies have shown that estradiol can induce rapid changes in the response of striatal neurons to D1 and D2 agonists (Demotes-Mainard et al. 1990). Furthermore, estradiol can act directly on intrinsic striatal neurons. Results from whole cell clamp studies in acutely dissociated striatal neurons indicate that there are rapid effects of estradiol on L-type $Ca^{2+}$ channels in striatal neurons (Mermelstein et al. 1996). In whole-cell clamp recordings from acutely dissociated striatal neurons, acute application of 17β-estradiol decreases $Ca^{2+}$ currents. The effects are rapid (within seconds), reverse as soon as estradiol delivery ceases, are sex specific (cells from females > males), and are seen at physiologically relevant concentrations of estradiol (1-100 pM). As illustrated in Figure 5A, estradiol conjugated to bovine serum albumin (BSA, which prevents estradiol entry onto cells) is also effective at blocking calcium current. Furthermore, estradiol applied internally to cells through the electrode is not effective at reducing $Ca^{2+}$ currents; neither does it block the effect of 1 pM estradiol applied externally, demonstrating that estradiol is acting at the exterior of the cell membrane to produce this effect (Fig. 5C; Mermelstein et al., 1996).

Collectively, these results indicate that the effect of estradiol occurs at the external membrane surface. In the presence of GTPγS (which prevents inactivation of G-protein-mediated events), the effect of 17β-estradiol does not reverse when hormone delivery ceases (Mermelstein et al. 1996). Thus, the effect of estradiol is dependent upon a G-protein coupled receptor. Finally, the effect of 17β-estradiol is stereospecific, as 17α-estradiol does not mimic the modulation, and steroid-specific, as 100 pM estrone and 3-methoxyestriol were ineffective whereas estriol and 4-hydroxy-estradiol mimic the effect of 17β-estradiol (Mermelstein et al. 1996). We conclude that estradiol has rapid stereospecific effects on striatal neurons that alter signaling pathways by acting at a receptor on the extracellular membrane. It is hypothesized that estradiol inhibition of calcium current in GABA neurons results in decreased GABA neurotransmission (Becker 1999). Since GABA neurons are known to have recurrent collaterals that synapse on presynaptic DA terminals in the striatum, a decrease in GABA release results in a decrease in inhibition and increased DA release when the axons fire. Experiments are in progress to directly test this hypothesis.

## Conclusions

We have shown that estradiol has rapid effects on the striatum and NAcc that induce an enhancement in stimulated DA release and DA-mediated behaviors. We propose that the mechanism mediating this effect of estradiol in striatum and NAcc is through inhibition of GABA release from medium spiny neurons that have recurrent collaterals that synapse on GABA-B receptors on pre-synaptic DA terminals. Thus, there is a release of inhibition in the presence of estradiol that enhances DA release. This effect results in greater behavioral activation when these DA systems are stimulated in the presence of estradiol. For the behavior of the animal, this activation means enhanced sexual motivation during behavioral estrus and enhanced effects of drugs that act on dopaminergic systems.

## References

Adler NT (1978) On the mechanisms of sexual behavior and their evolutionary constraints. In: Hutchison JB (ed) Biological determinants of sexual behavior New York: Wiley and Sons, pp 657-694.

Arbuthnott GW, Crow TJ (1971) Relation of contraversive turning to unilateral release of dopamine from the nigrostriatal pathway in rats. Exp Neurol 30:484-491.

Bazzett TJ, Becker JB (1994) Sex differences in the rapid and acute effects of estrogen on striatal D2 dopamine receptor binding. Brain Res 637:163-172.

Beatty WW, Holzer GA (1978) Sex differences in stereotyped behavior in the rat. Pharmacol Biochem Behav 9:777-785.

Beatty WW, Dodge AM, Traylor KL (1982) Stereotyped behavior elicited by amphetamine in the rat: organizational and activational effects of the testes. Pharmacol Biochem Behav 16:565-568.

Becker JB (1990a) Direct effect of 17β-estradiol on striatum: sex differences in dopamine release. Synapse 5:157-164.

Becker JB (1990b) Estrogen rapidly potentiates amphetamine-induced striatal dopamine release and rotaional behavior during microdialysis. Neurosci Lett 118:169-171.

Becker JB (1999) Gender differences in dopaminergic function in striatum and nucleus accumbens. Pharmacol Biochem Behavior 64:803-812.

Becker JB, Ramirez VD (1981a) Experimental studies on the development of sex differences in the release of dopamine from striatal tissue fragments in vitro. Neuroendocrinology 32:168-173.

Becker JB, Ramirez VD (1981b) Sex differences in the amphetamine stimulated release of catecholamines from rat striatal tissue in vitro. Brain Res 204:361-372.

Becker JB, Beer ME (1986) The influence of estrogen on nigrostriatal dopamine activity: behavioral and neurochemical evidence for both pre- and postsynaptic components. Behav Brain Res 19:27-33.

Becker JB, Cha J (1989) Estrous cycle-dependent variation in amphetamine-induced behaviors and striatal dopamine release assessed with microdialysis. Behav Brain Res 35:117-125.

Becker JB, Rudick CN (1999) Rapid effects of estrogen or progesterone on the amphetamine-induced increase in striatal dopamine are enhanced by estrogen priming: A microdialysis study. Pharmacol Biochem Behavior 64:53-57.

Becker JB, Robinson TE, Lorenz KA (1982) Sex differences and estrous cycle variations in amphetamine-elicited rotational behavior. Eur J Pharmacol 80:65-72.

Becker JB, Molenda HA, Hummer DL (2001a) Gender differences in the behavioral responses to cocaine and amphetamine: implications for mechanisms mediating gender differences in drug abuse. Ann NY Acad Sci 937:172-187.

Becker JB, Rudick CN, Jenkins WJ (2001b) The role of dopamine in the nucleus accumbens and striatum during sexual behavior in the female rat. J Neurosci 21:3236-3241.

Bowman BP, Vaughan SR, Walker QD, Davis SL, Little PJ, Scheffler NM, Thomas BF, Kuhn CM (1999) Effects of sex and gonadectomy on cocaine metabolism in the rat. J Pharmacol ExpTherap 290:1316-1323.

Camp DM, Becker JB, Robinson TE (1986) Sex differences in the effects of gonadectomy on amphetamine-induced rotational behavior in rats. Behav Neural Biol 46:491-495.

Castner SA, Becker JB (1990) Estrogen and striatal dopamine release: a microdialysis study. Soc Neurosci Abstr 16.

Conney AH (1967) Pharmacological implications of microsomal enzyme induction. Pharmacol Rev 19:317-366.

Costall B, Naylor RJ (1977) Mesolimbic and extrapyramidal sites for the mediation of stereotyped behavior patterns and hyperactivity by amphetamine and apomorphine in the rat. In: Ellinwood EH, Kilbey MM (eds) Cocaine and other stimulants. New York: Plenum Press, pp 47-76.

Crombag HS, Mueller H, Browman KE, Badiani A, Robinson TE (1999) A comparison of two behavioral measures of psychomotor activation following intravenous amphetamine or cocaine: dose- and sensitization-dependent changes. Behav Pharmacol 10:205-213.

Damsma G, Pfaus JG, Wenkstern D, Phillips AG, Fibiger HC (1992) Sexual behavior increases dopamine transmission in the nucleus accumbens and striatum of male rats: comparison with novelty and locomotion. Behav Neurosci 106:181-191.

Demotes-Mainard J, Arnauld E, Vincent JD (1990) Estrogens modulate the responsiveness of in vivo reorded striatal neurons to iontophoretic application of dopamine in rats: role of D1 and D2 receptor activation. J Neuroendocrinol 2:825-832.

Dluzen DE, Ramirez VD (1984) Bimodal effect of progesterone on in vitro dopamine function of the rat corpus striatum. Neuroendocrinology 39:149-155.

Dluzen DE, Ramirez VD (1987) Intermittent infusion of progesterone potentiates whereas continuous infusion reduces amphetamine-stimulated dopamine release from ovariectomized estrogen-primed rat striatal fragments superfused in vitro. Brain Res 406:1 9.

Dluzen DE, Ramirez VD (1989) Progesterone effects upon dopamine release from the corpus striatum of female rats. I. Evidence for interneuronal control. Brain Res 476:332-337.

Dluzen DE, Ramirez VD (1990) In vitro progesterone modulates amphetamine-stimulated dopamine release from the corpus striatum of castrated male rats treated with estrogen. Neuroendocrinology 52:517-520.

Dluzen DE, Ramirez VD (1991) Modulatory effects of progesterone upon dopamine release from the corpus striatum of ovariectomized estrogen-treated rats are stereo- specific. Brain Res 538:176-179.

Fink JS, Smith GP (1980) Relationships between selective denervation of dopamine terminal fields in the naterior forebrain and behavioral responses to amphetamine and apomorphine. Brain Res 201:107-127.

Fiorino DF, Phillips AG (1999) Facilitation of sexual behavior and enhanced dopamine efflux in the nucleus accumbens of male rats after D-amphetamine-induced behavioral sensitization. J Neurosci 19:456-463.

Fog R (1972) On stereotypy and catalepsy: studies on the effect of amphetamines and neuroleptics in rats. Acta Neurol Scand [Suppl] 50:3-66.

Griffin ML, Weiss RD, Lange U (1989) A comparison of male and female cocaine abuse. Arch Gen Psychiat 46:122-126.

Hruska RE, Pitman KT (1982) Hypophysectomy reduces the haloperidol-induced changes in striatal dopamine receptor density. Eur J Pharmacol 85:201-205.

Hruska RE, Ludmer LM, Pitman KT, De Ryck M, Silbergeld EK (1982) Effects of estrogen on striatal dopamine receptor function in male and female rats. Pharmacol Biochem Behav 16:285-291.

Hu M, Becker JB (2003) Effects of sex and estrogen on behavioral sensitization to cocaine in rats. J Neurosci 23:693-699.

Hu M, Crombag HS, Robinson T, Becker JB (2003) The biological basis for sex differences in the propensity to self-administer cocaine. Neuropsychopharmacology advance online publication Sept. 3, 2003: 1300301.

Jenkins WJ, Becker JB (2001) Role of the striatum and nucleus accumbens in paced copulatory behavior in the female rat. Behav Brain Res 121:119-128.

Jenkins WJ, Becker JB (2003a) Dynamic increases in dopamine during paced copulation in the female rat. Eur J Neurosci 18:1997-2001.

Jenkins WJ, Becker JB (2003b) Female rats develop conditioned place preferences for sex at their preferred interval. Horm Behav 43:503-507.

Kandel DB, Warner MPP, Kessler RC (1995) The epidemiology of substance abuse and dependence among women. In: Wetherington CL, Roman AR (eds) Drug addiction research and the health of women. (Rockville, MD: U.S. Department of Health and Human Services, pp 105-130.

Ke FC, Ramirez VD (1990) Binding of progesterone to nerve cell membranes of rat brain using progesterone conjugated to 125I-bovine serum albumin as a ligand. J Neurochem 54: 467-472.

Kosten TA, Gawin FH, Kosten TR, Rounsaville BJ (1993) Gender differeces in cocaine use and treatment response. J Subst Abuse Treat 10:63-66.

Levesque D, Di Paolo T (1988) Rapid conversion of high into low striatal D2-dopamine receptor agonist binding states after an acute physiological dose of 17 beta- estradiol. Neurosci Lett 88:113-118.

Lynch WJ, Carroll ME (1999) Sex differences in the acquisition of intravenously self-administered cocaine and heroin in rats. Psychopharmacology 144:77-82.

Lynch WJ, Roth ME, Carroll ME (2002) Biological basis of sex differences in drug abuse: preclinical and clinical studies. Psychopharmacology 164:121-137.

Maus M, Cordier J, Glowinski J, Premont J (1989a) 17β-Oestradiol pretreatment of mouse striatal neurons in culture enhances the responses to adenylate cyclase sensitive tobiogenic amines. Eur J Neurosci 1:1.

Maus M, Bertrand P, Drouva S, Rasolonjanahary R, Kordon C, Glowinski J, Premont J, Enjalbert A (1989b) Differential modulation of D1 and D2 dopamine-sensitive adenylate cyclases by 17β-estradiol in cultures styriatal neurons and anterior pituitary cells. J Neurochem 52:410-418.

McCarthy MM, Becker JB (2002) Neuroendocrinology of sexual behavior in the female. In: Becker JB, Breedlove SM, Crews D, McCarthy MM (eds) Behavioral endocrinology. 2nd Edition. . Cambridge, MA: MIT Press/ Bradford Books, pp 117-151

McClintock MK (1984) Group mating in the domestic rat as context for sexual selection: consequences for the analysis of sexual behavior and neuroendocrine responses. Adv Study Behav 14:1-50.

Meisel RL, Camp DM, Robinson TE (1993) A microdialysis study of ventral striatal dopamine during sexual behavior in female Syrian hamsters. Behav Brain Res 55:151-157.

Mendelson JH, Weiss R, Griffin M, Mirin SM, Teoh SK, Mello NK, Lex BW (1991) Some special considerations for treatment of drug abuse and dependence in women. NIDA Res Monogr 106:313-327.

Mermelstein PG, Becker JB (1995) Increased extracellular dopamine in the nucleus accumbens and striatum of the female rat during paced copulatory behavior. Behav Neurosci 109: 354-365.

Mermelstein PG, Becker JB, Surmeier DJ (1996) Estradiol reduces calcium currents in rat neostriatal neurons through a membrane receptor. J Neurosci 16:595-604.

Mislow JF, Freidhoff AJ (1973) A comparison of chlorpromazine-induced extrapyramidal syndrome in male and female rats. In: Lissak K (ed) Hormones and brain function. New York: Plenum Press, pp 315-326.

Paredes RG, Vazquez B (1999) What do female rats like about sex? Paced mating. Behav Brain Res 105:117-127.

Pfaus JG, Damsma G, Nomikos GG, Wenkstern DG, Blaha CD, Phillips AG, Fibiger HC (1990) Sexual behavior enhances central dopamine transmission in the male rat. Brain Res 530: 345-348.

Phillips AG, Pfaus JG, Blaha CD (1991) Dopamine and motivated behavior: insights provided by in vivo analyses. In: Willmer P, Scheel-Kruger J (eds) The mesolimbic dopamine system: from motivation to action. New York: John Wiley, pp 199-224.

Pleim ET, Matochik JA, Barfield RJ, Auerbach SB (1990) Correlation of dopamine release in the nucleus accumbens with masculine sexual behavior in rats. Brain Res 524:160-163.

Robbins SJ, Ehrman RN, Childress AR, OíBrien CP (1999) Comparing levels of cocaine cue reactivity in male and female outpatients. Drug Alcohol Depend 53:223-230.

Robinson TE, Berridge KC (2001) Incentive-sensitization and addiction. Addiction 96:103-114.

Robinson TE, Becker JB, Ramirez VD (1980) Sex differences in amphetamine-elicited rotational behavior and the lateralization of striatal dopamine in rats. Brain Res Bull 5: 539-545.

Robinson TE, Camp DM, Becker JB (1981) Gonadectomy attenuates turning behavior produced by electrical stimulation of the nigrostriatal dopamine system in female but not male rats. Neurosci Lett 23:203-208.

Robinson TE, Camp DM, Jacknow DS, Becker JB (1982) Sex differences and estrous cycle dependent variation in rotational behavior elicited by electrical stimulation of the mesostriatal dopamine system. Behav Brain Res 6:273-287.

Savageau MM, Beatty WW (1981) Gonadectomy and sex differences in the behavioral responses of amphetamine and apomorphine of rats. Pharmacol Biochem Behav 14:17-23.

Thompson TL (1999) Attenuation of dopamine uptake in vivo following priming with estradiol benzoate. Brain Research 834:164-167.

Thompson TL, Moss RL (1994) Estrogen regulation of dopamine release in the nucleus accumbens: genomic- and nongenomic-mediated effects. J Neurochem 62:1750-1756.

Thompson TL, Moss RL (1995) In vivo stimulated dopamine release in the nucleus accumbens: Modulation by prefrontal cortex. Brain Res 686:93-98.

Thompson TL, Moss RL (1997) Modulation of mesolimbic dopaminergic activity over the rat estrous cycle. Neurosci Lett 229:145-148.

Thompson TL, Moore CC, Smith B (2000) Estrogen priming modulates autoreceptor-mediated potentiation of dopamine uptake. Eur J Pharmacol 401:357-363.

Thompson TL, Bridges SR, Weirs WJ (2001) Alteration of dopamine transport in the striatum and nucleus accumbens of ovariectomized and estrogen-primed rats following N-(p-isothiocyanatophenethyl) spiperone (NIPS) treatment. Brain Res Bull 54:631-638.

Ungerstedt U (1971) Striatal dopamine release after amphetamine or nerve degeneration revealed by rotational behavior. Acta Physiol Scand 82 (Suppl. 367):49-68.

van Haaren F, Meyer M (1991) Sex differences in the locomotor activity after acute and chronic cocaine administration. Pharmacol Biochem Behav 39:923-927.

Verimer T, Arneric SP, Long JP, Walsh BJ, Abou Zeit-Har MS (1981) Effects of ovariectomy, castration, and chronic lithium chloride treatment on stereotyped behavior in rats. Psychopharmacology 75:273-276.

Walker QD, Cabassa J, Kaplan KA, Li ST, Haroon J, Spohr HA, Kuhn CM (2001) Sex differences in cocaine-stimulated motor behavior: Disparate effects of gonadectomy. Neuropsychopharmacology 25:118-130.

Wetherington CL, Roman AR (eds) (1995) Drug addiction research and the health of women. Rockville, MD: U.S. Department of Health and Human Services.

Wong M, Thompson TL, Moss RL (1996) Nongenomic actions of estrogen in the brain: physiological significance and cellular mechanisms. Crit Rev Neurobiol 10:189-203.

Xiao L, Becker JB (1994) Quantitative microdialysis determination of extracellular striatal dopamine concentrations in male and female rats: effects of estrous cycle and gonadectomy. Neurosci Lett 180:155-158.

Xiao L, Becker JB (1997) Hormonal activation of the striatum and the nucleus accumbens modulates paced mating behavior in the female rat. Horm Behav 32:114-124.

Xiao L, Jackson LR, Becker JB (2003) The effect of estradiol in the striatum is blocked by ICI 182,780 but not tamoxifen: pharmacological and behavioral evidence. Neuroendocrinology 77:239-245.

# Behavioral Effects of rapid Changes in Aromatase Activity in the Central Nervous System

J. Balthazart[1], M. Baillien[1], C.A. Cornil[1], T.D. Charlier[1],
H.C. Evrard [1*], and G.F. Ball[2]

## Summary

In many vertebrate species, male sexual behavior is activated by the action in the preoptic area of estrogens produced by the local aromatization of testosterone. Estrogens bind to intracellular receptors, which then act as transcription factors to activate the behavior. In parallel, changes in aromatase activity (AA) result from steroid-induced modifications of enzyme transcription. The transcription of aromatase is regulated in a synergistic manner by estrogenic and androgenic metabolites of testosterone. Regulatory proteins such as the steroid receptor coactivator-1 modulate steroid action in the brain, and an increasing amount of data now indicate that this mode of control is also implicated in the activation by steroids of sexual behavior and of aromatase transcription. More recently, rapid non-genomic effects of estrogens have been described in a variety of animal models, and evidence has accumulated in Japanese quail indicating that AA in the preoptic area is modulated by rapid (minute to hour) non-genomic mechanisms in addition to the slower (hours to days) transcriptional changes. Conditions that enhance protein phosphorylation, such as the presence of high concentrations of calcium, magnesium and ATP, rapidly (within min) downregulate AA in hypothalamic homogenates. Similarly, the pharmacological mobilization of intracellular calcium with thapsigargin or stimulation of various glutamate receptors (AMPA, kainate, NMDA) that lead to increased intracellular calcium concentrations depresses within minutes the AA that is measured in quail preoptic explants. Protein kinase inhibitors interfere with the calcium-induced inhibition of AA, and multiple phosphorylation consensus sites are present on the deduced amino acid sequence of quail aromatase. Fast changes in the local availability of estrogens in the brain can thus be caused by aromatase phosphorylations that rapidly regulate neuronal physiology and behavior. Recent studies suggest that the pharmacological blockade of AA by specific

[1] University of Liège, Center for Cellular and Molecular Neurobiology, Research Group in Behavioral Neuroendocrinology, Liège, Belgium
[2] Department of Psychological and Brain Sciences, Johns Hopkins University, Baltimore, MD 21218, USA
* Current address: Department of Biology, Boston University, Boston, MA 02215, USA

Kordon et al.
Hormones and the Brain
© Springer-Verlag Berlin Heidelberg 2005

inhibitors rapidly down regulates motivational and consummatory aspects of male sexual behavior in quail and decreases responsiveness to painful stimuli within minutes. The rapid and slower changes of AA in the central nervous system thus match well with the genomic and non-genomic actions of estrogens and potentially provide temporal variations in the bioavailability of estrogens that can support the entire range of established effects for this steroid.

## Introduction

### Assumptions about hormonal signaling versus neural signaling systems can still bias our thinking about neuroendocrine systems

Although the concept of neurosecretion and the need to think about neuroendocrine interactions from a "systems" perspective have been articulated to varying degrees for decades, our scientific thinking can still be hindered by assumptions about distinctions between endocrine signaling systems (involving hormones) and neural signaling systems (involving neurotransmitters). These biases in our thinking have clear historical origins. For example, the field of endocrinology, narrowly defined but still in a modern sense, goes back to Bayliss and Starling (1902), who observed that chemical messengers called hormones are released by ductless glands and have dramatic biological effects. The importance of these "internal secretions" on many physiological processes was stressed by endocrinologists working in the early 20th century, and distinctive aspects of how these messengers worked as compared to neurotransmission were often stressed (Medvi 1982). However, by the mid-20th century, the importance of the brain as an endocrine organ that can regulate the endocrine system in profound ways was slowly recognized (Harris 1955). With the development of the concept of neurosecretion, the field of neuroendocrinology was truly born. However, despite the recognition that the nervous system and the endocrine system need to be understood as one integrated physiological system, distinctions in thinking about the two systems persisted. One such distinction related to the action of steroid hormones. Steroids are released by ductless glands, such as the gonads and the adrenals, and then act on "target sites," such as various effector organs and muscles. However, it was recognized early on that the brain is such a target site. One of the primary functions of steroid hormones acting on neural targets is for negative and positive feedback effects on the hypothalamo-pituitary-gonadal axis, but the importance of the regulation of behavior was recognized as well (Beach 1948). The notion was that steroids acted in a relatively slow manner via intracellular receptors (McEwen and Pfaff 1985). These receptors then acted as transcription factors that enhanced the transcription of proteins related to neurotransmission that changed signaling patterns in the brain. Subsequently it was discovered that some hormones released by endocrine glands, such as testicular testosterone, were actually prohormones and were subsequently transformed at targets sites to more effective metabolites (Naftolin et al. 1975; MacLusky et al. 1984). The aromatization hypothesis articulated by Naftolin and colleagues provided us with a critical advance in our understanding of testosterone action in the brain. The hypothesis states that testosterone is first converted locally in specific brain regions via the enzyme aromatase (estrogen synthase) to an estrogenic metabolite before it exerts its biological effects via the binding to an estrogen receptor (Naftolin et al. 1975). These findings highlighted the fact that the brain is much more than just a target site of steroids but is an active participant in setting up an environment that can modulate the effectiveness of steroid hormone action.

With the identification of neurosteroids (steroids synthesized de novo by the brain), the notion that the brain can itself synthesize steroids and use them as messengers of some sort was proposed (Baulieu and Robel 1990; Baulieu et al. 1999). But distinctions in our thinking about how steroids act as opposed to traditional neurotransmitters persisted. The role these neurosteroids might play in many physiological functions of the brain remained obscure. Evidence has been accumulating for membrane effects of neurosteroids and neuroactive steroid hormones in the brain (usually assumed to be of peripheral origin; see McEwen 1991) that have a time course more akin to what has been observed for neurotransmitters. The complete acceptance of this concept of rapid steroid hormone effects in brain should finally clarify how steroid hormone action can be considered as a type of neuromodulation/neurotransmission akin to other messengers, such as neuropeptides and catecholamine transmitters, which act more slowly via metabotropic receptors as compared to amino acids, acting quickly and directly on ion channel receptors. In this review, we will discuss the rapid behavioral effects of testosterone and its metabolites on reproductive behavior in Japanese quail and the concomitant, possible rapid regulation of the synthesis of estrogens via actions on the metabolizing enzyme aromatase. We will argue that one can now view a part of steroid hormone actions in the brain as another neural signaling system that can act rapidly, be fine-tuned in response to environmental and experiential changes and play an essential role in the regulation of certain behavioral systems.

## Preoptic aromatase and sexual behavior in quail

In quail as in other vertebrate species, testosterone (T) can be irreversibly metabolized into a variety of compounds within the central nervous system, and these transformations play a key role in the activation of male sexual behavior (Schlinger and Callard 1987; Balthazart 1989). The enzyme 5α-*reductase* transforms T into 5α-*dihydrotestosterone*, a potent androgen (like T) that appears to be responsible for the development of male secondary sexual characteristics such as the growth of the cloacal gland in quail or the growth of the comb and wattles in chickens. In contrast, 5β-*reductase*, the enzyme that transforms T into *5β-dihydrotestosterone*, represents an inactivation pathway for the androgen at least as far as reproductive behavior is concerned. A third enzyme, aromatase (or estrogen synthase or $P450_{AROM}$) metabolizes T into estradiol. This enzyme is a member of the P450 enzyme family encoded by gene CYP19 (Simpson et al. 1994; Lephart 1996). In Japanese quail and in many other species such as the laboratory rat, brain aromatase activity (AA) plays a critical limiting role in the activation of male sexual behavior by T (Balthazart 1989). This conclusion was derived from a variety of experiments in which either AA was blocked by specific inhibitors or access of locally formed estrogens to their receptor was blocked by drugs known as anti-estrogens (e.g., nitromifene citrate or tamoxifen). In either case, pharmacological interference with the production or activity of estrogens almost completely suppressed the behavioral effects of T (Balthazart and Foidart 1993).

Morphometric analyses of the preoptic area (POA), a brain region known to be involved in the control of male-typical copulatory behavior in most, if not all, vertebrate species, identified the presence of a sexually dimorphic nucleus in quail. This structure, called the medial preoptic nucleus (POM), is significantly larger in males than in females (Viglietti-Panzica et al. 1986). The POM volume is sensitive to the circulating levels of androgens: it regresses in castrated birds and is restored to the volume typical of sexually mature males by a two-week treatment with exogenous T (Panzica et al. 1987, 1991). Lesions of the POM decrease or abolish the expression of male copulatory behavior and the behavioral deficits are proportional to the volume of POM lesioned but not to the absolute size of the lesion. Furthermore, stereotaxic implantation of T within the cytoarchitectonic boundaries of the POM activates male copulatory behavior in castrated males but implants located elsewhere in the POA are behaviorally ineffective. Stereotaxic implants of an aromatase inhibitor or of an antiestrogen within the POM substantially decrease or suppress the activating effects of a systemic treatment with T in castrated males (see Panzica et al. 1996 for review). Taken together, these data indicate that T must be aromatized and the locally produced estrogens must act within the POM to activate male copulation. The preoptic aromatase in quail thus plays a key role in the control of male reproductive behavior; therefore, a number of studies were devoted to the analysis of the neuroanatomical distribution of this enzyme and of the mechanisms that control its activity (Panzica et al. 1996; Balthazart and Ball 1998a,b; Ball and Balthazart 2002).

## Control by testosterone of aromatase transcription in the preoptic area

In all vertebrates studied so far, castration reduces the AA in the POA to basal levels and T restores the enzymatic activity to normal levels (Steimer and Hutchison 1981; Roselli et al. 1985, 1988; Connolly et al. 1990; Roselli and Resko

2001). In quail specifically, treatment of castrated males with Silastic™ implants filled with T produced a five- to six-fold increase in enzyme activity (Schumacher and Balthazart 1986; Balthazart et al. 1990a). In the quail brain, aromatase-containing neurons can also be readily visualized by immunocytochemistry (Balthazart et al. 1990b,c). Quantitative studies showed that, after five days, treatment of castrates with T-filled Silastic™ implants increased the number of aromatase-immunoreactive cells (ARO-ir) approximately five-fold by comparison with untreated castrates (see Fig. 1A; Balthazart et al. 1992, 1996; Harada et al. 1993). Given that the classification of cells as immunopositive or immunonegative largely depends on the concentration of the antigen protein in these cells, these data strongly suggest that T increases aromatase concentration in the POA. This notion is further supported by more recent studies indicating that similar changes in aromatase mRNA concentration, as measured by reverse transcription- polymerase chain reaction (RT-PCR), are observed following T treatment (Harada et al. 1992, 1993). These results therefore demonstrate that the control by T of AA takes place at least in part at the pretranslational level. Although these data do not exclude a regulation based on an increase in the stability of the aromatase mRNA, it is extremely likely that T enhances the transcription of the aromatase messenger. Figure 1A clearly indicates that the same treatment with T (exposure to 40-mm Silastic™ implants) produces changes in AA, in the number of ARO-ir cells and in the concentration of aromatase mRNA that are in the same order of magnitude. The observed percentage increase in AA is, however, slightly higher (645%) than the increase in the number of immunoreactive cells (497%), which is itself larger than the

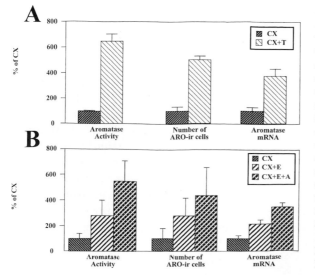

Fig. 1. Effect of treatments of castrated (CX) male quail with testosterone (T) or with estrogens (E) alone or in combination with non-aromatizable androgens (A) on aromatase activity (AA), on the number of aromatase-immunoreactive (ARO-ir) cells and on the concentration of the aromatase mRNA in the quail preoptic area. All data are expressed as percentages of values obtained in CX birds to allow direct comparisons. Redrawn from data in Schumacher and Balthazart 1986; Schumacher et al. 1987; Balthazart et al. 1992, 1994; Harada et al. 1992, 1993).

increase in the concentration of ARO mRNA (372%). These differences possibly reflect experimental errors in finding their origin, for example, in the different techniques employed or in individual differences between groups of birds used for the different measures. Alternatively, it is also interesting to note that the percentage increase following exposure to T becomes higher when the dependent variable is functionally more distant from the original DNA expression. Besides regulating aromatase transcription, it is thus possible that T also enhances the translation of the ARO mRNA and/or modulates the activity of the aromatase enzyme (see below).

## Effects of testosterone on aromatase activity are mimicked by estradiol in quail

Many effects of T in the brain are actually caused by the action of androgenic or estrogenic metabolites of this steroid (see Balthazart 1989; Ball and Balthazart 2002 for review). This conclusion also applies to aromatase induction in quail. Because the induction by T of AA in the POA appears to be a limiting step in the production of the behavioral effects of T (Balthazart et al. 1990a), we researched whether the induction of aromatase displayed the same hormonal specificity as the activation of copulatory behavior. During a series of independent experiments, castrated male quail were chronically treated with estrogens or with non-aromatizable androgens such as 5α-dihydrotestosterone or the synthetic androgen R1881 (methyltrienolone), alone or in combination (Schumacher et al. 1987; Harada et al. 1993; Balthazart et al. 1994). Effects of these treatments on AA were assessed by in vitro radioenzyme assays. We also assessed in parallel experiments the amount of enzymatic protein (semi-quantitative evaluation of immunoreactive aromatase) and the amount of aromatase mRNA (by RT-PCR).

Together, the results of these experiments indicate that, in quail, non-aromatizable androgens have by themselves very little or no effect on the preoptic AA. Estrogens in contrast (estradiol or the synthetic compound diethylstilbestrol) largely mimic the effects of testosterone on the enzyme, and the increase can be observed at the levels of the enzymatic activity, of the semiquantitative estimate of the enzymatic protein and of the corresponding mRNA concentration (Fig. 1B). At all three levels of analysis, a clear synergism between androgenic and estrogenic steroids could also be identified. Although non-aromatizable androgens did not affect aromatase expression by themselves, they significantly increased the effects of estrogens. A similar situation has been reported in another avian species, the ring dove (*Streptopelia risoria*; Hutchison and Steimer 1986). A similar synergism in the induction of aromatase by androgens and estrogens has also been reported in rats but the effect appears in this species to be mediated mostly by the activation of androgen receptors (Roselli and Resko 1984; Roselli et al. 1987).

In summary, in all species that have been studied in detail so far, there is a clear synergism between non-aromatizable androgens and estrogens in the mechanism that regulates aromatase, and this synergism can be observed at the three different levels at which aromatase has been studied (the mRNA, the protein and the enzyme activity). However, in rats, this effect appears to be largely mediated by the interaction of steroids with androgen receptors, whereas in quail and doves, the action of locally produced estrogens appears to be quantitatively the most important.

## Cellular basis of the synergism between androgens and estrogens in the activation of aromatase

The most parsimonious model that could explain this synergistic control of aromatase synthesis by estrogens and androgens assumes that, when entering its target cells, T acts as such or is aromatized in the cytoplasmic compartment into an estrogen and that both types of steroids then bind to androgen or estrogen receptors (AR/ER) to activate the transcription of the aromatase gene (Balthazart and Ball 1998a). Double label immunocytochemical studies have accordingly shown that AR are expressed in a large proportion of the preoptic aromatase cells (Balthazart et al. 1998a). Parallel immunocytochemical studies revealed, however, that, although estrogen receptors are expressed in the same brain areas as aromatase (e.g., the POA, the bed nucleus striae terminalis, the ventro-medial nucleus of the hypothalamus; Foidart et al. 1995), they are not generally co-localized in the same neurons (Balthazart et al. 1991). If a large fraction (70- 80%) of the ARO-ir neurons in the ventro-medial hypothalamus contain immunoreactive ER, the percentage of cells exhibiting such a co-localization is far lower in the POM (approximately 18%) and bed nucleus striae terminalis (approximately 4%). Similar results (ER co-localized with aromatase in the ventro-medial hypothalamus but not in the POA) have been reported in the neonatal mouse and rat brain (Tsuruo et al. 1995, 1996). This suggests that, in many cases, estrogens cannot act genomically, and in particular cannot control aromatase expression, by interacting with ER within the cells where they are produced. Other modes of estrogen action on AA should thus be considered.

A second type of estrogen receptor, called estrogen receptor beta (ERβ; Kuiper et al. 1996, 1998) to distinguish it from the previously identified receptor now renamed ERα, was recently identified in mammals. ERβ was also cloned and its neuroanatomical distribution was analyzed by in situ hybridization in the quail brain (Foidart et al. 1999). The ERβ mRNA was detected throughout the rostral-caudal extent of the hypothalamus, in the mesencephalic nucleus intercollicularis and in the telencephalic nucleus taeniae of the amygdala. An intense hybridization signal was, in particular, found in the POM and in the nucleus striae terminalis (BST) as defined by Aste and collaborators (1998), the two brain nuclei that contain the largest densities of ARO-ir neurons

(Foidart et al. 1995; Balthazart et al. 1996). ERβ could therefore be colocalized with aromatase in the POM and BST, allowing estrogens to control aromatase synthesis in an intracrine manner after binding to ERβ. However, the coexistence of ERβ and aromatase in the same brain area does not necessarily prove that these two antigens are colocalized in the same cells, as already observed for ERα. Additional studies combining on the same sections a detection of ERβ by in situ hybridization with the visualization of the aromatase protein or mRNA are thus needed to determine whether this mode of aromatase control is compatible with the anatomical organization of the enzyme and the receptor. If ARO-ir cells do not contain estrogen receptors (of the alpha or beta subtypes), alternative mechanisms mediating the control of aromatase synthesis must be contemplated. Locally produced estrogens could diffuse to adjacent cells that contain ER but alternatively estrogens could also modify AA by affecting inputs to aromatase cells in a manner reminiscent of what has been described in much more detail for the regulation of GnRH neurons. Although steroids exert a strong influence on the synthesis and release of GnRH, neurons producing this peptide usually contain no estrogen receptors α (Shivers et al. 1983; Herbison and Theodosis 1992; Herbison et al. 1993;see, however, Skynner et al. 1999; Herbison and Pape 2001), and they are controlled by an estrogen-sensitive neuronal network that involves several neurotransmitters and neuropeptides (Barraclough and Wise 1982; Weiner et al. 1988; Herbison 1998). This suggestion is supported by anatomical and pharmacological results, implying in particular a role of estrogen-dependent catecholaminergic inputs in the control of aromatase activation (see Absil et al. 2001; Balthazart et al. 2002 for review).

## Steroid receptors co-regulators and aromatase expression

Research during the past decades has characterized responses to steroids in a diversity of species and has clearly documented the reliability of their action on behavior. However, at the same time, a number of discrepancies (more or less dramatic changes in sensitivity to steroid action) have been identified. Recent biochemical and molecular work indicates that steroid co-activators and co-repressors markedly modify the physiological and behavioral responses to steroids and could therefore explain these discrepancies (Fig. 2A; McKenna et al. 1999; McKenna and O'Malley 2002; Molenda et al. 2003). We therefore decided to investigate the possible role of these proteins in the control of aromatase expression and initial experiments completed so far have focussed on the co-regulator that has been best characterized to this date, the steroid receptor co-activator 1 or SRC-1.

The lack of suitable specific antibodies to study the distribution and regulation of coactivators in birds led us to clone SRC-1 to design probes for in situ hybridization. We isolated and sequenced a full-length cDNA for quail SRC-

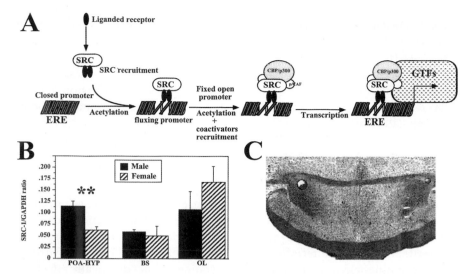

**Fig. 2.** The steroid receptor co-activator-1 (SRC-1) is implicated in steroid action in the quail brain. **A.** Model illustrating the involvement of SRC-1 (SRC) and other co-regulators during estrogen receptor (ER)–dependent transcription. Upon ligand fixation, ERs dimerize, recruit SRC-1 and bind to a specific recognition site on DNA (estrogen response element, ERE). This complex then extents with the fixation of other co-regulatory proteins such as CBP/p300 and p/CAF. The interaction of the different co-activators and ER promotes the conformational change of the chromatin through histone acetylation and methylation and the stabilization of the transcriptional machinery (general transcription factors, GTFs), thereby enhancing the transcription of ERE-associated genes. **B.** Real time quantitative PCR demonstrates a significantly higher expression of SRC-1 in the preoptic area-hypothalamus (POA-HYP) of male quail as compared to females. No significant difference is found in other brain areas (brain stem, BS; optic lobes, OL). **C.** In situ hybridization demonstrates a denser expression of SRC-1 transcripts in the quail medial preoptic nucleus by comparison with adjacent areas. From data in Charlier et al. 2002.

1, which shows a high degree of homology with the chicken, mouse and human SRC-1 (Charlier et al. 2002). RT-PCR experiments showed that SRC-1 transcripts are broadly expressed in a large number of quail tissues including several brain areas (e.g., telencephalon, diencephalon, optic lobes, brain stem, spinal cord, pituitary gland, liver, kidney, adrenal glands, heart, lung, epididymis, testis, ovary and oviducts). Analysis with real time quantitative PCR showed that in some brain regions (e.g., brain stem, optic lobes) SRC-1 expression is similar in males and females (Fig. 2B). In contrast, SRC-1 expression in the preoptic area-hypothalamus was significantly higher in males than in females (Charlier et al. 2002). In situ hybridization with oligoprobes labeled by digoxigenin further showed that SRC-1 mRNA expression can be broadly detected in the brain but is particularly high in many areas that contain high densities of steroid receptors (Charlier et al. 2002). An intense hybridization signal was namely observed in several hypothalamic and limbic nuclei, including the medial preoptic nucleus and the nucleus stria terminalis, two steroid targets that are involved in the control of reproductive behavior and express high densities of aromatase (Fig. 2C). The potential co-localization between aromatase and the co-regulator is currently under investigation. Experiments in progress are also evaluating the effects of a disruption of SRC-1 expression by injection of anti-sense oligonucleotides on the induction by steroids of preoptic aromatase and of male copulatory behavior.

## Faster changes in aromatase activity observed in phophorylating condition

In addition to the slow variations that result from changes in their concentration, the activity of many enzymes can be rapidly modified by conformational changes in the enzyme molecule. For example, phosphorylations catalyzed by specific kinases that transfer the terminal phosphate group from ATP to the hydroxyl moiety of amino acid residues (tyrosine, threonine, serine) drastically affect the activity of tyrosine hydroxylase, the rate limiting enzyme in catecholamine – synthesis (Albert et al. 1984; Daubner et al. 1992). ATP and $Mg^{2+}$ are required for this reaction which makes kinase activity critically dependent on the $Mg^{2+}$ intracellular concentration. Given that previous studies have implicated divalent cations in the control of AA ($Ca^{2+}$: Hochberg et al. 1986; Onagbesan and Podie 1989; $Mg^{2+}$: Steimer and Hutchison 1991) and because several consensus sites of phosphorylation are present in the mammalian and avian aromatase sequences (e.g., Corbin et al. 1988; Harada 1988; McPhaul et al. 1988; Means et al. 1989; Harada et al. 1992; Shen et al. 1994; Balthazart et al. 2003a), we investigated whether $Ca^{2+}$ concentrations or ATP and $Mg^{2+}$ concentrations such as those

---

**Fig. 3.** Effects of calcium-dependent kinases on the AA measured in quail preoptic homogenates (A-C) or in preoptic explants maintained in vitro (D-F). **A.** A 15-min  preincubation of preoptic homogenates in the presence of ATP, $Mg^{2+}$ and $Ca^{2+}$ markedly inhibited A A, where these compounds alone have little or no effect. This effect is blocked by EGTA, a compound that chelates divalent ions such as $Ca^{2+}$. **B.** The inhibition of AA produced in preoptic homogenates by the addition of ATP, $Mg^{2+}$ and $Ca^{2+}$ (Ctr vs Tot) is largely blocked in the presence of staurosporine (STAU, a serine-threonine kinase inhibitor) or genistein (GEN, a tyrosine kinase inhibitor). A significant blockade of the decrease is also observed after addition of a protein kinase C (PKC) inhibitor (BIS, Bisindolylmaleimide), a protein kinase A (PKA) inhibitor (H89) or of the myosin light chain kinase 7 inhibitor (ML7). Other kinase inhibitors have little or no effect. The specificity of each compound is indicated in the bar. **C.** Effect of increasing doses of staurosporine on the AA measured in the presence or absence (+ or - ATP) of 1 mM ATP, 1 mM $Mg^{2+}$ and 0.50 mM $Ca^{2+}$. **D-E.** AA in paired POA-hypothalamus explants incubated in vitro in which one explant is exposed [between 20 (up arrow) and 30 (down arrow) min] to increased intracellular $Ca^{2+}$ by the addition of $K^+$ (non-specific depolarization leading to $Ca^{2+}$ entry in the cells; **D**) or of thapsigargin, a compound that mobilizes the intracellular $Ca^{2+}$ stores (**E**). A rapid and transient decrease in aromatase activity was observed. **F.** Similar effects were observed after addition of agonists of the excitatory amino-acid receptors (in this case, kainate was added from 20 to 30 min). CON, control. Adapted from data in Balthazart et al. 2001a, 2003a, b.

used to obtain maximal changes in tyrosine hydroxylase activity (Ames et al. 1978) would affect AA in male quail brain homogenates. In the presence of suitable physiological concentrations of ATP, $Mg^{2+}$ and $Ca^{2+}$, a profound (80-90%) inhibition of AA was observed in quail brain homogenates (Fig. 3A). This inhibition was prevented by agents that chelate divalent ions, such as EGTA or EDTA (Balthazart et al. 2001a). These data indicate that AA is almost completely suppressed in conditions that promote protein phosphorylation. That this enzymatic inhibition is actually mediated by phosphorylation processes is indicated by the observation that the inhibitory effects of ATP/Mg/Ca are blocked in the presence of kinase inhibitors.

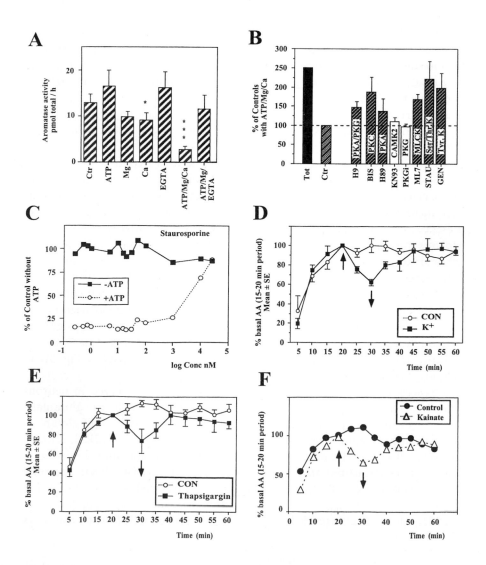

Inhibitors of serine/threonine (staurosporine) as well as of tyrosine kinase (genistein) were found to inhibit the inhibition of AA by ATP/Mg/Ca, and additional pharmacological experiments further pointed to the involvement of protein kinase C (PKC), protein kinase A (PKA) and one of several calmodulin (CAM) kinases (possibly MLCK) in the control of enzyme activity (Balthazart et al. 2001b, 2003a; Fig. 3B). The effects of the compounds that seemed to have the most specific effects on AA were further analyzed in dose-response experiments. The two general kinases inhibitors, staurosporine and genistein, clearly did not modify AA in the absence of ATP/Mg/Ca. However, increasing concentrations of these compounds progressively decreased the ATP/Mg/Ca-induced inhibition of enzymatic activity so that no inhibition remained at the highest doses (10-100 μM; see example in Fig. 3C; Balthazart et al. 2003a). These results clearly indicate that staurosporine and genistein exert their effects on AA by specifically interacting with the ATP/Mg/Ca-dependent phosphorylations of the enzyme. The identification by Western blotting of phosphorylated amino acid residues on the aromatase protein purified by immunoprecipitation and electrophoresis further supports this interpretation (Balthazart et al. 2003a). Available results also clearly point to the existence of a complex profile with multiple phosphorylation sites on aromatase that play a significant regulatory role.

*In vitro* experiments on explants of preoptic area-hypothalamus further demonstrated that $Ca^{2+}$-dependent inhibitions of aromatase also take place in intact neurons. Paired left and right explants of preoptic area-hypothalamus were incubated in vitro at 37°C in 300 μl of oxygenated glucose-saline in the presence of 25 nM [1β-$^3$H]-androstenedione, and cumulative AA in these explants was measured every 30 or every 5 min by quantifying the amount of tritiated water that had been released (see Balthazart et al. 2001a for techniques). After reaching steady state conditions (after approximately 20-30 min), AA remained relatively stable in these conditions for several hours, but conditions that affected the intracellular $Ca^{2+}$ concentration, such as a depolarization by addition of potassium in the incubation medium or the exposure to thapsigargin, a lactone known for its capacity to mobilize intracellular pools of $Ca^{2+}$ rapidly (within 5 min) and reversibly inhibited the enzymatic activity (see Fig. 3D-E; Balthazart et al. 2001a).

Changes in intracellular $Ca^{2+}$ concentration are also observed in neurons following stimulation by various neurotransmitters such as glutamate. Accordingly, other experiments showed that the 10-min addition of glutamate agonists such as amino-methyl-4-isoxazole propionic acid [AMPA], kainate or N-methyl-D-aspartic acid [NMDA] to the incubation medium significantly depressed AA measured in these explants (Fig. 3F). These effects are fully reversible following washing of these agents from the medium, indicating that they are likely physiological (Absil et al. 2001; Balthazart et al. 2001b; Baillien et al. 2003). These effects are likely mediated by direct actions of the transmitters on aromatase-expressing cells; electrophysiological studies indeed indicate that most ARO-ir cells are directly sensitive to dopamine, AMPA, kainate and NMDA (Balthazart et al. 2003b; Cornil et al., submitted for publication). Taken together, these experiments demonstrate that AA can be regulated rapidly in the brain as a function of changes in neurotransmitter activity. This regulation should result in changes in the local bioavailability of estrogens within minutes or even seconds, i.e., in a time frame that is compatible with the induction of membrane effects of estrogens. Estrogens indeed modify the electrical activity of the neurons within seconds after their application, which essentially rules out the possibility of a classical steroid receptor-mediated effect on protein synthesis (for additional discussion see Schumacher 1990; McEwen 1994; Ramirez et al. 1996; McEwen and Alves 1999; Kelly and Ronnekleiv 2002). Behaviorally relevant effects of estrogens on brain functioning that appear to be independent of their binding to intracellular receptors have also been described (e.g., Blaustein and Olster 1989; Thompson and Moss 1994; Pasqualini et al. 1995; Mermelstein et al. 1996; Küppers et al. 2000, 2001). These rapid changes in estrogen synthase activity address the conceptual gap existing between the well-documented, rapid non-genomic effects of estrogens in the brain and the apparent lack of mechanisms capable of rapidly modifying estrogen availability in specific brain areas. Experiments currently in progress clearly indicate that these rapid changes in brain AA have important behavioral consequences (see below).

## Cellular and subcellular distribution of aromatase

*Cellular*
Aromatase has been known for many years to be present in the limbic system in various species, including human (Naftolin et al. 1972, 1975). With the advent of immunocytochemical techniques and, later, of in situ hybridization, the neuroanatomical distribution of the enzyme has been studied with a cellular level of resolution. This distribution has been particularly well characterized by immunocytochemistry in the Japanese quail brain. High densities of ARO-ir cells were originally identified in various diencephalic and limbic structures such as the medial preoptic nucleus, ventromedial nucleus of the hypothalamus and bed nucleus of the stria terminalis (Balthazart et al. 1990b, 1990c; Foidart et al. 1995). More recently, however, aromatase was found to also be expressed throughout the rostrocaudal extent of the spinal cord, in the laminae I, II and III of the dorsal (or sensory) horn (Evrard et al. 2000). Radioenzyme assays based on measurement of the tritiated water released during aromatization of tritiated androstenedione confirmed the presence of substantial levels of AA throughout the rostrocaudal extent of the spinal cord. Interestingly, contrary to what is observed in the brain, the spinal AA and the number of ARO-ir cells in five representative segments of the spinal cord are not different in sexually mature males or females and are not influenced in males by castration, associated

or not with a treatment with testosterone (Evrard et al. 2000). Laminae I-III receive abundant sensory and, in particular, pain inputs arising from the periphery and contain estrogen receptors; recently it has been found that spinal aromatase plays a significant role in the estrogenic control of the spinal mechanisms of pain (Evrard and Balthazart 2002a, 2003b, 2004 c; see below). The presence of ARO-ir structures in the sensory part of the spinal cord extends in the hindbrain to other sensory nuclei (trigeminal, solitary tract, vestibular, optic tectum) as well as to nuclei primarily characterized by their integrative function (parabrachial, periaqueductal, cerulean, raphe nuclei; Evrard et al. 2004). The presence of aromatase in these nuclei where estrogen receptors were also previously identified suggests a role for locally produced estrogens in the control of sensory and integrative functions. The identification of ARO-ir cells in hindbrain sensory nuclei also allows us to extend the concept of spinal sensory aromatase to the much broader idea of a sensory aromatase that would be implicated in the modulation of most, if not all, sensory inputs (Horvath and Wikler 1999; Evrard et al. 2004).

*Subcellular*
Immunocytochemistry clearly demonstrates that brain aromatase is essentially localized in the neuronal perikarya. However, several studies have revealed that, in the diencephalon and limbic system, this immunoreactive material is also present in cell processes, including dendrites and the full length of axons (Foidart et al. 1994). Immunoreactive punctuate structures representing presumptive synaptic boutons were also described in this study. Dense to scattered networks of immunoreactive fibers were also found quasi-ubiquitously in the hindbrain and, in particular, in its most rostral and dorsal parts (Evrard et al. 2004). To a lesser extent, they were also present throughout the premotor nuclei of the reticular formation and in various fiber tracts.

Pre-embedding immunocytochemistry and electron microscopy confirmed that numerous axons and synaptic boutons containing ARO-ir material are indeed present in the preoptic area of the quail brain but also in zebra finches, rats, monkeys and even humans (Naftolin et al. 1996; Saldanha et al. 2003). Biochemical studies performed in quail, zebra finches and rats (Steimer 1988; Schlinger and Callard 1989; Roselli 1995) further indicate the presence of high levels of AA in synaptosomes ("pinched off" synaptic terminals) prepared by differential centrifugation. Two of these studies even demonstrated that AA is enriched in purified synaptosomal fractions by comparison with crude homogenates (Steimer 1988; Schlinger and Callard 1989), which indicates that the immunoreactive aromatase identified in pre-synaptic boutons is functionally active. These data thus suggest that significant amounts of estrogens are produced at the presynaptic level. This local production of estrogens in the close vicinity of synapses may provide steroid signals that could affect brain activity, independent of the binding to nuclear receptors acting as transcription factors (i.e., by non-genomic mechanisms).

The presence of aromatase in terminals located in brain regions that are often devoid of intracellular estrogen receptors provides anatomical evidence suggesting that estrogens locally produced in the brain may affect neuronal physiology by mechanisms that are independent of their action at the transcription level. Evidence that this is actually the case is progressively accumulating in quail, as described in the following sections.

## Functional significance of rapid changes in estrogen bioavailability

*Sexual behavior*
Although steroids are traditionally thought to exert their effects through relatively slow genomic mechanisms, evidence has accumulated during the last decade indicating that more rapid effects of steroids, and in particular of estrogens, can be observed in the brain (see above). Cross and Roselli (1999) recently showed that, in castrated male rats, systemic injections of estradiol increase within 35 min the expression of a variety of reproductive behaviors, including anogenital olfactory investigations and mounts by the male of the female. Rapid effects of estrogens could thus be relevant to the control of sexual behavior. We are currently testing this notion in quail by evaluating the acute effects of single injections of Vorozole$^{TM}$ (VOR), a nonsteroidal aromatase inhibitor (Wouters et al. 1989, 1994; De Coster et al. 1990), or of estradiol on male sexual behavior.

Several studies demonstrated that a single i.p. injection of VOR (30 mg/kg) in gonadally intact, sexually mature males or in castrates treated with 40 mm T implants (CX+T40), which are sufficient to induce a full copulatory behavior, significantly reduced most aspects of male copulatory behavior. Maximal effects were observed between 30 and 45 min after injection (Cornil et al. 2003; Fig 4A). Similar treatments with VOR also rapidly inhibited the expression of appetitive sexual behavior, as assessed by the frequency of rhythmic cloacal sphincter movements (RCSM). These movements are markedly increased when a sexually motivated male is presented with the view of a female (Balthazart et al. 1998b; Seiwert and Adkins-Regan 1998). This increase in RCSM frequency induced by the view of the female was markedly inhibited in males that had been injected with VOR (30 mg/kg; Fig 4B) 30 min before the test, and the effect was apparently vanishing after 60 min (Cornil et al. 2003). Interestingly, no effect of VOR was detected on the lower rate of RCSM displayed during the pretest period, when the female was not visible. Single VOR injections also did not affect the locomotor and exploratory behavior of the males tested in an open field. These data thus suggest that rapid changes in estrogen bioavailability resulting from acute inhibition of brain aromatase rapidly inhibit most, if not all, aspects of male sexual behavior.

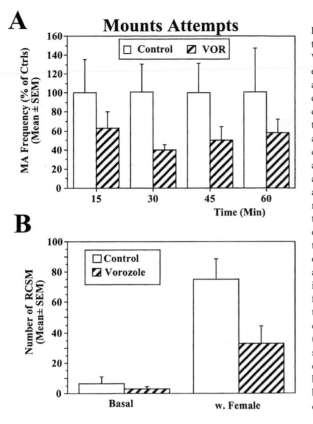

**Fig. 4.** Rapid effects of the aromatase inhibitor, Vorozole™ (VOR), on the expression of consummatory and appetitive components of male sexual behavior in quail. **A.** Injection of Vorozole to gonadally intact sexually active males decreases copulatory behavior (mount attempts). Maximal effects are observed 30 to 45 min after injection. All data were normalized as percentage of the behavioral frequencies observed in control subjects to allow direct comparison of the behavioral inhibitions at different latencies after injection. **B.** The view of a female drastically increases the frequency of rhythmic cloacal sphincter movements (RCSM) in gonadally intact sexually active males, and this effect is significantly inhibited by Vorozole injected 30 min before testing. Adapted from data in Cornil et al. 2003.

This conclusion is also supported by independent experiments in which the effects of a single systemic injection of estradiol on male copulatory behavior were studied in castrated males that had previously received a small, 2 mm-long Silastic™ implant filled with T (CX+T2). This dose of T is by itself insufficient to fully activate sexual behavior but induces expression of a weak sexual activity. Estradiol (500 µg/kg) injected i.p. 15 min before testing significantly stimulated copulatory behavior in castrated birds chronically treated with this low dose of T. This stimulation was no longer significant when birds were tested 30 or 45 min after the injection (Cornil et al. 2003). Given that similar results were previously reported in rats (Cross and Roselli 1999), the behavioral effects of rapid changes in estrogen availability appear to be of general significance.

### Estrogenic modulation of pain
As mentioned above, recent work in our laboratory identified the presence of active aromatase in numerous neurons all along the dorsal (sensory) horn of the spinal cord in quail (Evrard et al. 2000). Many of these neurons are localized in

laminae I-III, an important area for the processing of nociceptive inputs, and they express receptors for substance P, a neuropeptide released in laminae I-III from primary afferent fibers in response to painful stimulations (Evrard et al. 2003). To assess whether spinal aromatase could be implicated in the modulation of pain, we developed and validated in quail measures of the behavioral responsiveness to painful stimuli, including hot water (Evrard and Balthazart 2002b). Focusing first on the genomic effects of estrogens, we then showed that castration markedly increases, but a two-week treatment with T decreases, the latency of foot withdrawal from a mildly painful stimulus (54°C hot water bath; Evrard and Balthazart 2003a). This effect of T is mediated by its aromatization into estradiol, as indicated by the fact that a chronic treatment with estradiol has the same behavioral effects as T and the anti-estrogen tamoxifen blocks the effects of both steroids, whereas a specific aromatase inhibitor selectively inhibits the action of T, but not of estradiol (Fig. 5A-B).

Interestingly, more recent work indicates that similar effects on the foot withdrawal latency are also observed within a few minutes after an acute treatment with steroids or aromatase inhibitors (Evrard and Balthazart 2003a, b). In one experiment, we assessed whether an acute i.p injection of the aromatase inhibitor Vorozole™ could alter foot withdrawal latency from a 54°C hot water bath in castrated males treated with subcutaneous implants filled with testosterone or estradiol or left empty. As expected based on data reviewed above (Evrard and Balthazart 2004), the chronic treatments with T or estradiol decreased the foot withdrawal latency by comparison with castrates treated with empty implants. However, a single i.p. injection of Vorozole™ markedly and rapidly (within 20 min) increased the foot withdrawal latency in subjects chronically supplemented with T but not in subjects treated with empty or estradiol-filled implants that were used as controls (Fig. 5C). Based on these observations, it appears that changes in AA are able to rapidly and specifically alter nociception in male quail. Because aromatase has been identified in the dorsal horn of the spinal cord (Evrard et al. 2000), it is likely that these rapid effects of Vorozole™ take place, at least in part, at the spinal level. This conclusion is supported by recent unpublished experiments showing that a single injection of Vorozole™ directly into the spinal subarachnoid space of gonadally intact male quail, at the level where the nerves from the foot enter the spinal cord, increases within one minute the foot withdrawal latency in the hot water test. This effect vanishes within 30 minutes and is not observed if the aromatase inhibitor is co-injected with a dose of exogenous estradiol or if it is injected directly in the brain at the level of the third ventricle (Evrard and Balthazart 2003a, b). Taken together, these data suggest that estrogens modulate pain, as they do sexual behavior, through two different mechanisms. On the one hand, estradiol exerts long-term effects on pain processes through the activation of nuclear receptors. Previous immunocytochemical data in quail indicate that these effects could depend, at least in part, on the spinal aromatization of

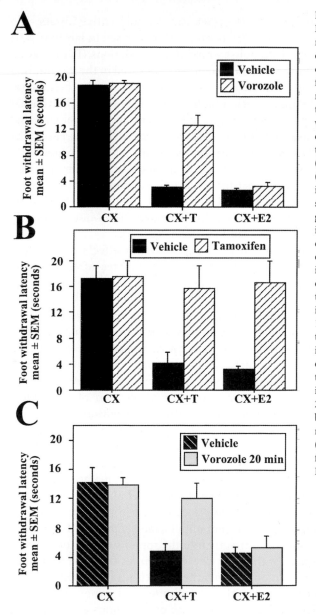

**Fig. 5.** Slow genomic (A-B) and rapid (presumably non-genomic, **C**) effects of estrogens on pain in male quail. The bars illustrate the foot withdrawal latencies measured with the hot water test at 54°C in male quail that were either castrated (CX) or castrated and chronically treated with testosterone (CX+T) or 17β-estradiol (CX+E2) subcutaneous implants. **A.** Half of the subjects in each of the three groups received a daily i.p. injection of Vorozole™ for 10 days (hatched bars) while the other half received vehicle injections (black bars). **B.** Half of the subjects in each of the three groups received a daily i.p. injection of tamoxifen for 10 days (hatched bars) while the other half received vehicle injections (black bars). **C.** Half of the subjects in each of the three groups received a single i.p. injection of Vorozole™ for 20 min before the test (gray bars) while the other half received vehicle injections (black hatched bars). Redrawn from data in Evrard and Balthazart 2003a, c.

androgens into estrogens and on the activation of nuclear estrogen receptors found in the vicinity of ARO-ir in the spinal dorsal horns (Evrard and Balthazart 2002a). On another hand, pain processes may also be subjected to rapid changes driven by estrogens produced in a tonic fashion locally in the spinal cord. This hypothesis would explain why a brief inhibition of spinal aromatase resulting in a rapid diminution of the local estrogen concentration can disrupt the response to painful stimuli within one minute. Rapid effects of estrogens have now been described in a variety of experimental models. They involve the activation of intracellular transduction cascades and appear to depend on the interaction of estrogens with the neuronal membrane rather than with nuclear receptors (Kelly and Ronnekleiv 2002). Additional studies are now needed and have been initiated in quail to clarify at the cellular level how rapid changes in AA and consequently in estrogen bioavailability, modulate the expression of male sexual behavior as well as behavioral responses to nociceptive stimuli.

## Cellular responses

### Phosphorylation of the cyclic AMP response element binding protein

The stimulation of adenylyl cyclase, leading to increased cAMP concentration and, as a consequence, to an increased phosphorylation of the cyclic AMP response element binding protein (pCREB) is a well-established cellular consequence of the rapid action of estrogens (Küppers et al. 2000; Kelly and Ronnekleiv 2002). Zhou et al. (1996) demonstrated that injection of estradiol leads to a rapid increase (after 15-30 min) in the number of pCREB-immunoreactive cells in the rat medial preoptic area. We are currently investigating whether similar effects can be detected in the quail diencephalon and limbic system and could eventually be modulated by endogenous rapid changes in AA. Castrated male quail were injected i.p. with estradiol (100 μg/bird, n = 12) or with the solvent (n = 8). Fifteen or 30 minutes later, half of the subjects in each group were perfused and coronal brain sections were stained by immunocytochemistry for pCREB. Basal levels of pCREB expression were detected in control birds. In contrast, high numbers of pCREB-immunoreactive (ir) cell nuclei were observed in E2-injected subjects (Fig. 6A-B). pCREB-ir nuclei were namely observed throughout the medial preoptic area and in the nucleus taeniae of the amygdala, where they largely overlapped with aromatase cell groups. Rapid changes of estrogen concentration can thus rapidly lead to localized variations in the level of CREB phosphorylation in brain areas implicated in the control of reproductive behavior. The behavioral significance of these cellular changes should now be investigated.

### Phosphorylation of tyrosine hydroxylase

The phosphorylation of Ser 40 in tyrosine hydroxylase (TH), the rate-limiting step in catecholamine synthesis, markedly enhances the activity of this enzyme by changing its maximal velocity (Albert et al. 1984; Waymire and Craviso 1993). In rats, TH phosphorylation can be rapidly induced by estrogens in brain areas that do not expresss significant levels of intracellular estrogen receptors (Pasqualini et al. 1995). Changes in the phosphorylation status of TH thus represent another potentially useful cellular marker for changes in

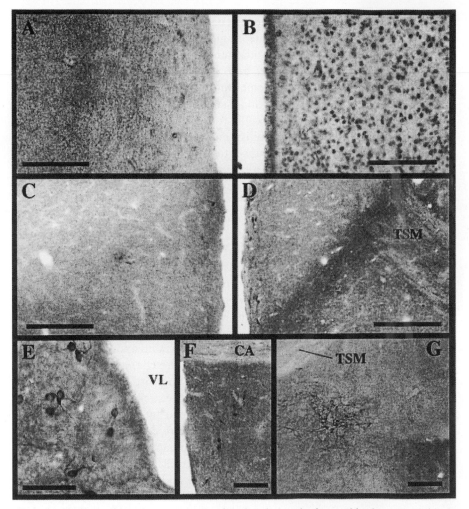

**Fig. 6.** Rapid effects of estrogens on protein phosphorylations in the quail brain. **A-B.** Within 15 minutes, a single injection of estradiol (E2) induces in the medial preoptic area a marked increase in the number of nuclei showing immunoreactivity for the phosphorylated form of the cAMP response element binding protein (pCREB; **A**, control oil-injected bird; **B**, E2-treated bird). **C-G.** Effects of a single injection of E2 15 minutes before sacrifice on the phosphorylation of tyrosine hydroxylase (TH). **C** and **D** illustrate matched sections in the rostral preoptic area at the level of the tractus septomesencephalicus (TSM) in a control oil-injected bird (**C**) and in an E2-injected subject (**D**). **E-G**, respectively, illustrate phosphorylated TH-immunoreactive structures at the levels of the septum adjacent to the ventriculus lateralis (VL) and the medial preoptic area ventral to the commissura anterior (CA) and in a fiber tract just ventral to the TSM.

estrogen availability in specific brain sites. We are currently investigating these changes by immunocytochemistry with antibodies that selectively recognize the phosphorylated (pTH) form of this enzyme (THS40P).

In castrated birds, THS40P labels, as expected, only a small fraction of the cells that express TH. The density of fibers and the number of cells labeled by THS40P are, however, markedly higher in birds that were injected with estradiol 15 minutes before sacrifice than in control, oil-injected subjects (see Fig. 6C-G). These data thus indicate that rapid changes in estrogen levels can affect the level of TH phosphorylation and, presumably, the activity of the enzyme. Given the prominent role played by dopaminergic transmission in the control of male copulatory behavior in all vertebrate species investigated so far (Hull 1995; Hull et al. 2002), and in quail in particular (Balthazart et al. 1997, 2002; Ball and Balthazart 2002), this enzymatic change could represent one way through which estradiol could rapidly affect male sexual behavior (by increasing DA synthesis). This hypothesis should now be experimentally explored.

## Conclusion

Recent research in quail has  illustrated that, besides their genomic effects mediated through binding to intracellular receptors that then act as transcription factors, steroids, in particular estrogens, can exert rapid behavioral effects, presumably via non-genomic mechanisms. It is interesting to note that estrogen synthesis in the brain also appears to change rapidly as a consequence of rapid changes in the phosphorylation status of the enzyme aromatase, controlled by neurotransmitter-dependent changes in neuronal calcium concentration. These effects, documented in greater detail in quail than in any other species to date, almost assuredly apply to other species, at least among endothermic vertebrates. Consensus phosphorylation sites are, for example, conserved in all mammalian and avian aromatase sequences that have been cloned to date, and rapid effects of estrogen injections have also been identified in other species, such as rats.

The analysis of steroid action in the brain is currently in a state of rapid evolution. It appears  that estrogens should be considered simultaneously as classic endocrine signals and signaling molecules with properties similar to those of neurotransmitters or at least neuromodulators. What is needed now is a balanced approach to this field, in which the roles of both of these actions of steroids can be appreciated. Such a balanced approach is more apt to be adopted if one approaches the question of steroid hormone action in the brain from the perspective of understanding how steroids regulate a functional end point such as behavior. It is fashionable in science today to focus on only one aspect of the cellular or molecular mechanisms of a signaling system. As useful as this approach might be, it is important to consider how a system can act in a multi-modal way to regulate an organism-level phenomenon. This approach is necessary both for a complete scientific understanding of steroid action in the brain and for an appreciation of the clinical significance of such action.

## Acknowledgments

Research described in this review was supported by grants from the National Institutes of Health (MH50388) to JB and GFB and grants from the French Community of Belgium (ARC99/04- 241), the Belgian FRFC (2.4555.01) and the Fonds Spéciaux pour la Recherche to JB. CAC is a FNRS Research Fellow. TDC is a FRIA Grant recipient.

## References

Absil P, Baillien M, Ball GF, Panzica G, Balthazart J (2001) The control of preoptic aromatase activity by afferent inputs in Japanese quail. Brain Res Rev 37: 38-58

Albert KA, Helmer-Matyjek E, Nairn AA, Müller TH, Haycock JW, Greene LA, Goldstein M, Greengard P (1984) Calcium/phospholipid-dependent protein kinase (protein kinase C) phosphorylates and activates tyrosine hydroxylase. Proc Natl Acad Sci USA 81: 7713-7717

Ames MM, Lerner P, Lovenberg W (1978) Tyrosine hydroxylase: activation by protein phosphorylation and end product inhibition. J Biol Chem 253: 27-31

Aste N, Balthazart J, Absil P, Grossmann R, Mülhbauer E, Viglietti-Panzica C, Panzica GC (1998) Anatomical and neurochemical definition of the nucleus of the stria terminalis in Japanese quail (Coturnix japonica). J Comp Neurol 396: 141-157

Baillien M, Ball GF, Bakker J, Balthazart J (2003) Calcium, calmodulin and aromatase: a key trio in the rapid control of estrogen concentration in the brain. Soc Neurosci Abstr 33: 726.3

Ball GF, Balthazart J (2002) Neuroendocrine mechanisms regulating reproductive cycles and reproductive behavior in birds. In: Pfaff DW, Arnold AP, Etgen AM, Fahrbach SE, Rubin RT (eds) Hormones, brain and behavior. Academic Press, San Diego, CA, pp 649-798

Balthazart J (1989) Steroid metabolism and the activation of social behavior. In: Balthazart J (ed) Advances in comparative and environmental physiology. Vol 3. Springer Verlag, Berlin, pp 105-159

Balthazart J, Foidart A (1993) Brain aromatase and the control of male sexual behavior. J Steroid Biochem Mol Biol 44: 521-540

Balthazart J, Ball GF (1998a) New insights into the regulation and function of brain estrogen synthase (aromatase). Trends Neurosci 21: 243-249

Balthazart J, Ball GF (1998b) The Japanese quail as a model system for the investigation of steroid-catecholamine interactions mediating appetitive and consummatory aspects of male sexual behavior. Ann Rev Sex Res 9: 96-176

Balthazart J, Foidart A, Hendrick JC (1990a) The induction by testosterone of aromatase activity in the preoptic area and activation of copulatory behavior. Physiol Behav 47: 83-94

Balthazart J, Foidart A, Harada N (1990b) Immunocytochemical localization of aromatase in the brain. Brain Res 514: 327-333

Balthazart J, Foidart A, Surlemont C, Vockel A, Harada N (1990c) Distribution of aromatase in the brain of the Japanese quail, ring dove, and zebra finch: An immunocytochemical study. J Comp Neurol 301: 276-288

Balthazart J, Foidart A, Surlemont C, Harada N (1991) Neuroanatomical specificity in the co-localization of aromatase and estrogen receptors. J Neurobiol 22: 143-157

Balthazart J, Stoop R, Foidart A, Harada N (1994) Synergistic control by androgens and estrogens of aromatase in the quail brain. Neuroreport 5: 1729-1732

Balthazart J, Foidart A, Surlemont C, Harada N, Naftolin F (1992) Neuroanatomical specificity in the autoregulation of aromatase-immunoreactive neurons by androgens and estrogens: An immunocytochemical study. Brain Res 574: 280-290

Balthazart J, Tlemçani O, Harada N (1996) Localization of testosterone-sensitive and sexually dimorphic aromatase-immunoreactive cells in the quail preoptic area. J Chem Neuroanat 11: 147-171

Balthazart J, Castagna C, Ball GF (1997) Differential effects of D1 and D2 dopamine receptor agonists and antagonists on appetitive and consummatory aspects of male sexual behavior in Japanese quail. Physiol Behav 62: 571-580

Balthazart J, Foidart A, Houbart M, Prins GS, Ball GF (1998a) Distribution of androgen receptor-immunoreactive cells in the quail forebrain and their relationship with aromatase immunoreactivity. J Neurobiol 35: 323-340

Balthazart J, Absil P, Gérard M, Appeltants D, Ball GF (1998b) Appetitive and consummatory male sexual behavior in Japanese quail are differentially regulated by subregions of the preoptic medial nucleus. J Neurosci 18: 6512-6527

Balthazart J, Baillien M, Ball GF (2001a) Rapid and reversible inhibition of brain aromatase activity. J Neuroendocrinol 13: 61-71

Balthazart J, Baillien M, Ball GF (2001b) Phosphorylation processes mediate rapid changes of brain aromatase activity. J Steroid Biochem Mol Biol 79: 261-277

Balthazart J, Baillien M, Ball GF (2002) Interactions between aromatase (estrogen synthase) and dopamine in the control of male sexual behavior in quail. Comp Biochem Physiol [B] 132: 37-55

Balthazart J, Baillien M, Charlier TD, Ball GF (2003a) Calcium-dependent phosphorylation processes control brain aromatase in quail. Eur J Neurosci 17: 1591-1606

Balthazart J, Baillien M, Charlier TD, Cornil CA, Ball GF (2003b) Multiple mechanisms control brain aromatase activity at the genomic and non-genomic level. J Steroid Biochem Mol Biol 86: 367-379

Barraclough CA, Wise PM (1982) The role of catecholamines in the regulation of pituitary luteinizing hormone and follicle stimulating-hormone secretion. Endo Rev 3: 91-119

Baulieu E-E, Robel P (1990) Neurosteroids: A new brain function? J Steroid Biochem 37: 395-403

Baulieu EE, Robel P, Schumacher M (1999) Neurosteroids. A new regulatory function in the nervous system. Humana Press, Totowa, NJ

Bayliss WM, Starling EH (1902) The mechanism of pancreatic secretion. J Physiol London 28: 325-353

Beach FA (1948) Hormones and behavior. Paul B. Hoeber, Inc., New York

Blaustein JD, Olster DH (1989) Gonadal steroid hormone receptors and social behaviors. In: Balthazart J (ed) Advances in comparative and environmental physiology. Vol 3. Springer Verlag, Berlin, pp 31-104

Charlier TD, Lakaye B, Ball GF, Balthazart J (2002) Steroid receptor coactivator SRC-1 exhibits high expression in steroid-sensitive brain areas regulating reproductive behaviors in the quail brain. Neuroendocrinology 76: 297-315

Connolly PB, Roselli CE, Resko JA (1990) Aromatase activity in adult guinea pig brain is androgen dependent. Biol Reprod 43: 698-703

Corbin CJ, Graham-Lorence S, McPhaul M, Mason JI, Mendelson CR, Simpson ER (1988) Isolation of a full-length cDNA insert encoding human aromatase system cytochrome P-450 and its expression in nonsteroidogenic cells. Proc Natl Acad Sci USA 85: 8948-8952

Cornil CA, Evrard HC, Ball GF, Balthazart J (2003) Rapid effects of 17β - Estradiol and vorozole, an aromatase inhibitor, on male sexual behavior in Japanese quail. Soc Neurosci Abstr 33: 726.5

Cross E, Roselli CE (1999) 17beta-estradiol rapidly facilitates chemoinvestigation and mounting in castrated male rats. Am J Physiol Regul Integr Comp Physiol 276: R1346-R1350

Daubner SC, Lauriano C, Haycock JW, Fitzpatrick PF (1992) Site-directed mutagenesis of serine 40 of rat tyrosine hydroxylase. J Biol Chem 267: 12639-12646

De Coster R, Wouters W, Bowden CR, Vanden Bossche H, Bruynseels J, Tuman RW, Van Ginckel R, Snoeck E, Van Peer A, Janssen PAJ (1990) New non-steroidal aromatase inhibitors: Focus on R76713. J Steroid Biochem 37: 335-341

Evrard HC, Balthazart J (2002a) Localization of oestrogen receptors in the sensory and motor areas of the spinal cord in Japanese quail (Coturnix japonica). J Neuroendocrinol 14: 894-903

Evrard HC, Balthazart J (2002b) The assessment of nociceptive and non-nociceptive skin sensitivity in the Japanese quail (Coturnix japonica). J Neurosci Meth 116: 135-146

Evrard HC, Balthazart J (2003a) Spinal estrogen synthesis rapidly increases responsiveness to noxious stimuli. Abst 4th Congress of the EFIC

Evrard HC, Balthazart J (2003b) Long term and short term aromatase inhibitions result in slow and rapid alterations of pain. Trabajos del Instituto Cajal 79: 122-123

Evrard H, Baillien M, Foidart A, Absil P, Harada N, Balthazart J (2000) Localization and controls of aromatase in the quail spinal cord. J Comp Neurol 423: 552-564

Evrard HC, Willems E, Harada N, Balthazart J (2003) Specific innervation of aromatase neurons by substance P fibers in the dorsal horn of the spinal cord in quail. J Comp Neurol 465: 309-318

Evrard HC, Balthazart J (2004) Aromatization of androgens into estrogens reduces response latency to a noxious thermal stimulus in male quail. Horm Behav 45:181-189

Evrard HC, Harada H, Balthazart J (2004) Immunocytochemial localization of aromatase in sensory and integrating nuclei of the hindbrain in Japanese quail (Coturnix japonica). J Comp Neurol 473:194-212

Foidart A, Harada N, Balthazart J (1994) Effects of steroidal and non steroidal aromatase inhibitors on sexual behavior and aromatase-immunoreactive cells and fibers in the quail brain. Brain Res 657: 105-123

Foidart A, Reid J, Absil P, Yoshimura N, Harada N, Balthazart J (1995) Critical re-examination of the distribution of aromatase-immunoreactive cells in the quail forebrain using antibodies raised against human placental aromatase and against the recombinant quail, mouse or human enzyme. J Chem Neuroanat 8: 267-282

Foidart A, Lakaye B, Grisar T, Ball GF, Balthazart J (1999) Estrogen receptor-beta in quail: Cloning, tissue expression and neuroanatomical distribution. J Neurobiol 40: 327-342

Harada N (1988) Novel properties of human placental aromatase as cytochrome P-450: purification and characterization of a unique form of aromatase. J Biochem 103: 106-113

Harada N, Yamada K, Foidart A, Balthazart J (1992) Regulation of aromatase cytochrome P- 450 (estrogen synthetase) transcripts in the quail brain by testosterone. Mol Brain Res 15: 19-26

Harada N, Abe-Dohmae S, Loeffen R, Foidart A, Balthazart J (1993) Synergism between androgens and estrogens in the induction of aromatase and its messenger RNA in the brain. Brain Res 622: 243-256

Harris GW (1955) Neural control of the pituitary gland. Edward Arnold and Company, London

Herbison AE (1998) Multimodal influence of estrogen upon gonadotropin-releasing hormone neurons. Endocrinol Rev 19: 302-330

Herbison AE, Theodosis DT (1992) Localization of oestrogen receptors in preoptic neurons containing neurotensin but not tyrosine hydroxylase, cholecystokinin or luteinizing hormone-releasing hormone in the male and female rat. Neuroscience 50: 283-298

Herbison AE, Pape JR (2001) New evidence for estrogen receptors in gonadotropin-releasing hormone neurons. Frontiers Neuroendocrinol 22: 292-308

Herbison AE, Robinson JE, Skinner DC (1993) Distribution of estrogen receptor immunoreactive cells in the preoptic area of the ewe: Co-localization with glutamic acid decarboxylase but not luteinizing hormone-releasing hormone. Neuroendocrinology 57: 751-759

Hochberg Z, Bick T, Pelman R, Brandes JM, Barzilai D (1986) The dual effect of calcium on aromatization by cultured human trophoblast. J Steroid Biochem 24: 1217-1219

Horvath TL, Wikler KC (1999) Aromatase in developing sensory systems of the rat brain. J Neuroendocrinol 11: 77-84

Hull EM (1995) Dopaminergic influences on male rat sexual behavior. In: Micevych PE, Hammer RPJ (eds) Neurobiological effects of sex steroid hormones. Cambridge University Press, Cambridge, pp 234-253

Hull EM, Meisel RL, Sachs BD (2002) Male sexual behavior. In: Pfaff DW, Arnold AP, Etgen AM, Fahrbach SE, Rubin RT (eds) Hormones, brain and behavior. Academic Press, San Diego, CA, pp 1-137

Hutchison JB, Steimer TH (1986) Formation of behaviorally effective 17beta-estradiol in the dove brain: steroid control of preoptic aromatase. Endocrinology 118: 2180-2187

Kelly MJ, Ronnekleiv OK (2002) Rapid membrane effects of estrogen in the central nervous system. In: Pfaff DW, Arnold AP, Etgen AM, Fahrbach SE, Rubin RT (eds) Hormones, brain and behavior. Academic Press, San Diego, pp 361-380

Kuiper GGJM, Enmark E, Pelto Huikko M, Nilsson S, Gustafsson JÅ (1996) Cloning of a novel estrogen receptor expressed in rat prostate and ovary. Proc Natl Acad Sci USA 93: 5925-5930

Kuiper GGJM, Shughrue PJ, Merchenthaler I, Gustafsson J-Å (1998) The estrogen receptor β, subtype: a novel mediator of estrogen action in neuroendocrine systems. Frontiers Neuroendocrinol 19: 253-286

Küppers E, Ivanova T, Karolczak M, Beyer C (2000) Estrogen: a multifunctional messenger to nigrostriatal dopaminergic neurons. J Neurocytol 29: 375-385

Küppers E, Ivanova T, Karolczak M, Lazarov N, Föhr K, Beyer C (2001) Classical and nonclassical estrogen action in the developing midbrain. Horm Behav 40: 196-202

Lephart ED (1996) A review of brain aromatase cytochrome P450. Brain Res Rev 22: 1-26

MacLusky NJ, Philip A, Hurlburt C, Naftolin F (1984) Estrogen metabolism in neuroendocrine structures. In: Celotti F, Naftolin F, Martini L (eds) Metabolism of hormonal steroids in the neuroendocrine structure., Raven Press, New York, pp 103-116

McEwen BS (1991) Non-genomic and genomc effects of steroids on neural activity. Trends Pharmacol Sci 12: 141-147

McEwen BS (1994) Steroid hormone actions on the brain: When is the genome involved? Horm Behav 28: 396-405

McEwen BS, Pfaff DW (1985) Hormone effects on hypothalamic neurons: analysing gene expression and neuromodulator action. Trends Neurosci 08: 105-110

McEwen BS, Alves SE (1999) Estrogen actions in the central nervous system. Endocrinol Rev 20: 279-307

McKenna NJ, O'Malley BW (2002) Minireview: Nuclear receptor coactivators – An update. Endocrinology 143: 2461-2465

McKenna NJ, Lanz RB, O'Malley BW (1999) Nuclear receptor coregulators: cellular and molecular biology. Endocrinol Rev 20: 321-344

McPhaul MJ, Noble JF, Simpson ER, Mendelson CR, Wilson JD (1988) The expression of a functional cDNA encoding the chicken cytochrome P-450arom (aromatase) that catalyzes the formation of estrogen from androgen. J Biol Chem 263: 16358-16363

Means GD, Mahendroo MS, Corbin CJ, Mathis JM, Powell FE, Mendelson CR, Simpson ER (1989) Structural analysis of the gene encoding human aromatase cytochrome P-450, the enzyme responsible for estrogen biosynthesis. J Biol Chem 264: 19385-19391

Medvi VC (1982) A history of endocrinology. MTP Press Limited, Boston, MA

Mermelstein PG, Becker JB, Surmeier DJ (1996) Estradiol reduces calcium currents in rat neostriatal neurons via a membrane receptor. J Neurosci 16: 595-604

Molenda HA, Kilts CP, Allen RL, Tetel MJ (2003) Nuclear receptor coactivator function in reproductive physiology and behavior. Biol Reprod 69: 1449-1457

Naftolin F, Ryan KJ, Petro Z (1972) Aromatization of androstenedione by the anterior hypothalamus of adult male and female rats. Endocrinology 90: 295-298

Naftolin F, Ryan KJ, Davies IJ, Reddy VV, Flores F, Petro Z, Kuhn M, White RJ, Takaoka Y, Wolin L (1975) The formation of estrogens by central neuroendocrine tissues. Rec Prog Horm Res 31: 295-319

Naftolin F, Horvath TL, Jakab RL, Leranth C, Harada N, Balthazart J (1996) Aromatase immunoreactivity in axon terminals of the vertebrate brain - an immunocytochemical study on quail, rat, monkey and human tissues. Neuroendocrinology 63: 149-155

Onagbesan OM, Podie MJ (1989) Calcium-dependent stimulation of estrogen secretion by FSH from theca cells of the domestic hen (Gallus domesticus). Gen Comp Endocrinol 75: 177-186

Panzica GC, Viglietti-Panzica C, Calcagni M, Anselmetti GC, Schumacher M, Balthazart J (1987) Sexual differentiation and hormonal control of the sexually dimorphic preoptic medial nucleus in quail. Brain Res 416: 59-68

Panzica GC, Viglietti-Panzica C, Sanchez F, Sante P, Balthazart J (1991) Effects of testosterone on a selected neuronal population within the preoptic sexually dimorphic nucleus of the Japanese quail. J Comp Neurol 303: 443-456

Panzica GC, Viglietti-Panzica C, Balthazart J (1996) The sexually dimorphic medial preoptic nucleus of quail: a key brain area mediating steroid action on male sexual behavior. Frontiers Neuroendocrinol 17: 51-125

Pasqualini C, Olivier V, Guibert B, Frain O, Leviel V (1995) Acute stimulatory effect of estradiol on striatal dopamine synthesis. J Neurochem 65: 1651-1657

Ramirez VD, Zheng JB, Siddique KM (1996) Membrane receptors for estrogen, progesterone, and testosterone in the rat brain: Fantasy or reality. Cell Mol Neurobiol 16: 175-198

Roselli CE (1995) Subcellular localization and kinetic properties of aromatase activity in rat brain. J Steroid Biochem Mol Biol 52: 469-477

Roselli CE, Resko JA (1984) Androgens regulate brain aromatase activity in adult male rats through a receptor mechanism. Endocrinology 114: 2183-2189

Roselli CE, Resko JA (2001) Cytochrome P450 aromatase (CYP19) in the non-human primate brain: distribution, regulation, and functional significance. J Steroid Biochem Mol Biol 79: 247-253

Roselli CE, Horton LE, Resko JA (1985) Distribution and regulation of aromatase activity in the rat hypothalamus and limbic system. Endocrinology 117: 2471-2477

Roselli CE, Horton LE, Resko JA (1987) Time-course and steroid specificity of aromatase induction in rat hypothalamus-preoptic area. Biol Reprod 37: 628-633

Roselli CE, Stormshak F, Resko JA (1998) Distribution and regulation of aromatase activity in the ram hypothalamus and amygdala. Brain Res 811: 105-110

Saldanha CJ, Peterson RS, Yarram L, Schlinger BA (2003) The synaptocrine hypothesis: a novel mechanism of estrogen delivery. Horm Behav 44: 74

Schlinger BA, Callard GV (1987) A comparison of aromatase, 5α-and 5 β-reductase activities in the brain and pituitary of male and female quail (Coturnix c. Japonica). J Exp Zool 242: 171-180

Schlinger BA, Callard GV (1989) Localization of aromatase in synaptosomal and microsomal subfractions of quail (Coturnix coturnix japonica) brain. Neuroendocrinology 49: 434-441

Schumacher M (1990) Rapid membrane effects of steroid hormones: an emerging concept in neuroendocrinology. Trends Neurosci 13: 359-362

Schumacher M, Balthazart J (1986) Testosterone-induced brain aromatase is sexually dimorphic. Brain Res 370: 285-293

Schumacher M, Alexandre C, Balthazart J (1987) Interactions des androgènes et des oestrogènes dans le contrôle de la reproduction. C R Acad Sci Paris,Série III 305: 569-574

Seiwert CM, Adkins-Regan E (1998) The foam production system of the male Japanese quail: characterization of structure and function. Brain Behav Evol 52: 61-80

Shen P, Campagnoni CW, Kampf K, Schlinger BA, Arnold AP, Campagnoni AT (1994) Isolation and characterization of a zebra finch aromatase cDNA: in situ hybridization reveals high aromatase expression in brain. Mol Brain Res 24: 227-237

Shivers BD, Harlan RE, Morrell JI, Pfaff DW (1983) Absence of oestradiol concentration in cell nuclei of LHRH-immunoreactive neurones. Nature 304: 345-347

Simpson ER, Mahendroo MS, Means GD, Kilgore MW, Hinshelwood MM, Graham-Lorence S, Amarneh B, Ito Y, Fisher CR, Michael MD, Mendelson CR, Bulun SE (1994) Aromatase cytochrome P450, the enzyme responsible for estrogen biosynthesis. Endocrinol Rev 15: 342-355

Skynner MJ, Sim JA, Herbison AE (1999) Detection of estrogen receptor alpha and beta messenger ribonucleic acids in adult gonadotropin-releasing hormone neurons. Endocrinology 140: 5195-5201

Steimer T (1988) Aromatase activity in rat brain synaptosomes. Is an enzyme associated with the neuronal cell membrane involved in mediating non-genomic effects of androgens? Eur J Neurosci Suppl 1988: 9

Steimer T, Hutchison JB (1981) Androgen increases formation of behaviorally effective oestrogen in dove brain. Nature 292: 345-347

Steimer T, Hutchison JB (1991) Micromethods for the in vitro study of steroid metabolism in the brain using radiolabelled tracers. In: Greenstein B (ed) Neuroendocrine research methods. Vol 2. Harwood Academic Publishers, Chur, Switzerland, pp 875-919-870

Thompson TL, Moss RL (1994) Estrogen regulation of dopamine release in the nucleus accumbens: genomic- and nongenomic-mediated effects. J Neurochem 62: 1750-1756

Tsuruo Y, Ishimura K, Osawa Y (1995) Presence of estrogen receptors in aromatase-immunoreactive neurons in the mouse brain. Neurosci Lett 195: 49-52

Tsuruo Y, Ishimura K, Hayashi S, Osawa Y (1996) Immunohistochemical localization of estrogen receptors within aromatase-immunoreactive neurons in the fetal and neonatal rat brain. Anat Embryol (Berl) 193: 115-121

Viglietti-Panzica C, Panzica GC, Fiori MG, Calcagni M, Anselmetti GC, Balthazart J (1986) A sexually dimorphic nucleus in the quail preoptic area. Neurosci Lett 64: 129-134

Waymire JC, Craviso GL (1993) Multiple site phosphorylation and activation of tyrosine hydroxylase. Adv Prot Phosphatases 7: 501-513

Weiner RI, Findell PR, Kordon C (1988) Role of classic and peptide neuromediators in the neuroendocrine regulation of LH and prolactin In: Knobil E, Neill J (eds) The physiology of reproduction. Raven Press, New York, pp 1235-1281

Wouters W, De Coster R, Krekels M, Van Dun J, Beerens D, Haelterman C, Raeymaekers A, Freyne E, Van Gelder J, Venet M, Janssen PAJ (1989) R 76713, a new specific nonsteroidal aromatase inhibitor. J Steroid Biochem 32: 781-788

Wouters W, Snoeck E, De Coster R (1994) Vorozole, a specific non-steroidal aromatase inhibitor. Breast Cancer Res Treat 30: 89-94

Zhou Y, Watters JJ, Dorsa DM (1996) Estrogen rapidly induces the phosphorylation of the cAMP response element binding protein in rat brain. Endocrinology 137: 2163-2166

# Modulators of Endogenous Neuroprotection: Estrogen, Corticotropin-releasing Hormone and Endocannabinoids

*Christian Behl**

## Summary

Age-associated neurodegenerative disorders are among the most challenging problems of our aging society. Alzheimer's disease is affecting people with increasing frequency, since there is a clear relationship between the incidence of this detrimental disorder and age. Other neurodegenerative disorders, including Parkinson's disease, stroke and amyotrophic lateral sclerosis, are also frequently observed in our aging society. For most of these diseases, no causal therapy has yet been identified. Many of the treatments given to patients that are affected by these disorders have different side effects, and therefore the search is on to identify novel molecular approaches that may lead to a more effective therapy. In addition to treatment after the onset of these disorders, preventive strategies are of great importance. The brain itself may lead us to such novel preventive avenues, since large areas of the brain and the central nervous system in general resist detrimental processes and remain functional, even in late stages of the disorders mentioned. Such intrinsic neuroprotective and neuropreventive signals may indeed help to stabilize brain function and to make the central nervous system more resistant to the development of neurodegenerative disorders. Among these signals, we identified a potent neuroprotective role for the female sex hormone, estrogen, the corticotropin-releasing hormone (CRH) and endogenously produced and secreted cannabinoids (endocannabinoids). These hormones are powerful neuroprotective compounds when applied in paradigms of oxidative nerve cell death. Oxidative stress is a major hallmark of many neurodegenerative processes and of aging in general. The identification of common downstream pathways induced by these hormones may be the basis for the development of novel molecular strategies for neuroprevention.

* Institute for Physiological Chemistry and Pathobiochemistry, Johannes Gutenberg University, Medical School, D-55099 Mainz, Germany

Kordon et al.
Hormones and the Brain
© Springer-Verlag Berlin Heidelberg 2005

## Introduction

In the last hundred years, the average life expectancy in our society has dramatically increased. In 1900 the average life expectancy was approximately 37 years; in the year 2000 it was around 73 years, with the tendency toward a further increase. Consequently, research into the elucidation of the aging process in general and of age-associated degenerative disorders is *the* challenge of modern medical research. Taking a closer look into diseases of the nervous system, it becomes clear that a rise in the incidence of Alzheimer's disease (AD) can be expected. AD is a detrimental and deadly disorder that is the most frequent cause of dementia in the elderly population. AD is a neurodegenerative disorder that is progressive and is the paradigm of a *chronic* neurodegenerative event. One important example of an *acute* neurodegenerative insult is stroke in humans. Looking into the pathogenesis of both disorders, many differences can be observed but also many common pathways. One of the major hallmarks of the pathogenesis of both disorders is the occurrence of an increased level of oxidations. Oxidative stress is characterized by the accumulation of free oxygen and nitrogen species that can oxidize the molecules in the cells, with detrimental consequences. Oxidative stress occurs when the balance between the formation of oxidants and the detoxification by antioxidants is disturbed. At any time, cells produce free oxygen and nitrogen radicals, but cells have powerful antioxidative defense systems, including antioxidant enzymes, such as superoxide dismutase and catalase, and free radical scavenging compounds, such as the hydrophilic vitamin C (ascorbate) and the lipophilic vitamin E (α-tocopherol). With an overflow of free radical species, oxidative stress occurs, inducing either rapid necrotic processes or delayed apoptosis or both. It is now well acknowledged that oxidations may occur very early in the development of certain neurodegenerative disorders and are not just late, and rather downstream, effects (for review, see Moosmann and Behl 2002; Dawson and Dawson 2003).

A variety of neuroprotective strategies are proposed in the literature. These approaches include the prevention of excitotoxicity by antagonizing glutamate receptors, the inhibition of apoptosis with caspase inhibitors, as well as the application of neurotrophins. In addition, antioxidant molecules and anti-inflammatory drugs, as well as neurotransplantation and preconditioning approaches, have been successfully applied in a variety of experimental paradigms of neurodegeneration. All of these neuroprotection measures have been reported to be very effective in certain model systems in vitro and in vivo, but there are still many open questions with respect to treatment of AD and stroke as well as of other neurodegenerative syndromes.

The discussion presented here focuses mainly on the pathogenic role of oxidative stress and of oxidative stress-induced nerve cell death in the development of neurodegenerative disorders and on the intrinsic and endogenous signals that counteract the destructive activities of oxidative stress. Indeed, the

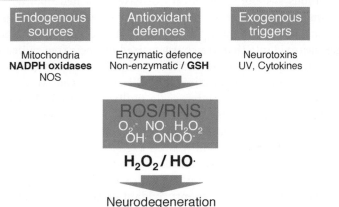

## OXIDATIVE STRESS
## as final common pathway in neurodegeneration

| Endogenous sources | Antioxidant defences | Exogenous triggers |
|---|---|---|
| Mitochondria<br>**NADPH oxidases**<br>NOS | Enzymatic defence<br>Non-enzymatic / **GSH** | Neurotoxins<br>UV, Cytokines |

ROS/RNS
$O_2^-$  NO  $H_2O_2$
OH  ONOO$^-$

$H_2O_2$ / HO·

Neurodegeneration

**Alzheimer's Disease**, Amyotrophic Lateral Sclerosis, Demyelinating Diseases, Diabetic Polyneuropathy, Down Syndrome, HIV Neuropathy, Huntington's Disease, Multiple System Atrophy, Parkinson's Disease, Prion Diseases **Stroke**, Tardive Dyskinesia, Tauopathies, Traumatic Brain Injury, **Aging**

**Fig. 1.** Oxidative stress occurs when the balance between free radical production and free radical removal and detoxification by antioxidants is disturbed. Reactive oxygen and nitrogen species are formed and, frequently, neurodegeneration is induced. Oxidations can be found in a variety of disorders and processes including Alzheimer's disease, stroke and the aging process, in general. (From Moosmann and Behl 2002).

accumulation of reactive oxygen and nitrogen species (ROS, RNS) is a major hallmark of various neurodegenerative disorders (Fig. 1). More specifically, in AD many players of pathogenetic importance do induce oxidative events, leading to the generation of a general, overall oxidative micro-environment. Consequently, the oxidation of biomolecules leads to dysfunction and to nerve cell death. DNA, proteins and lipids can be affected by oxidations. One of the key proteins that is believed to be of central importance for the development of AD, the amyloid beta protein, has been shown to induce a cascade of oxidative events, leading to rapid necrosis or delayed apoptosis. Thereby, amyloid beta protein itself can interact with neuronal membranes, inducing intracellular oxidases. In addition, amyloid beta protein that is deposited as protein aggregates (senile plaques) in AD brain can attract mediators of inflammation and can even induce an inflammatory response that leads to the generation of ROS and RNS.

In stroke that is characterized by a phase of ischemia followed by reperfusion, even more cascades of oxidations are activated through a variety of signals. A close look at the literature indicates that many different and completely unrelated neurodegenerative disorders are characterized by the accumulation of oxidations, which may, indeed, not only play a role in downstream events but may also be active in upstream processes. In some circumstances, oxidations are cited as the cause of neurodegenerative destruction. In addition to AD and stroke, there are other disorders that are associated with oxidative stress of the human nervous system: Parkinson's disease, HIV neuropathy, Huntington's disease, amyotrophic lateral sclerosis, prion diseases and aging in general. Due to the importance of oxidations in neurodegenative disorders, many different anti-oxidants that are characterized by their free radical-scavenging and free radical-preventing activities have been tested in various cellular and animal models, as well as in clinical studies of AD and stroke. With respect to AD, the most important, large-scale multicenter study is a clinical study employing vitamin E as a therapeutic drug in AD patients; it has shown some beneficial effects with respect to certain parameters (for review, see Sano 2003). Other anti-oxidant structures have been used and are reviewed in more detail elsewhere (for review, see Moosmann and Behl 2002). Since the pharmacokinetic of vitamin E as well as of other anti-oxidant structures is not well described, we have focused on molecules with anti-oxidant capacity that are known to enter the brain. Indeed, we have been successful in assigning estradiol/estrogen, the female sex hormone, an anti-oxidant role that is described in more detail below. In general, estrogen has many functions in the brain and enters the brain through the blood-brain passage quite easily. Moreover, the brain has an intrinsic capacity to synthesize estrogen.

## Estrogen:
## the female sex hormone as neuroprotective compound

Due to its chemical structure, estradiol has been identified as an antioxidant compound that is quite similar to vitamin E ($\alpha$-tocopherol) in its antioxidant activities. Both compounds are phenolic structures that can scavenge upcoming free radicals with unpaired electrons by donating a hydrogen atom to the toxic radical (Fig. 2). Indeed, we and others found that estradiol can act as a direct chemical antioxidant by interacting with accumulating radicals. In paradigms of oxidative nerve cell death, estradiol has been demonstrated to be a neuroprotective antioxidant (Behl et al., 1995; Behl et al., 1997; Prokai et al., 2003). Of course, the hormone estradiol is not *the* ideal antioxidant, due to its possible and expected feminizing side effects. Therefore, we concentrated on the development and identification of compounds that still carry the antioxidant phenolic structure that is intrinsic to estradiol but lack the hormonal estrogenic activity. By screening through chemical libraries, we identified a couple of such chemical structures, and we present 2,4,6-trimethylphenol (TMP) as such a compound. TMP has no estrogen receptor binding affinity and no activity on estrogen receptor-dependent gene transcription. Nevertheless, it acts as a potent antioxidant molecule and is more effective than estradiol itself but does not display any estrogenic or hormonal activities. Due to its small molecular

# α-Tocopherol and 17β-estradiol are monophenolic antioxidants

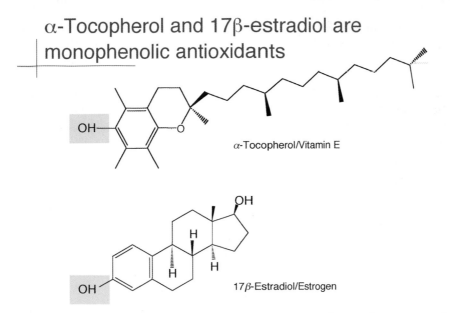

**Fig. 2.** α-Tocopherol and 17β-estradiol are monophenolic antioxidants and can scavenge free radicals. Both structures carry a radical scavenging phenolic group as well as a lipophilic tail.

size, improved permeability of the blood-brain barrier can be expected. This compound is under investigation in a variety of neurodegenerative model systems in vivo, and initial results on the effectiveness of this compound are expected soon.

Of course, estradiol (17β-estradiol) is an intrinsic physiological hormone that actsivate on the activation of estrogen receptors. This hormonal activity by activating gene transcription is the major function of estrogen in the various tissues throughout the body where estrogen receptors are expressed. Estrogen is well known to have essential roles in the development and maintenance of brain function. Estrogen acts on dendritic plasticity, neurotrophin signalling and synaptic connectivity, to mention just a few of the most important functions of estrogen on nerve cells (for review, see McEwen 2001).

Estrogen receptors, the targets of estrogen, come in two types, as estrogen receptor alpha and as estrogen receptor beta. Both receptors are expressed throughout the brain, with regional differences in density. In those areas that are highly affected in neurodegenerative disorders, such as the neocortex and the hippocampus, both estrogen receptors are expressed and are therefore primary targets of estrogen functions. Among the extra-hypothalamic sites where estrogen receptors are expressed are the neocortex, hippocampus, cholinergic system, serotonergic system, and catecholaminergic system. Estrogen receptors are also expressed in endothelial and glial cells, blood-brain barrier tissue and  spinal cord (for review, see McEwen 2001; Behl 2002). One of our major experimental goals in the search for novel neuroprotective targets is the identification of genes and signalling mechanisms that are specifically regulated by either estrogen receptor alpha or estrogen receptor beta. To identify such receptor subtype-specific target genes, we established a simple neuronal cell system. Human neuroblastoma cells (SK-N-MC) have been permanently transfected with either estrogen receptor alpha or estrogen receptor beta and these cells have been applied in gene expression profiling experiments employing gene chip analysis. In a first set of experiments, the estrogen receptor alpha-dependent gene transcription was investigated. As expected, a variety of genes have been shown to be up regulated in their expression. Most interestingly,  very high numbers of genes are also repressed in their transcription by the presence and activation of estrogen receptor alpha in neuroblastoma cells. Among those suppressed genes are  various caspases, the executors of apoptosis and the central players of the apoptosis network. This finding is consistent with an idea that estrogen and estrogen receptors improve nerve cell survival by blocking the apoptosis machinery.

Most interestingly, in our cellular model system, a group of genes that was previously shown to be related to estrogen receptor function is highly repressed in their transcription. These genes belong to the family of caveolin proteins. We have shown that the expression of caveolin 1 and of caveolin 2 is suppressed up to 6- to 20-fold in the estrogen receptor alpha-overexpressing neuroblastoma cells (Zschocke et al. 2002). Caveolins are the major protein constituents of membrane invaginations, the caveolae, which play a major function in exocytosis and endocytosis as well as in cholesterol transport. In addition, caveolae appear to be central signalling points in this membrane, by attracting and concentrating various cell signalling modulators at one site in the cell. Caveolins have also been shown to act as tumor suppressors, and the overexpression of caveolin 1 is an apoptotic signal. In the neuroblastoma cells that have been investigated in more detail, we found a specific downregulation of caveolin 1 and caveolin 2 in estrogen receptor alpha-overexpressing cells, whereas estrogen beta-overexpressing cells still showed a normal level of caveolin expression. Interestingly, when both types of estrogen receptors are expressed in one cell, the expression of caveolin is maintained, indicating a dominant effect of estrogen receptor alpha versus estrogen receptor beta at least with respect to caveolin expression. Therefore, caveolins are examples of proteins that are differentially regulated in their expression by estrogen receptors. Interestingly enough, when both estrogen receptors are expressed, caveolin expression is still maintained, suggesting a dominant effect of estrogen receptor alpha compared to estrogen receptor beta, an idea that is intensively elaborated on in the laboratory at the moment. The suppression of caveolin expression by estrogen receptor alpha occurs via the hypermethylation of the promoter, as we have shown for caveolin 1 (Zschocke et al. 2002). DNA hypermethylation is a well-known mechanism for

# Estrogen protects neurons:
# SUMMARY OF MODES OF ACTION

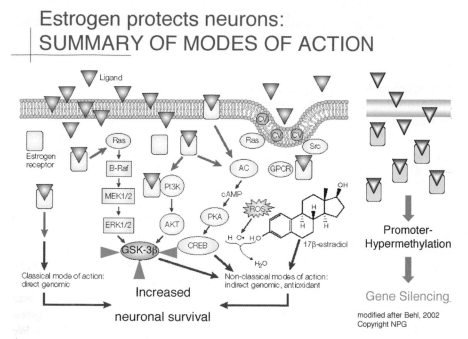

**Fig. 3.** Estrogen can act as a neuroprotectant via many different pathways. Estrogen controls the transcription of potent neuroprotective factors such as BDNF via the classical mode of action through activation and translocation of estrogen receptors. In addition, activated estrogen receptors can interact with intracellular signalling pathways such as MAPK and PI3K, leading to the down-stream phosphorylation of the survival factor GSK-3β. Estrogen receptors that are associated with the membrane via caveolae or that are even integrated in the neuronal membrane have been postulated. Such receptors can induce rapid down-stream signalling events. Moreover, estrogen receptors may mediate the long-term gene silencing that may also ultimately introduce protective pathways. Finally, the intrinsic antioxidant structure of estradiol can directly mediate protection against oxidations. Taken together, many potential cross-talks between estrogen, estrogen receptors and intracellular signalling pathways still need to be elucidated.

silencing genes in certain tissues where the expression needs to be suppressed permanently.

In summary, estrogen displays various modes of action that can mediate a neuroprotective function of this hormone. It is well known that estrogen targets directly the transcription of various neurotrophic factors (e.g., BDNF). Moreover, estrogen can interact with a variety of intracellular signal transduction pathways that may also activate neuroprotective genes that are not directly targeted by estrogen receptors. Also the antioxidant activity of estradiol, due to its phenolic structure, needs to be considered, especially in lipophilic environments, where estradiol can accumulate in high concentration. Finally, the targeting of certain genes and their repression by DNA hypermethylation, leading to direct gene silencing, can also be considered a potential neuroprotective mode of action.

Therefore, estrogen is a multifunctional neuroprotective hormone and much more work needs to be done to clarify this picture (Fig. 3).

## Corticotropin-releasing hormone, the modulator of the hypothalamic-pituitary-adrenal stress axis, as neurotrophic factor

The neuropeptide corticotropin-releasing hormone (CRH), which is the central modulator of the human stress axis, was discovered more than two decades ago (Vale et al. 1981). This 41-amino acid peptide was found to have a key role in mediating neuroendocrine effects that occur in response to stressful stimuli, through modulation of the hypothalamic-pituitary-adrenal (HPA) axis (for review, see Holsboer 2003). CRH also affects synaptic plasticity and promotes memory and learning, and the CRH system is affected during the progression of AD (for review, see Behan et al. 1996). In addition, to the link between CRH levels and AD, CRH has been discussed in association with stress-associated disorders, including anxiety and depression. In fact, increased levels of CRH have been directly linked to the onset and progression of these psychiatric disorders. A hyperdrive of the HPA axis is a well-acknowledged process that may be the cause of mood disorders and depressive syndromes. This type of stress is referred to as "pathological stress." Since the activity of the HPA stress axis is of central importance for the survival of the body, a functional stress system is the prerequisite for survival strategies under stress conditions, including energy recruitment and escape. Consequently, the physiological activation of the body's stress system ("physiological stress") is absolutely necessary for the survival of the organism and can be therefore called protective. Based on early work from De Souza and colleagues (for review, see Behan et al. 1996), we started a molecular investigation of the effects of CRH on nerve cell survival under oxidative stress. At that time we found that CRH is indeed a protective factor and prevents oxidative stress-induced neurodegeneration. Interestingly, in the brain, one major receptor for CRH, CRH receptor type 1, is not equally distributed; rather, there are hot spots of expression, i.e., in the cerebellum. The cerebellum is not affected in many neurodegenerative disorders, including AD. Consequently, one may hypothesize that specific intrinsic protective mechanisms are activated in this brain area. And, in fact, physiological levels of CRH protect cerebellar neurons cultured from embryonic mice and rats against the type of AD-associated neurodegeneration induced by amyloid beta protein toxicity (Lezoualc'h et al. 2000). But the protective activity of CRH is not equally distributed throughout the brain, since the cerebellar neurons and hippocampal neurons are highly protected against amyloid beta protein toxicity and cortical neurons are not protected when CRH is used in physiological concentrations (Bayatti et al. 2003). To identify the molecular basis of this differential protective effect, we focused on downstream signalling of the CRH receptor type 1, which is a well-described, G-protein coupled seven transmembrane receptor. Interestingly we found a direct correlation of cAMP response element binding protein (CREB) activation and glycogen synthase kinase-3 beta (GSK-3-beta) inactivation with the neuroprotective activities of CRH. CREB was activated and GSK-3-beta was inactivated only in the cerebellum and the hippocampus, areas that are highly protected by CRH (Bayatti et al. 2003). It will be of great interest to now look for downstream target genes that are differentially activated in the different brain areas. Moreover, it is of great importance to also study these protective effects of CRH in in vivo mouse models. Taking these findings together, CRH represents an intrinsic neuroprotective factor that shields neurons in certain brain areas but not in others. Targeting the CRH receptor type 1 could therefore be a powerful approach to identify novel neuroprotective pathways.

## Endocannabinoids, endogenous activators of the cannabinoid receptor, deliver on-demand protection against excitotoxicity

Similar to the female sex hormone, cannabinoids represent a family of compounds that affect a variety of neuronal functions, including feeding behavior, reward, sleep, and other activities. Interestingly, cannabinoids also affect learning and memory (for review, see Lutz 2002) and may mediate neuroprotection. The major target of exogenous cannabinoids, such as tetra-hydrocannabinol, the psychoactive compound of the plant *Cannabis sativa*, and of endogenous cannabinoids (endocannabinoids) is the cannabinoid receptor type 1 (CB1), which is expressed in the brain. Again, the cerebellum is one hot spot of cannabinoid receptor expression. Exogenous and endogenous ligands bind to CB1, which signals through G-proteins that are in contrast to the CRH receptor type 1 linked to inhibitory G-protein signalling. We investigated the effects of acute excitotoxic and oxidative insult in an in vivo mouse model that had been genetically modified to carry no functional CB1 receptor (CB1 knock-out mouse). Employing the well-known model of kainate injections into mice, which first induce epileptic-type seizures followed by nerve cell death in defined areas of the hippocampus, we investigated CB1 knock-out mice and control mice (wild-type) side by side. We found that the epileptic seizure response was significantly increased in those mice lacking a functional CB1. This enhanced responsiveness of mice to kainate could be mimicked by administering specific antagonists of CB1 to wild-type mice. In a detailed investigation of the molecular course of this increased sensitivity for epileptic seizure upon knock-out of CB1, we revealed that, upon kainate challenge, wild-type mice carrying a functional CB1 responded with an enhanced release of the endocannabinoid anandamide into the hippocampus. Anandamide may therefore be the intrinsic

## The endogenous cannabinoid system protects (on-demand) against excitotoxicity

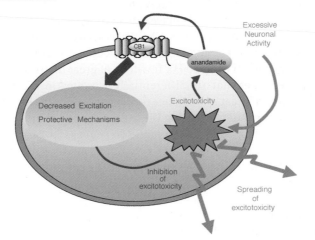

**Fig. 4.** Challenge of neurons by excitotoxic stimuli induces the on-demand release of the endogenous cannabinoid (endocannabinoid) anandamide, which acts on the CB1 receptor. Consequently, this process leads to the dampening of the excitatory response of the nerve cells and ultimately to the prevention of neuronal cell death. (From Marciano et al. 2003)

factor that prevents long-term effects of excitotoxicity and downstream neurodegeneration when the system is challenged with excitotoxic stimuli (Fig. 4). Indeed we found enhanced apoptosis and an enhanced gliosis in CB1 knock-out mice after the kainate challenge, further supporting the presence of an effective endocannabinoid protection system under normal wild-type conditions (Marsicano et al. 2003). It will be of great importance to investigate the role of the endogenous cannabinoid protection system under conditions of chronic progressive neurodegeneration. In summary also the endocannabinoid system may be considered a potent target for neuroprotective pharmaceutical intervention and therefore needs to be studied in greater detail.

## Conclusion and outlook

By studying the brain's intrinsic maintenance and survival factors, we found that hormones that are well known for a variety of highly important neuronal functions also supply the brain with neuroprotective activities. The female sex hormone estrogen, the stress peptide corticotropin-releasing hormone, and endocannabinoids such as anandamide are just a few examples demonstrating the high potency of self-defense intrinsically expressed in the brain. It can be easily imagined that, without such maintenance factors, the brain is left highly vulnerable to any kind of exogenous insults and endogenous imbalances. One pharmacological strategy could be to increase the level and activity of the brain's self-defense systems to make the brain more resistant to neurodegeneration. In fact, this view is a paradigm shift away from treating an ongoing disease by administration of certain compounds to long-term preventive stabilization of endogenous protective mechanisms. In the long run, and given the dramatic detrimental changes in age-associated neurodegenerative disorders, this approach may pay off and may help to increase the number of people that are able to achieve healthy and successful aging.

## Acknowledgments

Due to space limitations, references given here do not reflect a complete list of work performed, but various reviews are cited where the interested reader can find additional references. I would like to thank the people of my laboratory for their contribution. Work of the Behl lab referred to in this overview is supported by the Deutsche Forschungsgemeinschaft, European Union, and the Peter Beate Heller Stiftung.

## References

Bayatti N, Zschocke J, Behl C (2003) Brain region-specific neuroprotective action and signaling of corticotropin-releasing hormone in primary neurons. Endocrinoloy 144: 4051-4060
Behan DP, Grigoriadis DE, Lovenberg T, Chalmers D, Heinrichs S, Liaw C, De Souza EB. (1996) Neurobiology of corticotropin releasing factor (CRF) receptors and CRF-binding protein: implications for the treatment of CNS disorders. Mol Psychiat 1:265-277
Behl C (2002) Estrogen as a neuroprotective hormone. Nature Rev Neurosci, 3: 433-442
Behl C, Widmann M, Trapp T, Holsboer F (1995) 17-beta estradiol protects neurons from oxidative stress-induced cell death in vitro. Biochem Biophys Res Commun 216: 473-82
Behl C, Skutella T, Lezoualc'h F, Post A, Widmann M, Newton C, Holsboer F (1997) Neuroprotection against oxidative stress by estrogens: structure-activity relationship. Mol Pharmacol 51: 535-541
Dawson TL, Dawson VL (2003) Molecular pathways of neurodegeneration in Parkinson's disease. Science 302: 819-822
Holsboer F (2003) The role of peptides in treatment of psychiatric disorders. J Neural Transm Suppl. 64: 17-34
Lezoualc'h F, Engert S, Berning B, Behl C (2000) Corticotropin-releasing hormone-mediated neuroprotection against oxidative stress is associated with the increased release of non-amyloidogenic amyloid beta precursor protein and with the suppression of nuclear factor-kappaB. Mol Endocrinol 14: 147-159
Lutz B (2002) Molecular biology of cannabinoid receptors. Prostaglandins Leukot Essent Fatty Acids 66 123-142
Marsicano G, Goodenough S, Monory K, Hermann H, Eder M, Cannich A, Azad SC, Cascio MG, Gutierrez SO, van der Stelt M, López-Rodriguez ML, Casanova E, Schütz G,

Zieglgänsberger W, Di Marzo V, Behl C, Lutz B (2003) CB1 cannabinoid receptors and on-demand defense against excitotoxicity. Science 302: 84-88

McEwen BS (2001) Estrogen's effects on the brain: multiple sites and molecular mechanisms. J Appl Physiol. 91: 2785-2801

Moosmann B, Behl C (2002) Antioxidants as treatment for neurodegenerative disorders. Expert Opin Invest Drugs 11: 1407-1435

Prokai L, Prokai-Tatrai K, Perjesi P, Zharikova AD, Perez EJ, Liu R, Simpkins JW (2003) Quinol-based cyclic antioxidant mechanism in estrogen neuroprotection. Proc Natl Acad Sci USA 100:11741-11746

Sano M (2003) Noncholinergic treatment options for Alzheimer's disease. J Clin Psychiat 64 Suppl 9: 23-28

Vale W, Spiess J, Rivier C, Rivier J (1981) Characterization of a 41-residue ovine hypothalamic peptide that stimulates secretion of corticotropin and beta-endorphin. Science 213:1394-1397

Zschocke J, Manthey D, Bayatti N, van der Burg B, Goodenough S, Behl C (2002) Estrogen receptor alpha-mediated silencing of caveolin gene expression in neuronal cells. J Biol Chem 277: 38772-38780

# Estrogens, Aging, and Neurodegenerative Diseases

*Caleb E. Finch, Todd Morgan, and Irina Rozovsky*

## Summary

Age is the greatest risk factor in Alzheimer's disease (AD) and Parkinson's disease (PD). Indications of a female bias in AD and of a male bias in PD have been often discussed but are not definitive. Moreover, evidence that estrogen replacement may be beneficial for AD and PD is also controversial. An unevaluated factor is how aging and cumulative estrogen exposure may modify brain responses to estradiol. Rodent models show that sustained exposure to estradiol can desensitize certain neuroendocrine responses.

## Introduction

This review addresses the controversies in Alzheimer's disease (AD) and Parkinson's disease (PD) that concern sex differences and estrogen replacement therapy (ERT). In this essay, we prefer to use the term *sex differences* rather than *gender differences*: the latter, while deriving from effects of genes on sex chromosomes, is also strongly influenced by the individual's self-representation. First, we consider evidence on sex differences in AD and PD. Next, we briefly review the state of ERT in relation to AD and PD. Third, we consider how biological aging may be important in evaluating animal model studies of ERT, with recent examples as well as early work from our laboratory.

## Age and sex in AD and PD

Age is the greatest risk factor in both AD and PD, this much is clear. Currently, the overall incidence and prevalence are better documented for AD than for PD. Both diseases are rare before the age of menopause.

Andrus Gerontology Center and Department of Biological Sciences, University of Southern California, Los Angeles, California 90089-0191, USA

Kordon et al.
Hormones and the Brain
© Springer-Verlag Berlin Heidelberg 2005

Dementia associated with AD is rare (<1%) before 60. Subsequently, the prevalence of dementia doubles about every five years and reaches the range of 5-50% by 85 years (Kawas and Katzman 1999; Kukull et al. 2002; Mayeux 2003; Suthers et al. 2003). This surprisingly wide range may be due to two major factors: heterogeneity within and between population (sociodemographic differences such as ethnicity, education, and income) and criteria for diagnosis. The dementia in AD can arise without stroke or cerebrovascular pathology (the "pure" cases). However, cerebrovascular-derived neuropathology (infarcts and lacunes) frequently co-exists with AD neuropathology in the same brains. For example, a large series with neuropathologically diagnosed AD had a 48% frequency of cerebrovascular pathology, versus 33% in non-AD brains (Jellinger and Mitter-Ferstl 2003). Hypertension is an important factor in stroke, varying widely between populations.

A general impression of female bias in dementia and AD is being challenged by better data on incidence and prevalence. Incidence refers to the frequency of new cases, whereas prevalence refers to the total number alive. Recent studies do not support early indications that women are at higher risk for dementia and AD than men (e.g., Kukull et al. 2002). Moreover, in Down' syndrome, males have a three-fold higher risk of dementia than females (Schupf et al. 1998), as discussed below. According to some studies, the greater prevalence of dementia in the general population of older women is mainly attributable to women's greater life expectancy, which at age 70 is about three years longer than for men in the industrial countries (Suthers et al. 2003). For example, at age 70, US women averaged 1.7 years with cognitive impairment, about 50% longer than the 1.1 years for men. This differential is compounded by the greater life expectancy of women at this age.

PD is about 90% less prevalent than dementia, but difficulties in diagnosis are well recognized (Tanner et al. 1997). Before 60 years of age, the prevalence of PD is <0.1%. Rapid increases after age 60 reach a prevalence of 1-3% by 85 years of age (de Rijk et al. 2000; Mayeux 2003; Tanner et al. 1997; Van Den Eeden et al. 2003). A male bias is found in many studies (Dluzen 2000; Horstink et al. 2003; Tanner et al. 1997; Van Den Eeden et al. 2003), but not in all (de Rijk et al. 2000; Diamond et al. 1990; Tanner et al. 1997). The sex effect may vary ethnically. In a large series from Kaiser Permanente, sex differences were absent in Asian/Pacific Islanders, whereas white, blacks and Hispanics showed a two-fold male bias (Van Den Eeden et al. 2003). Other studies also found ethnic differences (Mayeux 2003; Mayeux et al. 1995). We provisionally conclude that sex differences in AD and PD are smaller than population differences.

## Menopause and estrogen replacement

The risks and benefits of estrogen replacement after menopause are hotly controversial. We must keep in mind the extreme case of Mme. Jeanne Calment, who achieved the greatest documented human life span of 122 years, yet was considered to be neurologically healthy. At 118 years of age, Mme Calment tested for neuropsychological performance in the range expected for a healthy 80-year-old (Ritchie 1995). Although no specific tests were given, major motor impairments or Parkinsonism could hardly have escaped notice because of the great attention she received. Assuming a typical age at menopause, Mme Calment lived 70 years in the absence of estrogens, with at least 50 of those years in good physical health. Mme Calment's extraordinary life history cannot be generalized. We do not know whether her uniquely robust constitution also protected her from the effects of postmenopausal deficits that manifestly afflict a substantial fraction of older women.

In contrast to the example of Mme Calment's apparent insensitivity to menopausal estrogen deficits are the clear effects of menopause on cognitive decline in Down's syndrome. As is well known, trisomy chromosome 21 causes very early onset of AD neuropathology in most Down's patients' brains by age 30. However, there are huge individual differences in the onset of cognitive decline, and only a subset of patients show clinical declines (Lott and Head 2001). Of great interest is the finding that early menopause (before age 46) increased the risk of dementia by 2.7-fold (Schupf et al. 2003; Fig. 1). Demented female Down's patients had higher serum sex hormone binding globulin but similar total serum estradiol concentrations. This finding suggests that reductions in free estradiol are a specific factor in the onset of dementia. However, the full explanation

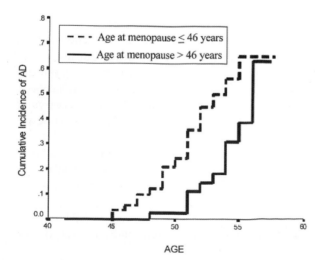

**Fig. 1.** Early menopause increases the risk of dementia by 2.7-fold (Schupf et al. 2003).

is likely to be more complex, because male Down's patients have a three-fold higher incidence of dementia overall than do females (Schupf et al. 1998).

Estrogen replacement therapy is highly controversial in relation to AD and vascular dementia. On one hand, numerous post hoc observational studies are consistent in citing the benefits of long-term ERT in reducing the risk of dementia (Paganini-Hill and Henderson 1994; Breitner and Zandi 2003; Lamberts 2003; Sherwin 2002). The benefits of ERT may also extend to stroke (Wise 2002). One of these studies is the Cache County (Utah) observational study of all drug use and dementia, which showed a duration-dependent benefit in women who, in the majority, were taking only estrogen (not ERT plus progesterone; Breitner and Zandi 2003). More than 10 years of ERT provided the greatest risk reduction. Animal model studies also generally show benefits of estrogen (Sherwin 2002; Wise 2002). In contrast, an interim report on the Women's Health Initiative Memory Study (WHIMS) showed statistically strong negative effects of an increased incidence of dementia (odds ratio, two-fold) during a randomized trial of equine estrogens plus medroxyprogesterone, with average exposure of four years (Shumaker et al. 2003). Most of the dementia was considered to be probable AD. The effect was equivalent to an increase of 23 cases of dementia/10, 000 women/ year. However, this study also clearly showed adverse cardiovascular effects that could be independent contributors to AD-type dementia, as discussed by Sparks et al. (2000). Many explanations are being considered: in brief, the necessity of prolonged replacement (Breitner and Zandi 2003); the special characteristics of women who voluntarily take estrogen and who tend to be highly educated and have high income, each of which is health promoting; but, also possible adverse effects of medroxyprogesterone, a synthetic progestin with adverse effects on neurons differing from natural progestins (Brinton and Nilsen 2003).

Discussions have also been held about possible benefits of ERT in PD, but much fewer data are available. Again, benefits are indicated by some observational studies of women taking ERT. In older PD patients, the following results were reported: ERT improved motor performance (Benedetti et al. 1998; Saunders-Pullman et al. 1999); ERT improved cognition, but not motor performance (Thulin et al. 1998); and ERT improved cognition in PD, but did not lower the risk of PD (Marder et al. 1998). So far, no controlled trial has been reported. In premenopausal PD patients, one study found sharp increases of motor symptoms just before menstruation, when estrogen and progesterone are dropping sharply (Quinn and Marsden 1986), whereas a more detailed study did not find any consistent relationship between motor symptoms and cycle stage (Kompoliti et al. 2000). Rodent models clearly show that estrogens are neuroprotective for dopaminergic neurotoxicity (MPTP and kainate; Dluzen 2000; Miller et al. 1998; Rostene et al. 2003).

It is fair to say that the divergent and perplexing findings on ERT imply a complex biology of estrogen's effects on different neural pathways and on the cerebro- and myocardial vascular systems. We suspect that several other factors are pertinent and have not been adequately considered: aging and the schedule of prior estrogen exposure.

## Aging modifies brain responses to estrogen

Neuronal plasticity is modulated by estradiol in many brain systems. Synaptic sprouting in the hippocampus is induced by perforant path lesions, which are models for degeneration of this pathway during AD (reviewed in Stone et al. 2000). In young adult rats (three months), ovariectomy decreased sprouting relative to intact or estradiol-replaced rats (Fig. 2). However, in middle-aged rats (18 months), sprouting was less and was not influenced by ovariectomy (Fig. 2). We are investigating the cellular basis for this age change using the "wounding-in-a-dish" model of sprouting. Astrocytic GFAP (the intermediate filament) has a negative effect on sprouting that is reversed by estradiol treatment, which represses GFAP transcription (Rozovsky et al. 2002). We hypothesize that the elevation of GFAP expression that occurs during normal aging (Finch et al. 2002; Miller et al. 1998; Morgan et al. 1999; Nichols et al. 1993) is a factor in impaired sprouting. Astrocytes derived from middle-aged rat cortex support notably less neurite outgrowth in the presence of estradiol, which implicates aging in astrocytes as a factor in the impairments of estradiol-sensitive sprouting (Fig. 2). Down regulation of GFAP by SiRNA restored the ability of aging astrocytes to support sprouting of E18 neurons (Rozovsky et al., manuscript in press). Further

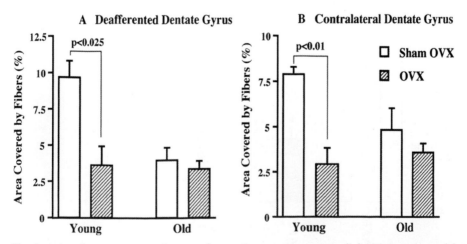

**Fig. 2.** Aging decreases responsiveness of synaptic sprouting to estradiol (E2) in a rat model of AD (perforant path lesion-induced sprouting, as observed in AD; Stone et al. 2000). OVX, ovariectomized.

studies are needed to establish the consequences on neuronal functions of the general induction of GFAP in most brain regions during aging.

Other brain regions also show age impairments in the responses of neurons to estradiol. In the olfactory bulb, estradiol induced the neurotrophin receptor TrkA in young, but not in middle-aged, female rats (Jezierski and Sohrabji 2001; Fig. 3). Moreover, BDNF mRNA and protein were induced in the olfactory bulb and its forebrain afferent by estradiol in the young, but not in the middle-aged; in the latter, a decrease was observed (Jezierski and Sohrabji 2001). The age impairments in estradiol regulation of trk receptors could alter neurotrophin transport and signal transduction pathways. Besides these modulations of synaptic plasticity, estradiol is also recognized as neuroprotectant to MPTP in dopaminergic neurons (model of drug-induced Parkinsonism; Miller et al. 1998; Rostene et al. 2003). In contrast to the neuroprotection to systemic MPTP shown in two-month-old mice, estradiol did not block the loss of dopamine in 24-month-old mice or the induction of GFAP (Miller et al. 1998; Fig. 4). These observations suggest that age changes in estradiol levels could reduce endogenous neuroprotection. Estrogens and estrogen receptor modulators are also neuroprotective to excitotoxins in glutamatergic neurons (O'Neill et al. 2004). Thus, the diminishing levels of estradiol in the cerebrospinal fluid (CSF) after menopause (Murakami et al. 1999) could be important in the increased risk of neurodegeneration. AD patients have lower CSF estradiol than controls (Schonknecht et al. 2001). If the age change in estradiol neuroprotection extends to other brain regions, then age may bring a double jeopardy to neurons:

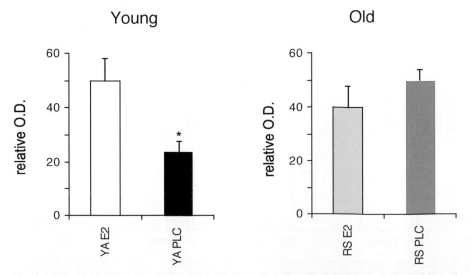

Fig. 3. Aging impairs the inducibility of Trk A in the olfactory bulb of the female rat (Jezierski and Sohrabji 2001).

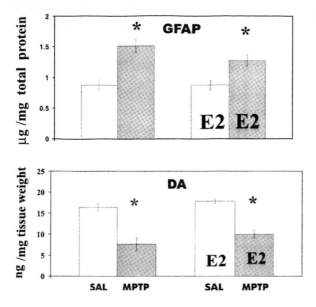

**Fig. 4.** Aging impairs neuroprotection by estradiol (E2) to MPTP neurotoxicity, a model of drug-induced PD (Miller et al. 1998). DA, dopamine. GFAP, Glial Fibrillary Acidic Protein.

decreased endogenous neuroprotection by estradiol with further adverse effects from the reduced neuroprotection.

## Estrogen exposure as a factor in aging of brain cells

The role of estrogen exposure in loss of estrogen responses during aging is indicated by studies on the neuroendocrinology of aging from two decades ago. Female rodents show a characteristic pattern of reproductive aging during their life spans of about 30 months (Fig. 5). (For general references on the following profile, see vom Saal et al. 1994; Wise et al. 1999; Gosden and Finch 2000). In rodents as in humans, the ovary has acquired its maximum store of oocytes and primary follicles before birth and no new oogenesis occurs during the rest of life. Oocyte depletion shows exponential decline from birth onwards, so that by puberty, about 50% of the original stock of oocytes is already lost. Fertility declines in rodents by eight months and in women after 30 years (long before the depletion of oocytes and hormone-producing follicles). Estrous cycles tend to become progressively longer and finally cease between 8 and 16 months. Nonetheless, the acyclic ovary has a substantial number of estrogen-secreting follicles that give a vaginal cytology described as "constant estrus." The basis for this loss of cycles in rodents is hypothalamic, because total depletion of ovarian oocytes and follicles does not occur for several more months (Gosden et al. 1983). Reciprocal ovarian transplants in still-cycling 12- and 3-month old mice show, at this intermediate stage of aging, impairments at both ovarian and

## REPRODUCTIVE CHANGES IN C57BL/6J MICE

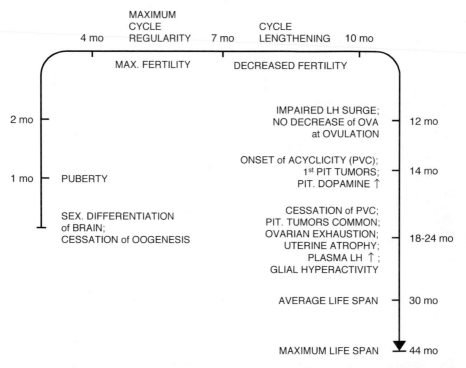

**Fig. 5.** Reproductive maturation and aging during the life span of inbred C57BL/6J mice. Original figure by Caleb E. Finch summarizing vom Saal et al. (1994). PIT, pituitary.

hypothalamic levels (Nelson et al. 1992). The hypothalamus shows a progressive loss of the preovulatory surge of gonadotrophins (LH, FSH), whether autogenous (in the presence of the aging animal's ovaries) or induced in ovariectomized animals with standard treatment of estrogen and progesterone.

These major hypothalamic impairments are further documented by the failure of young ovarian grafts to restore estrus cycles (Finch et al. 1984). However, if young ovaries are given to middle-aged mice just before cycles have ceased, then cycles continue for many more months (Fig. 6). Our hypothesis is that the hypothalamus becomes desensitized during the lengthened cycles as constant estrus is approached. This phase is characterized by sustained levels of estradiol and very low levels of progesterone. Similar estrogen-dominated prolonged cycles are observed before menopause (Santoro et al. 1996; Fig. 7). To model this phase, we developed a noninvasive administration of oral estradiol (Kohama et al. 1989; Fig. 8). Time-dose studies showed that 12 weeks of low physiological levels of estrogen in young mice caused permanent neuroendocrine

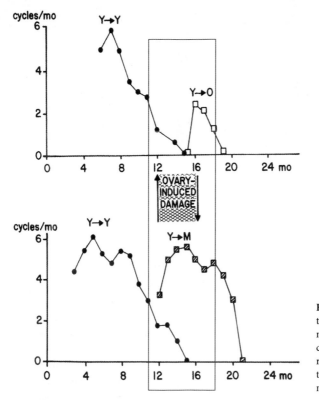

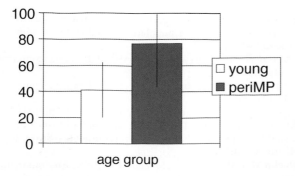

**Fig. 6.** Grafts of young ovaries to replace aging ovaries of middle-aged mice just before cycles have ceased allow regular ovulatory cycles to continue for many more months (Finch et al. 1984).

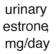

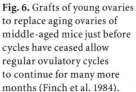

**Fig. 7.** Estrogen-dominated prolonged cycles are also observed before menopause (peri-MP; Santoro et al. 1996).

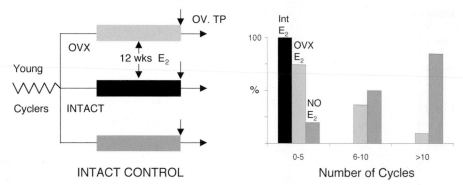

**Fig. 8.** Oral estrogens yield low physiological levels of estrogen in young mice and cause permanent neuroendocrine impairments. Redrawn from Kohama et al. (1989).

impairments, so that the LH/FSH surge could no longer be induced; neither could grafting of young ovaries from control mice restore cyclicity (Kohama et al. 1989). With a shorter exposure for six weeks to low-dose estradiol, mice regained cycling but then ceased prematurely. We estimate that 3500 pg-day/ml plasma is sufficient to cause permanent hypothalamic desensitization, within boundary levels of approximately 10-30 pg estradiol/ml plasma.

Of course, these rodent model studies cannot be simply extrapolated to humans. Nonetheless, the irreversible effect of sustained physiological levels of estradiol on the hypothalamic regulation of LH/FSH provides a model for studying specific cellular targets of estrogen regulation, such as age-related changes in estrogen-mediated synaptic sprouting (Fig. 2), TrkA induction (Fig. 3), and neuroprotection (Fig. 4).

## References

Benedetti M, Bower J, Maraganore D, McDonnell S, Rocca W (1998) Postmenopausal estrogen replacement therapy and Parkinson's disease: a population based study in Olmstead County, Minnesota. Mov Disord 13(Suppl 2):51.

Breitner JC, Zandi PP (2003) Effects of estrogen plus progestin on risk of dementia [comment]. JAMA 290:1706-1707; author reply, 1707-1708.

Brinton RD, Nilsen J (2003) Effects of estrogen plus progestin on risk of dementia [comment]. JAMA 290:1706; author reply, 1707-1708.

de Rijk MC, Launer LJ, Berger K, Breteler MM, Dartigues JF, Baldereschi M, Fratiglioni L, Lobo A, Martinez-Lage J, Trenkwalder C, Hofman A (2000) Prevalence of Parkinson's disease in Europe: A collaborative study of population-based cohorts. Neurologic Diseases in the Elderly Research Group. Neurology 54:S21-S23.

Diamond SG, Markham CH, Hoehn MM, McDowell FH, Muenter MD (1990) An examination of male-female differences in progression and mortality of Parkinson's disease. Neurology 40:763-766.

Dluzen DE (2000) Neuroprotective effects of estrogen upon the nigrostriatal dopaminergic system. J Neurocytol 29:387-399.

Finch CE, Felicio LS, Mobbs CV, Nelson JF (1984) Ovarian and steroidal influences on neuroendocrine aging processes in female rodents. Endocrine Rev 5:467-497.

Finch C, Morgan T, Rozovsky I, Xie Z, Weindruch R, Prolla T (2002). Microglia and aging in the brain. In: Streit W (ed) Microglia in the regenerating and degenerating central nervous system. New York: Springer-Verlag pp 275-305.

Gosden RG, Finch CE (2000) Definition and character of reproductive ageing. In: te Velde E, Pearson P, Broekmans F (eds) Female reproductive aging New York: Parthenon Publishing pp 11-26.

Gosden RG, Laing SC, Felicio LS, Nelson JF, Finch CE (1983) Imminent oocyte exhaustion and reduced follicular recruitment mark the transition to acyclicity in aging C57BL/6J mice. Biol Reprod 28:255-260.

Horstink MW, Strijks E, Dluzen DE (2003) Estrogen and Parkinson's disease. Adv Neurol 91: 107-14.

Jellinger KA, Mitter-Ferstl E (2003) The impact of cerebrovascular lesions in Alzheimer disease-a comparative autopsy study. J Neurol 250:1050-1055.

Jezierski MK, Sohrabji F (2001) Neurotrophin expression in the reproductively senescent forebrain is refractory to estrogen stimulation. Neurobiol Aging 22:309-219.

Kawas CH, Katzman R (1999) Epidemiology of dementia and Alzheimer disease. In: Morris J, Terry R, Katzman R, Bick K, Sisodia S (eds) Alzheimer disease. Philadelphia: Lippincott Williams & Wilkins pp 95-116.

Kohama SG, Anderson CP, Osterburg HH, May PC, Finch CE (1989) Oral administration of estradiol to young C57BL/6J mice induces age-like neuroendocrine dysfunctions in the regulation of estrous cycles. Biol Reprod 41:227-232.

Kompoliti K, Comella CL, Jaglin JA, Leurgans S, Raman R, Goetz CG (2000) Menstrual-related changes in motoric function in women with Parkinson's disease. Neurology 55: 1572-1575.

Kukull WA, Higdon R, Bowen JD, McCormick WC, Teri L, Schellenberg GD, van Belle G, Jolley L, Larson EB (2002) Dementia and Alzheimer disease incidence: a prospective cohort study. Arch Neurol 59:1737-1746.

Lamberts SW (2003) The endocrinology of gonadal involution: menopause and andropause. Ann Endocrinol 64:77-81.

Lott IT, Head E (2001) Down syndrome and Alzheimer's disease: a link between development and aging. Ment Retard Dev Disabil Res Rev 7:172-178.

Marder K, Tang MX, Alfaro B, Mejia H, Cote L, Jacobs D, Stern Y, Sano M, Mayeux R (1998) Postmenopausal estrogen use and Parkinson's disease with and without dementia. Neurology 50:1141-1143.

Mayeux R (2003) Epidemiology of neurodegeneration. Annu Rev Neurosci 26:81-104.

Mayeux R, Marder K, Cote LJ, Denaro J, Hemenegildo N, Mejia H, Tang MX, Lantigua R, Wilder D, Gurland B (1995) The frequency of idiopathic Parkinson's disease by age, ethnic group, and sex in northern Manhattan, 1988-1993[erratum appears in Am J Epidemiol 1996 143(5):528]. Am J Epidemiol 142:820-827.

Miller DB, Ali SF, O'Callaghan JP, Laws SC (1998) The impact of gender and estrogen on striatal dopaminergic neurotoxicity. Ann NY Acad Sci 844:153-165.

Morgan TE, Xie Z, Goldsmith S, Yoshida T, Lanzrein AS, Stone D, Rozovsky I, Perry G, Smith MA, Finch CE (1999) The mosaic of brain glial hyperactivity during normal ageing and its attenuation by food restriction. Neuroscience 89:687-699.

Murakami K, Nakagawa T, Shozu M, Uchide K, Koike K, Inoue M (1999) Changes with aging of steroidal levels in the cerebrospinal fluid of women. Maturitas 33:71-80.

Nelson JF, Felicio LS, Osterburg HH, Finch CE (1992) Differential contributions of ovarian and extraovarian factors to age-related reductions in plasma estradiol and progesterone during the estrous cycle of C57BL/6J mice. Endocrinology 130:805-810.

Nichols NR, Day JR, Laping NJ, Johnson SA, Finch CE (1993) GFAP mRNA increases with age in rat and human brain. Neurobiol Aging 14:421-429.

O'Neill K, Chen S, Brinton R (2004) Impact of the selective estrogen receptor modulator, raloxifene, on neuronal survival and outgrowth following toxic insults associated with aging and Alzheimer's disease. Exp Neurol. 185:63-80.

Paganini-Hill A, Henderson VW (1994) Estrogen deficiency and risk of Alzheimer's disease in women. Am J Epidemiol 140:256-261.

Quinn NP, Marsden CD (1986) Menstrual-related fluctuations in Parkinson's disease. Mov Disord 1:85-87.

Ritchie K (1995) Mental status examination of an exceptional case of longevity J. C. aged 118 years. Brit J Psych 166:229-235.

Rostene W, Callier S, D'astous M, Grandbois M, Lesaux M, Bedard P, Di Paolo T, Pelaprat D (2003) Sex steriods in normal and pathological aging: implication in dopaminergic neurodegeneration. Fondation IPSEN Symposium, abstract.

Rozovsky I, Wei M, Stone DJ, Zanjani H, Anderson CP, Morgan TE, Finch CE (2002) Estradiol (E2) enhances neurite outgrowth by repressing glial fibrillary acidic protein expression and reorganizing laminin. Endocrinology 143:636-646.

Rozovsky I, Wei M, Morgan TE, Finch CE (2004) Reversible age unpairments in neurite outgrowth by manipulations of astrocytic GFAP. Neurobiol Aging (in press).

Santoro N, Brown JR, Adel T, Skurnick JH (1996) Characterization of reproductive hormonal dynamics in the perimenopause. J Clin Endocrinol Metabol 81:1495-1501.

Saunders-Pullman R, Gordon-Elliott J, Parides M, Fahn S, Saunders HR, Bressman S (1999) The effect of estrogen replacement on early Parkinson's disease. Neurology 52:1417-1421.

Schonknecht P, Pantel J, Klinga K, Jensen M, Hartmann T, Salbach B, Schroder J (2001) Reduced cerebrospinal fluid estradiol levels are associated with increased beta-amyloid levels in female patients with Alzheimer's disease. Neurosci Lett 307:122-124.

Schupf N, Kapell D, Nightingale B, Rodriguez A, Tycko B, Mayeux R (1998) Earlier onset of Alzheimer's disease in men with Down syndrome. Neurology 50:991-995.

Schupf N, Pang D, Patel BN, Silverman W, Schubert R, Lai F, Kline JK, Stern Y, Ferin M, Tycko B, Mayeux R (2003) Onset of dementia is associated with age at menopause in women with Down's syndrome. Ann Neurol 54:433-438.

Sherwin BB (2002) Estrogen and cognitive aging in women. Trends Pharmacol Sci 23:527-34.

Shumaker SA, Legault C, Rapp SR, Thal L, Wallace RB, Ockene JK, Hendrix SL, Jones BN, 3rd, Assaf AR, Jackson RD, Kotchen JM, Wassertheil-Smoller S, Wactawski-Wende J, Whims Investigators (2003) Estrogen plus progestin and the incidence of dementia and mild cognitive impairment in postmenopausal women: the Women's Health Initiative Memory Study: a randomized controlled trial [see comment]. JAMA 289:2651-2662.

Sparks DL, Martin TA, Gross DR, Hunsaker JC, 3rd (2000) Link between heart disease, cholesterol, and Alzheimer's disease: a review. Microsc Res Tech 50:287-290.

Stone DJ, Rozovsky I, Morgan TE, Anderson CP, Lopez LM, Shick J, Finch CE (2000) Effects of age on gene expression during estrogen-induced synaptic sprouting in the female rat. Exp Neurol 165:46-57.

Suthers K, Kim JK, Crimmins E (2003) Life expectancy with cognitive impairment in the older population of the United States. J Gerontol B Psychol Sci Soc Sci. 58:S179-S186.

Tanner C, Hubble J, Chan P (1997) Epidemiology and genetics of Parkinson's disease. In; Watts R, Koller, W (eds) Movement disorders: neurologic principles and practice.. New York: McGraw-Hill, pp 137-152.

Thulin PC, Filoteo V, Roberts JW, O'Brien SA (1998) Effects of hormone replacement therapy on cognitive and motor function in women with Parkinson's disease. Neurology 50: A280.

Van Den Eeden SK, Tanner CM, Bernstein AL, Fross RD, Leimpeter A, Bloch DA, Nelson LM (2003) Incidence of Parkinson's disease: variation by age, gender, and race/ethnicity. Am J Epidemiol 157:1015-1022.

vom Saal F, CE F, Nelson J (1994). Natural history of reproductive aging in humans, laboratory rodents, and selected other vertebrates. In: Knobil E (ed) The physiology of reproduction New York: Raven Press, pp 1213-1214

Wise PM (2002) Estrogens and neuroprotection. Trends Endocrinol Metab 13:229-230.

Wise PM, Smith MJ, Dubal DB, Wilson ME, Krajnak KM, Rosewell KL (1999) Neuroendocrine influences and repercussions of the menopause. Endocrinol Rev 20:243-248.

... ... ...

# Hormones, Stress and Depression

*Marianne B. Müller[1] and Florian Holsboer[1]*

## Summary

Every disturbance of the body, either real or imagined, evokes a stress response. Essential to this stress response is the activation of the hypothalamic-pituitary-adrenocortical (HPA) system, finally resulting in the release of glucocorticoid hormones from the adrenal cortex. Glucocorticoid hormones, in turn, feed back to this system by central activation of two types of corticosteroid receptors: the glucocorticoid receptor (GR) and the mineralocorticoid receptor (MR). Whereas a brief period of controllable stress, experienced with general arousal and excitement, can be a challenge and might thus be beneficial, chronically elevated levels of circulating corticosteroid hormones are believed to enhance vulnerability to a variety of diseases, including human affective disorders.

The cumulative evidence makes a strong case implicating corticosteroid receptor dysfunction in the pathogenesis of affective disorders. Corticosteroid receptor dysfunction is followed by changes in the sensitivity of the system to the inhibitory effects of glucocorticoids on the synthesis of CRH and vasopressin in hypothalamic neurons. Changes in CRH and vasopressin levels, in turn, determine the responsiveness of the axis to subsequent stressors: increased production of these neuropeptides leads to increased HPA responses to stress and might be associated with an enhanced anxiety state. Although definitive controlled trials remain to be conducted, there is evidence indicating that cortisol-lowering or corticosteroid receptor antagonist treatments, as well as CRH type 1 receptor antagonists, may be of clinical benefit in individuals with major depression. Therefore, a more detailed knowledge of GR and CRH receptor signalling pathways will ultimately lead to the development of novel neuropharmacological intervention strategies.

[1] Max Planck Institute of Psychiatry, Kraepelinstrasse 2–10, 80804 Munich, Germany

Kordon et al.
Hormones and the Brain
© Springer-Verlag Berlin Heidelberg 2005

## Introduction

*The stress hormone (hypothalamic-pituitary-adrenocortical; HPA) system: corticosteroid hormones are the main actors in restoring homeostasis*
Every disturbance of the body, either real or imagined, either physical or psychological, evokes a stress response. This stress response involves a large number of mechanisms and processes which, all together, serve to restrain the body's defense reactions to stress, so as to restore homeostasis and to facilitate adaptation (Selye 1946). A brief period of controllable stress, experienced with general arousal and excitement, can be a challenge and might thus be beneficial. In contrast, lack of control and persistent uncertainty in prolonged stressful situations can lead to a chronic state of "distress," resulting in chronically elevated levels of circulating corticosteroid hormones ("stress hormones"), which is believed to enhance vulnerability to a variety of diseases. Chronic exposure to elevated corticosteroid levels has been associated with several pathophysiological conditions, such as dysfunction of the immune system, neurodegeneration in aging and human affective disorders (Chrousos and Gold 1992; Mc Ewen 2000).

Essential to the stress response are hypothalamic paraventricular neurons expressing corticotropin-releasing hormone (CRH) and other co-secretagogues, such as vasopressin. CRH is the primary hypothalamic hypophysiotropic factor regulating both basal and stress-induced release of pituitary corticotropin (ACTH; Vale et al. 1981; Owens and Nemeroff 1991; Aguilera 1998). CRH triggers the immediate release of ACTH from the anterior pituitary, which, in turn, potently stimulates the release of glucocorticoids from the zona fasciculata of the adrenal cortex.

Corticosteroids feed back to the HPA system via two major negative feedback routes, one directly at the level of the paraventricular nucleus of the hypothalamus, parvocellular part to control hypothalamic CRH expression (Erkut et al. 1998) and at the level of the anterior pituitary. This immediate negative feedback is a fundamental way in which the HPA system is restrained during stress and activity, and this restraint of HPA activation by glucocorticoids is rapid and profound (for review, see Herman and Cullinan 1997). In contrast, induction of CRH expression by increasing glucocorticoid levels has been described to occur at the level of the central amygdala and the bed nucleus of the stria terminalis (BNST; for review, see Watts 1996; Schulkin et al. 1998). The latter is derived embryologically from the amygdala and plays a fundamental role in the regulation of the HPA system during stress. This "paradoxical' elevation of CRH gene expression by glucocorticoids in the central nucleus of the amygdala and lateral BNST may underlie a number of functional as well as pathological emotional states in which elevated circulating levels of glucocorticoids are accompanied by increased anxiety, such as in human affective disorders (for review, see Holsboer 1995, 2000).

In concert with other components of the stress hormone system, the action of corticosteroid hormones displays two modes of operation (for review, see de Kloet et al. 1998). On the one hand, corticosteroids maintain basal activity of the HPA system and control the sensitivity or threshold of the system's response to stress. On the other hand, corticosteroid feedback helps to terminate stress-induced HPA system activation and to restrain the stress response. Corticosteroid hormones, therefore, facilitate an individual's ability to cope with, adapt to and recover from stress.

Due to their lipophilic nature, glucocorticoid hormones are able to easily penetrate through cell membranes into every cell of the body. Physiological control of the access of endogenous glucocorticoids into the brain is an important issue, all the more so as both glucocorticoid overexposure and glucocorticoid deficiency have been shown to potentially impair and endanger neuronal integrity and function. Accordingly, the potentially disruptive effects of corticosteroids in control of brain function and behaviour have received much attention over the last years (Uno et al. 1989; Lucassen et al. 2001; Müller et al. 2001). In this context, the recent findings that endogenous corticosteroid hormones are substrates of the multidrug-resistance gene 1-type P-glycoproteins are of particular importance (Meijer et al. 2000; Karssen et al. 2001; Müller et al. 2003a): mdr 1-type P-glycoproteins are highly expressed at the blood-brain-barrier to protect the central nervous system against the entry and accumulation of a wide range of toxic xenobiotics and drugs by actively transporting them against a concentration gradient.

Glucocorticoid receptors (GRs) occur everywhere in the brain but are most abundant in hypothalamic CRH neurons and pituitary corticotropes. Mineralocorticoid receptors (MRs), in contrast, are highly expressed in the hippocampus and, at lower expression levels, in hypothalamic sites involved in the regulation of salt appetite and autonomic outflow. Interestingly, the MRs and GRs are co-localized in those brain structures that are involved in the regulation of fear and anxiety, such as hippocampus, septum and amygdala. The two corticosteroid receptor types differ not only in their neuroanatomical distribution but also in their affinity and binding capacity for corticosteroids: the MR binds GCs with a t10-fold higher affinity than does the GR (Reul and de Kloet 1985). These findings on corticosteroid receptor diversity led to the working hypothesis that the tonic influences of corticosterone are exerted via hippocampal MRs, whereas the additional occupancy of GRs with higher levels of corticosterone, e.g., following stress, mediates feedback actions aimed to restrain HPA system activation. Thus, the balance in MR- and GR-mediated effects exerted by corticosterone seems to be critical for homeostatic control (de Kloet et al. 1997,1998).

*Impaired stress hormone regulation – a risk factor for depression?*
Several research groups formulated a hypothesis relating aberrant stress hormone regulation to causality of depression (for review, see Holsboer 1999, 2000). The reason for HPA hyperactivity and, in particular, for enhanced synthesis and release of CRH in depression is not yet clear. Genetic and experience-related factors may interact to induce manifold changes in corticosteroid receptor signaling, finally resulting in hypersecretion of both CRH and vasopressin (Raadsheer et al. 1994; Purba et al. 1996; de Kloet et al. 1998; Müller et al. 2000). A considerable amount of evidence has been accumulated suggesting that normalization of the HPA system might be the final step necessary for stable remission of the disease (Holsboer and Barden 1996; Zobel et al. 1999; Holsboer 2000). On the basis of these findings, it has been further hypothesized that antidepressants may act through normalization of HPA system function (for review, see Holsboer 2000).

Prominent HPA abnormalities among patients with major depression are increased numbers of ACTH and cortisol secretory pulses, which is also reflected in elevated urinary cortisol secretion rates (Rubin et al. 1987). These studies were complemented by different neuroendocrine function tests, including the dexamethasone suppression test (DST) and the combined dexamethasone-CRH-challenge test (dex-CRH test). This dex-CRH-test, combining the DST with CRH stimulation, has been shown to be a sensitive test for detecting HPA dysregulation in patients with affective disorders. In fact, Heuser and co-workers concluded from their studies that the sensitivity of this combined dex-CRH test (i.e., the likelihood to differentiate between normal and pathological states) is above 80%, depending on age and gender (Heuser et al. 1994). Whereas CRH-elicited ACTH response is blunted in depressives, dexamethasone pretreatment produces the opposite effect and paradoxically enhances ACTH release following CRH. Similarly, CRH-induced cortisol release is much higher in dexamethasone-pretreated patients than following a challenge with CRH alone. Moreover, the combined dex-CRH test has proved to be particularly useful as a predictor of increased risk for relapse: in those patients where the neuroendocrine abnormality persists, the risk of relapse or resistance to treatment is much higher (Holsboer et al. 1987; Heuser et al. 1996; Zobel et al. 1999).

Such a HPA disturbance in feedback control can be acquired as a result of stressful life experiences and can be compounded by age (Brunson et al. 2001), or it can be genetically predetermined at all levels involved in fine-tuned neuroendocrine regulation. Depressive and anxiety disorders are likely to have significant genetic components, as suggested by familial segregation of these disorders and twin and adoption studies. It is possible, however, that the genetic component is not an independent risk factor for the development of these disorders but rather a vulnerability factor predisposing for the development of affective disorders following stress exposure. Likewise, genetic factors may also protect an individual from stress-related illness. Genetic and experience-related factors may interact to induce manifold changes in corticosteroid receptor signaling, finally resulting in hypersecretion of both CRH and AVP (Raadsheer et al. 1994; Purba et al. 1996; de Kloet et al. 1998; Müller et al. 2000). In this context, the data from the Munich Vulnerability Study are of particular interest (Holsboer et al. 1995; Modell et al. 1997, 1998). This study investigated whether the HPA feedback disturbance observed among patients with major depression is present in otherwise healthy individuals who are at high risk for psychiatric disorders because they have a first-degree relative with an affective illness. The Munich Vulnerability Study revealed that subjects who never suffered from a psychiatric disorder, but belong to families with a considerably high genetic load for depression, may display abnormal responses to the combined dex-CRH-challenge test (Holsboer et al. 1995; Lauer et al. 1998; Modell et al. 1998). In the absence of any previous depression in these individuals, or other life events or lifestyles that would explain the functional corticosteroid receptor changes as an enduring adaptation to major stress, the findings from this study are best understood as indicating a genetically transmitted risk factor, possibly rendering these individuals susceptible to affective disorders. In a follow-up study, 14 of the initial 47 high-risk probands were re-examined about four years after the index investigation and showed surprisingly constant results in the combined dex-CRH challenge test, so that one of the requirements for a vulnerability marker is fulfilled (Modell et al. 1998).

Whereas genetic linkage studies so far reject the glucocorticoid receptor gene as a possible gene of inherited pathology (Detera-Wadleigh et al. 1992; Mirow et al. 1994; Morisette et al. 1999; Moutsatsou et al. 2000), the recent development of refined genetic technologies opens up the possibility for large-scale screening of single nucleotide polymorphisms (SNPs; Syvanen 2001; Cowan et al. 2002). These SNPs are highly abundant and are estimated to occur at one out of every 1,000 bases in the human genome. Depending on where a SNP occurs, it might have different consequences at the phenotypic level. The reason for the current interest in SNPs is the hope that they could be used as markers to identify genes that predispose individuals to complex, polygenic disorders. A recent investigation provided evidence that carriers of a specific polymorphism (ER22/23EK) in the GR gene are less sensitive to the suppressive effects of low-dose dexamethasone (van Rossum et al. 2002) and are suspected to be relatively more resistant to the effects of GC, with respect to the sensitivity of adrenal feedback mechanisms, than are non-carriers. Considering the aforementioned implications of HPA system dysregulation for the development and maintenance of affective disorder, those functionally relevant polymorphisms of the GR, therefore, may alter an innate setpoint for susceptibility to stress-associated psychiatric disorders (DeRijk et al. 2002).

As outlined above, there is robust evidence for a hyperactivtity of the HPA system in human affective disorders, and it has been proposed that hypercortisolemia is in some way integral to the pathogenesis and maintenance of psychopathology and cognitive deficits in these diseases. It is, therefore, not surprising that research into novel therapeutic approaches to depression has focused on strategies designed to modulate the effects of hypercortisolemia and/or the mechanisms underlying this phenomenon (Murphy 1997; McQuade and Young 2000). Antiglucocorticoid drugs and approaches in the treatment of human affective disorder include the administration of steroid-synthesis inhibitors, such as ketoconazole, metyrapone and aminogluthetimide (e.g., Ravaris et al. 1988; Malison et al. 1999; Wolkowitz et al. 1999) or GR antagonists, such as mifepristone (Belanoff et al. 2002).

Pathological anxiety is a frequent concomitant of major depression. Moreover, there is a longstanding debate about whether anxiety and depression constitute different aspects of the same disorder ("continuum hypothesis") or distinct, yet overlapping, conditions. Anxiety-related behavior is one of the most important, highly conserved behaviors among all kind of species that can be reliably measured in specific experimental paradigms in rodents. Increased CRH neuronal activity has been hypothesized both in major depression and anxiety disorders. The crucial role of CRHR1 in mediating anxiety-related behavior was confirmed in transgenic mice with a functional null mutation of CRHR1 (Smith et al. 1998; Timpl et al. 1998). Most recently, using a brain area-specific conditional knockout mouse line, researchers showed that limbic *Crhr1* neuronal circuitries mediate anxiety-related behavior, and that this anxiolytic effect is independent of HPA system activity (Müller et al. 2003b). These results, therefore, allow us to genetically dissect CRH/Crhr1 neuronal pathways modulating behavior from those regulating neuroendocrine function, underlining the importance of limbic CRH/Crhr1 neuronal pathways as a promising pharmacological target for the treatment of human affective disorders, such as major depression or the consequences of early-life stress (Holsboer 1999; Keck and Holsboer 2001).

One such selective CRHR1 antagonist, NBI-30775 (also referred to as R121919), was first shown to decrease anxiety- and fear-related behaviors in response to stress in rodents (Keck et al. 2001). In an open-label proof of concept study, 20 patients with major depression receiving NBI-30775 experienced significant reductions in depression and anxiety ratings, whereas neither basal nor CRH-stimulated HPA system activity was impaired (Zobel et al. 2000).

Besides pharmacological and other more traditional approaches to examine stress-anxiety interactions in animal models, an alternative way is to directly modify neurobiological systems involved in the stress response and to examine the effects of these manipulations on anxiety-related behaviors. As mentioned before, the primary candidates for these types of manipulations are the various components of the HPA system (for review, see Müller et al. 2002; Müller and Keck 2002). The ability to generate mice with specific mutations or complete deletions of certain genes of interest through homologous recombination in embryonic stem cells has facilitated the study of many biological processes, from embryogenesis to animal behavior. The generation of genetically engineered mice (e.g., "conventional" and "conditional" knock-outs) has allowed us to specifically target individual genes involved in stress hormone regulation. The identification and detailed characterization of these molecular pathways will ultimately lead to the development of novel neuropharmacological intervention strategies.

## References

Aguilera G (1998) Corticotropin releasing hormone, receptor regulation and the stress response. Trends Endocrinol Metab 9: 329-336.

Belanoff JK, Rothschild AJ, Cassidy F, De Battista C, Baulieu EE, Schold C, Schatzberg AF (2002) An open label trial of C-1073 (mifepristone) for psychotic major depression. Biol Psychiat 52: 386-392.

Brunson KL, Avishai-Eliner S, Hatalski CG, Baram TZ (2001) Neurobiology of the stress response early in life: evolution of a concept and the role of corticotropin-releasing hormone. Mol Psychiat 6: 647-656.

Chrousos PW, Gold PW (1992) The concepts of stress and stress system disorders. Overview of physical and behavioural homeostasis. JAMA 267: 1244-1252.

Cowan WM, Kopnisky KL, Hyman SE (2002) The human genome project and its impact on psychiatry. Ann Rev Neurosci 25: 1-50.

de Kloet ER, Vreugdenhil E, Oitzl MS, Joels M (1997) Glucocorticoid feedback resistance. Trends Endocrinol Metab 8: 26-33.

de Kloet ER, Vreugdenhil E, Oitzl MS, Joels M (1998) Brain corticosteroid receptor balance in health and disease. Endocrine Rev 19: 269-301.

DeRijk RH, Schaaf M, de Kloet ER (2002) Glucocorticoid receptor variants: clinical implications. J Steroid Biochem Mol Biol 81: 103-122.

Detera-Wadleigh SD, Berrettini WH, Goldin LR, Martinez M, Hsieh WT, Hoehe MR, Encio IJ, Coffman D, Rollins DY, Muniec D (1992) A systematic search for a bipolar predisposing locus on chromosome 5. Neuropsychopharmacology 6: 219-229.

Erkut ZA, Pool C, Swaab DF (1998) Glucocorticoids suppress corticotropin-releasing hormone and vasopressin expression in human hypothalamic neurons. J Clin Endocrinol Metab 83: 2066-2073.

Herman JP, Cullinan WE (1997) Neurocircuitry of stress: central control of the hypothalamic-pituitary-adrenocortical axis. Trends Neurosci 20: 78-84.

Heuser I, Yassouridis A, Holsboer F (1994) The combined dexamethasone/CRH test: a refined laboratory test for psychiatric disorders. J Psychiatr Res 28: 341-356.

Heuser IJE, Schweiger U, Gotthardt U, Schmider J, Lammers CH, Dettling M, Yassouridis A, Holsboer F (1996) Pituitary-adrenal system regulation and psychopathology during amitriptyline treatment in elderly depressed patients and in normal control subjects. Am J Psychiat 153: 93-99.

Holsboer F (1995) Neuroendocrinology of mood disorders. In: Bloom FE, Kupfer DJ (eds) Psychopharmacology: The fourth generation of progress. Raven Press, New York, pp. 957-968.

Holsboer F (1999) The rationale for the corticotropin-releasing hormone receptor (CRH-R) antagonists to treat depression and anxiety. J Psychiatr Res 33: 181-214.

Holsboer F (2000) The corticosteroid receptor hypothesis of depression. Neuropsychopharmacology 23: 477-501.

Holsboer F, Barden N (1996) Antidepressants and hypothalamic-pituitary-adrenocortical regulation. Endocrine Rev 17: 187-205.

Holsboer F, Von Bardeleben U, Wiedemann K, Müller OA, Stalla GK (1987) Serial assessment of corticotropin-releasing hormone response after dexamethasone in depression: implications for pathophysiology of DST nonsuppression. Biol Psychiat 22: 228-234.

Holsboer F, Lauer CJ, Schreiber W, Krieg J-C (1995) Altered hypothalamic-pituitary-adrenocortical regulation in healthy subjects at high familial risk for affective disorders. Neuroendocrinology 62: 340-347.

Karssen AM, Meijer OC, van der Sandt ICJ, Lucassen PJ, de Lange EC, de Boer AG, de Kloet ER (2001) Multidrug resistance P-glycoprotein hampers the access of cortisol but not of corticosterone to mouse and human brain. Endocrinology 142: 2686-2694.

Keck ME, Holsboer F (2001) Hyperactivity of CRH neuronal circuits as a target for therapeutic interventions in affective disorders. Peptides 22: 835-844.

Keck ME, Welt T, Wigger A, Renner U, Engelmann M, Holsboer F, Landgraf R (2001) The anxiolytic effect of the CRH1 receptor antagonist R121919 depends on innate emotionality in rats. Eur J Neurosci 13: 373-380.

Lauer CJ, Schreiber W, Modell S, Holsboer F, Krieg JC (1998) The Munich vulnerability study on affective disorders: overview of the cross-sectional observations at index investigation. J Psychiatric Res 32: 393-401.

Lucassen PJ, Müller MB, Holsboer F, Bauer J, Holtrop A, Wouda J, Hoogendijk WJG, de Kloet ER, Swaab DF (2001) Hippocampal apoptosis in major depression is a minor event and absent from subareas at risk for glucocorticoid overexposure. Am J Pathol 158: 453-468.

Malison RT, Anand A, Pelton GH, Kirwin P, Carpenter L, McDougle CJ, Heninger GR, Price LH (1999) Limited efficacy of ketoconazole in treatment-refractory major depression. J Clin Psychopharmacol 19: 466-470.

Mc Ewen BS (2000) The neurobiology of stress: from serendipity to clinical relevance. Brain Res 886: 172-189.

McQuade R, Young AH (2000) Future therapeutic targets in mood disorders: the glucocorticoid receptor. Br J Psychiat 177: 390-395.

Meijer OC, de Boer AG, van der Sandt ICJ, de Lange ECM, De Kloet ER (2000) The multidrug resistance 1A P-glycoprotein affects the penetration of glucocorticoids, except corticosterone, in the brain. Soc Neurosci Abstr 26: 419.

Mirow AL, Kristbjanarson H, Egeland JA, Shilling P, Helgason T, Gillin JC, Hirsch S, Kelsoe JR (1994) A linkage study of distal chromosome 5q and bipolar disorder. Biol Psychiat 36: 223-229.

Modell S, Yassouridis A, Huber J, Holsboer F (1997) Corticosteroid receptor function is decreased in depressed patients. Neuroendocrinology 65: 216-222.

Modell S, Lauer CJ, Schreiber W, Huber J, Krieg JC, Holsboer F (1998) Hormonal response pattern in the combined DEX-CRH test is stable over time in subjects at high familial risk for affective disorders. Neuropsychopharmacology 18: 253-262.

Morisette J, Villeenuve A, Lordeleau L, Rochette D, Laberge C, Gagné B, Laprise C, Bouchard G, Plante M, Gobeil L, Shink E, Weissenbach J, Barden N (1999) Genome-wide search for linkage of bipolar affective disorders in a very large pedigree derived from a homogenous population in Quebec points to a locus of major affect on chromosome 12q23-q24. Am J Med Genet 88: 567-587.

Moutsatsou P, Tsolakidou A, Trikkas G, Troungos C, Sekeris CE (2000) Glucocorticoid receptor alpha and beta isoforms are not mutated in bipolar affective disorder. Mol Psychiat 5: 196-202.

Müller MB, Keck ME (2002) Genetically engineered mice for studies of stress-related clinical conditions. J Psychiatr Res 36: 53-76.

Müller MB, Landgraf R, Sillaber I, Kresse AE, Keck ME, Zimmermann S, Holsboer F, Wurst W (2000) Selective activation of the hypothalamic vasopressinergic system in mice deficient for the corticotropin-releasing hormone receptor 1 is dependent on glucocorticoids. Endocrinology 141: 4262-4269.

Müller MB, Lucassen PJ, Hoogendijk WGJ, Holsboer F, Swaab DF (2001) Neither major depression nor glucocorticoid treatment affects the cellular integrity of the human hippocampus. Eur J Neurosci 14: 1603-1612.

Müller MB, Holsboer F, Keck ME (2002) Genetic modification of corticosteroid receptor signalling: Novel insights into pathophysiology and treatment strategies of human affective disorders. Neuropeptides 36: 117-131.

Müller MB, Keck ME, Binder EB, Kresse AE, Hagemeyer TP, Landgraf R, Holsboer F , Uhr M (2003a) ABCB1- (MDR1)-type P-glycoproteins at the blood-brain barrier modulate the activity of the hypothalamic-pituitary-adrenocortical system: implications for affective disorder. Neurospychopharmacology 28: 1991-1999.

Müller MB, Zimmermann S, Sillaber I, Hagemeyer TP, Deussing JM, Timpl P, Kormann MSD, Droste S, Kühn R, Reul JMHM, Holsboer F, Wurst W (2003b) Limbic corticotropin-releasing hormone receptor 1 mediates anxiety-related behavior and hormonal adaptation to stress. Nature Neurosci 6: 1100-1107.

Murphy BE (1997) Antiglucocorticoid therapies in major depression: a review. Psychoneuroendocrinology 22: 125-132.

Owens MJ, Nemeroff CB (1991) Physiology and pharmacology of corticotropin releasing factor. Pharmacol Rev 43: 425-473.

Purba JS, Hoogendijk WJG, Hofman MA, Swaab DF (1996) Increased number of vasopressin- and oxytocin-expressing neurons in the paraventricular nucleus of the hypothalamus in depression. Arch Gen Psychiat 53: 137-143.

Raadsheer FC, Hoogendijk WJG, Stam FC, Tilders FJH, Swaab DF (1994) Increased number of corticotropin-releasing hormone expressing neurons in the hypothalamic paraventricular nucleus of depressed patients. Neuroendocrinology 60: 436-444.

Ravaris CL, Sateia MJ, Beroza KW, Noordsy DL, Brinck-Johnsen T (1988) Effect of ketoconazole on a hypophysectomized, hypercortisolemic, psychotically depressed woman. Arch Gen Psychiat 45: 966-967.

Reul JMHM, de Kloet ER (1985) Two receptor systems for corticosterone in the rat brain: microdistribution and differential occupation. Endocrinology 117: 2505-2512.

Rubin RT, Poland RE, Lesser IM, Winston RA, Blodgett ALN (1987) Neuroendocrine aspects of primary endogenous depression. Arch Gen Psychiat 44: 328-336.

Schulkin J, Gold PW, McEwen BS (1998) Induction of corticotropin-releasing hormone gene expression by glucocorticoids: implication for understanding the states of fear and anxiety and allostatic load. Psychoneuroendocrinology 23: 219-243.

Selye H (1946) The general adaptation syndrome and the diseases of adaptation. J Clin Endocrinol 6: 117-196.

Smith GW, Aubry J-M, Dellu F, Contarino A, Bilezikijan LM, Gold LH, Chen R, Marchuk Y, Hauser C, Bentley CA, Sawchenko PE, Koob GF, Vale W, Lee K-F (1998) Corticotropin releasing factor receptor 1-deficient mice display decreased anxiety, impaired stress response, and aberrant neuroendocrine development. Neuron 20: 1093-1102.

Syvanen AC (2001) Accessing genetic variation: genotyping single nucleotide polymorphisms. Nature Rev Genet 2: 930-942.

Timpl P, Spanagel R, Sillaber I, Kresse A, Reul JMHM, Stalla GK, Blanquet V, Steckler T, Holsboer F, Wurst W (1998) Impaired stress response and reduced anxiety in mice lacking a functional corticotropin-releasing hormone receptor 1. Nature Genet 19: 162-166.

Uno H, Tarara R, Else JG, Suleman MA, Sapolsky RM (1989) Hippocampal damage associated with prolonged and fatal stress in primates. J Neurosci 9: 1705-1711.

Vale W, Spiess J, Rivier C, Rivier J (1981) Characterization of a 41-residue ovine hypothalamic peptide that stimulates secretion of corticotropin and b-endorphin. Science 213: 1394-1397.

van Rossum EF, Koper JW, Huizenga NA, Uitterlinden AG, Janssen JA, O. BA, Grobbee DE, de Jong FH, van Duyn CM, A. PH, Lamberts SW (2002) A polymorphism in the glucocorticoid receptor gene, which decreases sensitivity to glucocorticoids in vivo, is associated with low insulin and cholesterol levels. Diabetes 51: 3128-3134.

Watts AG (1996) The impact of physiological stimuli on the expression of corticotropin-releasing hormone (CRH) and other neuropeptide genes. Front Neuroendocrinology 17: 281-326.

Wolkowitz OM, Reus VI, Chan T, Manfredi F, Raum W, Johnson R, Canick J (1999) Antiglucocorticoid treatment of depression: double-blind ketoconazole. Biol Psychiat 45: 1070-1074.

Zobel AW, Yassouridis A, Frieboes R-M, Holsboer F (1999) Prediction of medium-term outcome by cortisol response to the comined dexamethasone-CRH test in patients with remitted depression. Am J Psychiat 156: 949-951.

Zobel AW, Nickel T, Künzel HE, Ackl N, Sonntag A, Ising M, Holsboer F (2000) Effects of the high-affinity corticotropin-releasing hormone receptor antagonist R121919 in major depression: the first 20 patients treated. J Psychiatr Res 34: 171-181.

# Subject Index

**A**

Acetylcholine  74, 127, 128, 134, 139
Activin  1–27
Addiction  156, 163–167
Adrenocorticotropic hormone (ACTH)  2, 228, 230
Aging  202–204, 213–225
Alzheimer's disease  138, 202–204, 208, 213–218
AMPA  52–53, 173, 185
Amphetamine  155–161
Amyotrophic lateral sclerosis  136, 203, 204
Analgesia  74, 75
Antioxidant (cf. free-radicals scavenger)
Antiprogestins  111–153
Anxiety  75, 228, 230, 232
Aromatase activity in the central nervous system  173–199

**B**

Barker hypothesis (cf. fetal origin hypothesis)
Behavioural effect of change in aromatase activity  173–199
Betaglycan  8–11
Bone morphogenetic protein  1, 5–7, 10, 11, 15
Brain-derived neurotrophic factor (BDNF)  134, 135, 207, 217

**C**

Cancer  12, 13, 82, 89, 123
Cannabinoid receptor  209, 210
Cerebellar Purkinje cell  121, 137, 138
Cocaine  156, 163–166
Corticosterone  125, 137, 229
Corticotrophin-releasing hormone (CRH)  201–212, 227–232
Cortisol  125, 227, 230
Cripto  13–16
Cyclic AMP response element binding protein (CREB)  191–193, 208, 209

**D**

Dehydroepiandrosterone  99–101, 105, 106
Depression  106, 227–236
Dopamine  155–164, 167, 168, 216
Down's syndrome  215

**E**

Endocannabinoids  201–212
Endocrine disruption  82–85
Endozepine  100–104, 106, 107
Enkephalin  55, 74, 75
Epidermal growth factor  14, 49
erbB  50–53
Estradiol  61–70, 73, 76, 93, 94, 155–172, 178, 179, 188–192, 204, 205, 213, 217–219
Estradiol and motivated behavior  155–177
Estrogen (cf. also estradiol)  73–75, 79–98, 173–180, 187–193, 201–225
Estrogen replacement therapy  213, 215–217

**F**

Fetal origin hypothesis  29–46
Fibroblast growth factor  4, 49
Follicle stimulating hormone (FSH)  2, 10, 14, 47, 80, 81, 84, 222
Follistatin  3, 9, 14, 15
Free-radical scavenger  138, 202, 204, 205

**G**

GABA  48, 49, 55, 56, 99, 100, 102–104, 106, 107, 127, 128, 130–133, 139, 168
Gene expression  53–56
Genetic  29–59, 230, 231
Genetic and environmental influences on growth and size  29–46
Genomic  47–59, 74, 75, 138, 174
Genomic routes activating functional modules  74–75
Glial control of GnRH neurons  49–52
Glucocorticoid receptor  137, 138, 227, 229
Glyceraldehydes-3-phosphate dehydrogenase  61–63, 66–70
Gonadotropin-releasing hormone (GnRH)  3, 47–56, 74, 75, 80, 81, 84, 85, 91, 180
Growth and twin study  29–46
Growth hormone  2

**H**

Huntington's disease  203, 204
Hypothalamic changes in gene expression  53–56
Hypothalamic-pituitary-adrenal stress axis  208, 209, 227–233

Hypothalamic-pituitary unit  79–98
Hypothalamus  3, 4, 53–56, 73–98, 179, 181, 182, 185, 186

**I**
Inhibin  1–27
Insulin-like growth factor  42, 49

**L**
Luteinizing hormone (LH)  10, 47, 49, 74, 80, 81, 84, 91, 222

**M**
Mechanisms of progesterone action  111–153
Mechanisms of steroid hormone actions  73–77
Menopause  88, 89, 213, 215–217, 221, 222
Microtubule  62–66
Mifepristone  111, 115, 119–123, 137, 138
Mineralocorticoid receptor  227, 229
Motivated behavior and estradiol  155–172
Myelination  111–153

**N**
Nell-2  49
Netherland Twin Register  29–46
Neuregulin  49–51, 53
Neurodegenerative disease  213–225
Neuropeptide  99–109, 189
Neuropeptide Y  55, 99, 100, 105–107
Neuroprotection  111–153, 201–212
Neurostéroïde  99–139, 175
Neurotransmitter  56, 70, 74, 99–109, 112, 127, 128, 139, 174, 175, 193
NMDA  49, 73, 85, 127, 133, 173, 185
Non-genomic action of sex steroids  61–72, 174, 185, 187, 190, 193
Nucleus accumbens  155–163

**O**
Osteoporosis  89, 90
Ovaryectomy  91–94, 155, 158–166, 217
Oxidative stress  132, 201–203
Oxytocin  75

**P**
Pain  189–191
Parkinson's disease  203, 204, 213, 214, 216, 217, 219
Pituitary  11, 79–98
Pregnane X receptor  123, 124
Preoptic area  175–184, 192
Prion diseases  203, 204
Progesterone  74, 99, 102, 111–139, 215
Progestins  111–153
Prolactin  2, 81, 91, 94

Prostaglandin E$_2$  50
Proteomic  47–59
Puberty  47–59

**R**
Raloxifen  88–92
Regulation of neurosteroid biosynthesis  99–107
Reproductive function  82, 83
Reproductive maturation and aging  220

**S**
Selective estrogen receptor modulator (SERM)  79–98
Selective progesterone receptor modulator (SPRM)  111–113, 119
Serine kinase superfamily  5, 6
Sex differences in drug abuse  156, 163–167
Sex differences in neurodegenerative disorders  213, 214
Sex steroids (cf. also estrogen, testosterone)  61–72, 80
Sexual behaviour  91, 106, 161–163, 175, 176, 187–189, 193
Sexual brain differentiation  81–83, 86, 88, 90–92, 95, 156–161
Signaling mechanisms  1–27
Size and twin study  29–46
Smad protein  7, 8, 10–12, 15
Somatostatin  4
Spinal cord injury  133–136
Spinal motoneuron degeneration  136, 137
Steroid  61–225
Steroid receptor coactivator-1  173, 180–182
Stress  227–236
Stroke  202, 203
SynCAM  52, 56

**T**
Tamoxifen  88–90, 163, 176
Testosterone  61–69, 80, 84, 125, 173, 175–179, 188–190
Transforming growth factor α  49, 50, 53
Transforming growth factor β  1, 5–13, 15, 16, 50
Transsynaptic control of GnRH neurons  48, 49
Tubulin  62–63, 66
Tyrosine hydroxylase  192, 193
Twin  29–46, 230

**V**
Vasopressin  227, 230

**X**
Xenosteroid  79–98